Mental Health, Racism, and Contemporary Challenges of Being Black in America

Mental Health, Racism, and Contemporary Challenges of Being Black in America

Edited by

Donna M. Norris, M.D.
Annelle B. Primm, M.D., M.P.H.

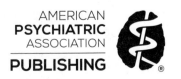

AMERICAN
PSYCHIATRIC
ASSOCIATION
PUBLISHING

Note: The authors have worked to ensure that all information in this book is accurate at the time of publication and consistent with general psychiatric and medical standards, and that information concerning drug dosages, schedules, and routes of administration is accurate at the time of publication and consistent with standards set by the U.S. Food and Drug Administration and the general medical community. As medical research and practice continue to advance, however, therapeutic standards may change. Moreover, specific situations may require a specific therapeutic response not included in this book. For these reasons and because human and mechanical errors sometimes occur, we recommend that readers follow the advice of physicians directly involved in their care or the care of a member of their family.

Books published by American Psychiatric Association Publishing represent the findings, conclusions, and views of the individual authors and do not necessarily represent the policies and opinions of American Psychiatric Association Publishing or the American Psychiatric Association.

If you wish to buy 50 or more copies of the same title, please go to www.appi.org/specialdiscounts for more information.

Copyright © 2024 American Psychiatric Association Publishing
ALL RIGHTS RESERVED
First Edition
Manufactured in the United States of America on acid-free paper
27 26 25 24 23   5 4 3 2 1

American Psychiatric Association Publishing
800 Maine Avenue SW, Suite 900
Washington, DC 20024-2812
www.appi.org

Library of Congress Cataloging-in-Publication Data
A CIP record is available from the Library of Congress.
ISBN: 9781615374700 (hardcover), 9781615374717 (ebook)

British Library Cataloguing in Publication Data
A CIP record is available from the British Library.

CONTENTS

PART II
Responding to the Realities of Racism

PART III
A Call to Research

PART IV
Racism, Leadership, and Organized Psychiatry

Contributors

June Jackson Christmas, M.D.
Professor Emeritus of Behavioral Science, City of New York Medical School, New York, New York

H. Westley Clark, M.D., J.D., M.P.H.
Dean's Executive Professor of Public Health, Santa Clara University, Santa Clara, California

Pamela Y. Collins, M.D., M.P.H.
Professor, Department of Psychiatry and Behavioral Sciences and Department of Global Health, University of Washington, Seattle, Washington

James P. Comer, M.D., M.P.H.
Maurice Falk Professor of Child Psychiatry, Yale Child Study Center, New Haven, Connecticut

Devin Cromartie, M.D., M.P.H.
Assistant Professor of Psychiatry, Boston University School of Medicine, Boston, Massachusetts

Michelle P. Durham, M.D., M.P.H., DFAPA, DFAACAP
Chief Behavioral Health Officer, Ibn Sina Foundation, Houston, Texas

Loma K. Flowers, M.D.
Clinical Professor of Psychiatry, University of California San Francisco Volunteer Faculty; President, EQDynamics, San Francisco, California

Keith Hermanstyne, M.D., M.P.H., M.S.H.P.M.
Former UCLA–Robert Wood Johnson Foundation Clinical Scholars Program Member, Los Angeles, California

William Lawson, M.D., Ph.D., DLFAPA
Clinical Professor, Department of Psychiatry and Behavioral Sciences, George Washington University, Washington, D.C.

Hassell H. McClellan, M.B.A.
Associate Professor of Finance and Policy (retired), Boston College Carroll School of Management, Chestnut Hill, Massachusetts

Stephen A. McLeod-Bryant, M.D.
Clinical Associate Professor, Department of Psychiatry and Behavioral Sciences, University of Miami Miller School of Medicine, Miami, Florida

Donna M. Norris, M.D.
Assistant Professor (part-time), Beth Israel Deaconess Medical Center, Department of Psychiatry, Harvard Medical School, Boston, Massachusetts

Nicola Park, M.D.
Psychiatry Resident, Department of Psychiatry and Behavioral Sciences, University of Washington, Seattle, Washington

Annelle B. Primm, M.D., M.P.H., DLFAPA
Senior Medical Director, The Steve Fund; Associate Professor (part-time, volunteer), The Johns Hopkins School of Medicine, Department of Psychiatry and Behavioral Sciences, Baltimore, Maryland

David Satcher, M.D., Ph.D.
16th U.S. Surgeon General; Founder and Senior Advisor, Satcher Health Leadership Institute, Morehouse School of Medicine, Atlanta, Georgia

Ruth S. Shim, M.D., M.P.H.
Luke and Grace Kim Professor in Cultural Psychiatry, Professor, Department of Psychiatry and Behavioral Sciences, and Associate Dean, Diverse and Inclusive Education, School of Medicine, University of California, Davis, Sacramento, California

Altha J. Stewart, M.D.
Senior Associate Dean for Community Health Engagement, University of Tennessee Health Science Center, Memphis, Tennessee

Johnny Williamson, M.D.
Clinical Instructor, Department of Psychiatry, University of Illinois Chicago; President, Spectrum Behavioral Health, Hinsdale, Illinois

Disclosures

The following contributors to this book have indicated a financial interest in or other affiliation with a commercial supporter, a manufacturer of a commercial product, a provider of a commercial service, a nongovernmental organization, and/or a government agency, as listed below:

Stephen A. McLeod-Bryant, M.D., owns shares of Pfizer common stock and NextEra Energy common stock and a partial investment share in Electronic Health Networks.

The following contributors have indicated that they have no financial interests or other affiliations that represent or could appear to represent a competing interest with their contributions to this book:

June Jackson Christmas, M.D.; H. Westley Clark, M.D., J.D., M.P.H.; Pamela Y. Collins, M.D., M.P.H.; Michelle P. Durham, M.D., M.P.H., DFAPA, DFAACAP; Loma K. Flowers, M.D.; Keith Hermanstyne, M.D., M.P.H., M.S.H.P.M.; William Lawson, M.D., Ph.D.; Hassell H. McClellan; Donna M. Norris, M.D.; Annelle B. Primm, M.D., M.P.H.; David Satcher, M.D., Ph.D.; Altha J. Stewart, M.D.; Johnny Williamson, M.D.

Preface

In this book, we establish the Solomon Carter Fuller Award lectures, named for the first Black psychiatrist in the United States, as a critical reference on African American history and mental health in the twentieth and twenty-first centuries. The editors undertook this book project as a tribute to the Solomon Carter Fuller awardees who have been honored by the Black Psychiatrists of America and the American Psychiatric Association (APA) Committee and Caucus of Black Psychiatrists since 1970. As we attended these lectures over the years, we became aware that there was no archive of this seminal collection of writings. We are passionate about documenting the insights offered by awardees during their lectures at the APA Annual Meeting. These lecturers used their voices and scholarship as tools for advocacy to increase awareness of the imprint of enslavement and racism on the lived experience of Black people in the United States as well as society on the whole. This body of knowledge is a treasure that needs to be recognized for its merit, celebrated for its impact, and shared with a wider audience.

Among the chapter authors are Solomon Carter Fuller lecturers from the past 30 years. In addition, several psychiatrists contributed chapters using the work of past awardees as inspiration. A scholar expert in finance developed a chapter on the role of economic disparities on mental health in Black communities.

The authors present a multidisciplinary cross-sectional look back in history and examine the contemporary environment in which Black people are living in the United States. Notable aspects of this environment include the law enforcement killing of unarmed Black people and horrific acts of mass violence. Mass shootings in a wide array of diverse communities have become more frequent in recent years, and the May 2022 murders in Buffalo, New York, were identified as a federal hate crime against Black people. This occurrence underscores that for a Black person, engaging in everyday activities such as attending church or grocery shopping may represent life-endangering events.

The authors of this volume also use the historical lens as a bridge to the future as it relates to mental health in Black communities. The areas covered intersect with a wide expanse of American life, including public health, public policy, health care inequities, racism, economic well-being, media, and education.

Thinking critically about the perspectives shared in this book will permit readers to gain insight into the biopsychosocial and political realities of life in Black and other communities of color. This material is clinically applicable in mental health practice. Furthermore, the pernicious aspect of racism is discussed as it relates to Black psychiatrists as clinicians and leaders within the profession. Each chapter offers salient takeaways that encourage hope in the face of adversity.

We give heartfelt thanks to all of the chapter authors for their perseverance in completing their contributions to the book during the COVID-19 pandemic. We are grateful to Alison Bondurant, M.A., CAPM, for her diligence and indispensable project management. To our distinguished psychiatrist colleague, Yvonne Ferguson, M.D., we express gratitude for her support. We greatly appreciate the artist Mr. Emmett Wigglesworth for granting us permission to use his vibrant original artwork on the cover of the book. We extend a special thank you to Ms. Erika Parker, Acquisitions Editor, American Psychiatric Association Publishing, who has been our guide throughout the process of developing the book.

We dedicate this book to our children, who are the future: Marlaina Norris, M.D., M.B.A.; Michael Norris, M.B.A., M.Fin.; and India Primm-Spencer, M.H.A.

PART I

Conditions Affecting Life in Black Communities

Public Health and Mental Health Disparities in Black Communities

CHALLENGES FOR AMERICAN PSYCHIATRY

June Jackson Christmas, M.D.
Donna M. Norris, M.D.
Annelle B. Primm, M.D., M.P.H., DLFAPA

June Jackson Christmas, M.D., a distinguished New York City–based psychiatrist, has had an illustrious career. She has held numerous significant leadership roles in psychiatry and public health, including vice president of the American Psychiatric Association in 1974; president of the American Public Health Association in 1980 (the first Black woman president of the organization); New York City commissioner of Mental Health, Mental Retardation, and Alcoholism Services in 1972; and professor emeritus, Behavioral Sciences, City University of New York Medical School (Christmas 1925–2008). Dr. Christmas was a professor of psychiatry at the Columbia University College of Physicians and Surgeons, and Columbia University has named the Dr. June Jackson Christmas Medical Student Program at the Department of Psychiatry in her honor. The numerous honors bestowed on Dr. Christmas include Distinguished Visitor, Distinguished Scholar, and Distinguished Lecturer at Vassar College, the University of Oklahoma, Boston University School of Medicine, and the Phelps Stokes Fund. In addition, Dr. Christmas has received honorary degrees from Boston University, Trinity College, and the University of Medicine and Dentistry of New Jersey, and she is a fellow of the New York Academy of Medicine.

In 1995, Dr. Christmas delivered the Solomon Carter Fuller Lecture at the Annual Meeting of the American Psychiatric Association (Christmas 1995). Nearly 30 years later, we (D.M.N. and A.B.P.) joined Dr. Christmas for a conversation to revisit aspects of her lecture pertaining to the social determinants of health and mental health and the structural forces and policies that undergird them. Our discussion served as a basis for this chapter, in which we consider historical issues viewed through the prism of the circumstances confronting the Black community and other communities of color in the contemporary period and their impact on well-being and quality of life.

Health and Mental Health Care Disparities

Regarding public health and mental health care disparities, policy changes over the past 50 years have only incrementally affected the health and mental health care that Black people receive. One major policy change was the enactment of the Patient Protection and Affordable Care Act of 2010 (also known as the Affordable Care Act [ACA]) and the move toward accessibility of health care for more people. However, disparities in access to health care between Black and white populations remain. A study published in 2020 found that in the years since the ACA was passed, insurance coverage increased more for non-Hispanic Black people and Hispanics than for non-Hispanic whites, and disparities in coverage decreased (Buchmueller and Levy 2020). However, "despite these improvements, a large number of adults remain uninsured, and the uninsurance rate among Blacks and Hispanics is substantially higher than the rate among whites" (Buchmueller and Levy 2020, p. 400). There has been a modicum of progress among Black people in gaining access, but access still lags behind that of white people, resulting in continued disparities (Taylor 2019).

The COVID-19 pandemic has highlighted the differences in access to care and the amount of money spent for services. For example, the New York City Department of Health, a leading department of public health, kept records of racial identity inconsistently in the first months of the pandemic. As a result of national inquiries about COVID-19 illness and mortality rates by race, the health department had to make a special effort to extract that data. The mandate to collect health-related data by race was a major policy change brought about by the ACA, which requires that federal health data collection efforts include information on race, ethnicity, sex, primary language, and disability status. As noted by a fact sheet from the U.S. Department of Health and Human Services (2012), "In the past, identifying disparities and effectively monitoring efforts to reduce them has been limited by a lack of specificity, uniformity, and quality in data collection and reporting procedures" (p. 1).

Lack of inclusion of Black people in COVID-19-related research has hindered the ability of researchers to collect reliable data on this critical issue. For example, a review of six studies early in the pandemic found underrepresentation of Black patients in all six in relation to the affected population in the cities in which the studies took place. The review authors made an urgent request: "It is essential that all investigators uniformly report race/ethnicity data as well as attempt, in earnest, to obtain representativeness among study participants in order to ensure that we do not develop a further widening of the treatment gap during this pandemic" (Borno et al. 2020).

Similarly, the documentation of mental health care data disaggregated by race and ethnicity is sporadic. The variation is due to geographical differences given that 12 states have not adopted Medicaid expansion (Kaiser Family Foundation 2022). Medicaid access may be higher for Black people than white people because of greater poverty. However, Medicaid access has not made a significant difference in health disparities between Black, white, American Indian, and Hispanic populations. A recent study of Medicaid recipients with depression found that African Americans were about half as likely as whites to receive treatment, Hispanics were about a third as likely, and people from other racial/ethnic groups were about a fifth as likely. Whites were more likely than any other group to receive medication only (Baumgartner et al. 2020; Cross-Call 2020; McGregor et al. 2020).

Black people, and Black men in particular, are overrepresented among people who have mental illness and are living on the street in large urban areas such as San Francisco, Los Angeles, New York City, and Washington, D.C., because of lack of adequate mental health care and follow-up. Deinstitutionalization, which had the goal of releasing people with mental illness from hospitals into communities, did not make adequate provisions for community-based outpatient mental health care (Frontline 2005). A street survey of unsheltered people in Manhattan found that about one-third had a mental illness, about two-thirds had had a substance use disorder in their lifetime, and just over half had a history of repeated trauma (Levitt et al. 2009). According to the Coalition for the Homeless (2021), the number of homeless single adults in New York City is 103% higher than it was 10 years earlier, and the large majority of unsheltered homeless people are living with mental illness or other severe health problems.

Since 1960, rehabilitation efforts to improve mental health and physical health equity and to increase access to Medicaid have not resulted in a significant reduction in the number of people with persistent mental illness who are unsheltered and homeless. A report from the Treatment Advocacy Center notes that "people with untreated serious mental illness comprise an estimated one-third of the total homeless population in the United States," and "in major cities from New York to San Diego, homeless people with severe mental illness are now an accepted part of the urban landscape" (Treatment Advocacy Center 2016).

Geographic differences in fiscal allotments for mental health care from the federal government (Medicaid) to the states have a differential impact on Black people and people living in poverty. States and counties choose the amount of money they will put into mental health. As an example, Kentucky was resistant to accepting funding for Medicaid for mental health care. As of September 2021, 7 of the 12 states that had not expanded Medicaid were in the Southeast: Alabama, Florida, Georgia, Kansas, Mississippi, North Carolina, and South Carolina (Commonwealth Fund 2021). An annual state-by-state ranking of mental health care by Mental Health America shows that 6 of those 7 states are among the lowest ranked (Reinert et al. 2021).

Whether in the North or the South in the United States, even areas of greater affluence, such as Dupont Circle in Washington, D.C., have people coping with addictions. This area, which was once a high-end neighborhood, now looks like any other urban area, with a triad of social conditions that often accompany each other: mental illness, addiction, and homelessness.

States are still making decisions that affect people locally. Very often the push has been to get homeless people out of sight and put them in housing, even if temporarily. Commonly, because of shifting political priorities, the promised objective to house homeless people becomes less of an imperative. As a result, financial support of these initiatives becomes a casualty of budgetary strain.

The Impact of the Political and Judicial Systems on Health Care in the Twenty-First Century

On June 17, 2021, the U.S. Supreme Court rejected a challenge to the ACA, marking the third time it had done so. This is an example of how policy is a determinant of health and health care (Dawes 2020). The health and mental health of Black people hinge on their access to health care, for which policy is a major driver.

It has been disappointing that policy changes have not been a difference maker as anticipated. Medicine, psychiatry, and public health must keep policy in the forefront—deliberating on processes even when progress is slow. Significantly, even with a new administration in 2020, the policy direction reflects aspirational goals in task force selection and gives hope that there will be advancement. Political leadership and community advocacy have driven significant increases in funding for mental health, addictions, housing, children, poverty, and job opportunities, which have the potential of significantly improving the quality of life of all Americans and, in particular, people living in poverty, of which disproportionate numbers are Black.

The focus now is on the intersectionality of the social-economic-political context currently affecting Black people in the United States today. These issues do not stand alone. Viewing them in isolation is inappropriate given the fact that they are interdependent.

Historically, Black people were the foundation of the economy of the United States, considered as chattel, goods, and services for purchase, sale, and discarding. Black people made the economy of this country. It was important then and continues to be important in this country today that there is a racial hierarchy in which Black people are at the bottom and white people are at the top. In the nineteenth century, being a Black person, whether enslaved or not, was a constant risk factor for an individual's well-being and safety.

In the twenty-first century, we see the emergence of questioning the value and applicability of democracy to all of the people in the United States. Case in point: even with the passage of civil rights legislation that guaranteed the right to vote in 1964, political leaders are now challenging these rights that are essential to citizenship. Therefore, Black people throughout the country are experiencing blatant efforts to disenfranchise them. Contemporary trends indicate that progress is retreating from the promise offered in the 1960s. During the first 9 months of

2021, 19 states enacted 33 laws making it more difficult to vote, according to a report from the Brennan Center. The report noted that state lawmakers are "justifying these measures with falsehoods steeped in racism about election irregularities and breaches of election security" (Brennan Center for Justice 2021).

Given the stark racial disparities in wealth that persist today, many Black people are not able to afford all the elements needed for good health care, such as medical visits, medication, and rehabilitation. Diabetes and obesity are known to be adverse effects of certain psychopharmacological treatments, but because of our limited repertoire of options, these medications are commonly prescribed. When medication is unaffordable, most people will not purchase it, or they will ration it, using less than the recommended dosage, which means they may not receive the full benefit of the treatment. For example, the cost of insulin has skyrocketed in recent years even though insulin is a medication that has been available since 1921, which should have made it more affordable for everyone. As a result, people went without insulin during the COVID-19 pandemic. Hawryluk (2020) pointed out that "Surveys conducted before the pandemic showed that 1 in 4 people with either Type 1 or Type 2 diabetes had rationed insulin because of the cost. Black people, Hispanics, and American Indians have disproportionately high rates of diabetes and are also more likely to face economic disparities that make insulin unaffordable." It is a sad commentary that the people who need this medication the most are the least able to afford it (Cefalu et al. 2018).

During the COVID-19 pandemic, on top of the mortality and medical morbidity of the virus itself, an economic crisis of unemployment, loss of housing, inability to pay rent, and food insecurity hit people of color the hardest. Given the high prevalence of chronic diseases such as diabetes, hypertension, end-stage renal disease, and asthma among Black people, they were more susceptible to COVID-19, increasing their risk of severe illness and death. These conditions are commonly regarded as "diseases of choice," meaning that their risk is determined by an individual's lifestyle choices. However, research has shown that the stress of racial discrimination contributes to high rates of hypertension among African Americans (Centers for Disease Control and Prevention 2021; Williams et al. 2019). Black people have higher rates of hypertension than other racial/ethnic groups—in 2017, the rate of hypertension among Black adults was 40% compared with 28% for whites, 28% for Hispanics, and 25% for Asians (Fryar et al. 2017). It is common for hypertension, diabetes, and other chronic diseases to be comorbid with mental illnesses such as depression. Furthermore, the psychological burden of racism can contribute to "self-medication" with food, resulting in obesity, diabetes, and heart disease, or with substances such as alcohol and illicit drugs, leading to addiction (Jackson et al. 1996). Placing blame on Black patients for the high prevalence of these diseases is a misrepresentation of the devastating impact of racism on health status, its maintenance, and emotional well-being (Williams et al. 2019).

Stereotypes About Black People That Lead to Disparities in Health Care

The myth of Black people being "happy-go-lucky" has contributed to the erroneous belief that they do not experience pain as compared with white people. In the nineteenth century, obstetrician-gynecologist J. Marion Sims conducted surgery on Black women without adequate anesthesia on the basis of his assumption that Black women were supposed to bear pain (Domonoske 2018; Lerner 2003). During medical school in the 1940s, one of the authors of this chapter noted that Black women did not receive painkillers (J. Christmas, personal communication, June 2021). The stereotype was that "they can take anything." It is unfortunate that this stereotype about pain management and these practices from the nineteenth century carried over into present-day medical education and affect Black men as well as women. Black people often do not receive adequate pain management because of a concern that they are inappropriately seeking drugs. A meta-analysis of 20 years of studies of disparities in pain management found that "Blacks/African Americans experienced both a higher number and magnitude of disparities than any other group in the analyses. In sub analyses, opioid treatment disparities for Blacks/African Americans remained consistent across pain types, settings, study quality, and data collection periods" (Meghani et al. 2012, p. 156).

　　Early in the COVID-19 crisis, it was common for Black people to choose to forego seeking timely medical care in hospitals for fear that they would die in those facilities. Currently, people with chronic conditions who went without care earlier in the pandemic are now presenting to hospitals with increased morbidity and poorer prognoses. This results in more extensive hospitalizations (Czeisler et al. 2020). When people severely ill with COVID-19 were hospitalized, they often encountered ventilator rationing and medication shortages. The presence of chronic illness in a given patient determined whether they would be eligible for certain treatment protocols. In a study of 2,217 adults hospitalized for COVID-19 in 2020, Black patients experienced the lowest physician follow-up after discharge and the longest delays in returning to work. Nonwhite (Black, Asian, Latinx) patients also were more likely to be readmitted to the hospital within 60 days of discharge (Robinson-Lane et al. 2021).

A study that looked at the convergence of poverty and race during the pandemic found that numerous impediments to safe housing and quality health care may have negative impacts on comorbidities (Duque 2021). For people living in poverty, it is cheaper to eat fast foods that are higher in fat, salt, and sugar that fill you up but have lower nutritional value and create risk for chronic disease. It is expensive to eat a healthier diet, and Black people commonly have limited access to fresh fruits and vegetables. Typically, grocery stores with higher-quality food, more choices, and lower prices are located at an inconvenient distance from their neighborhoods.

According to a 2021 study, during the pandemic, food insecurity increased significantly among low-income Black households enrolled in the Supplemental Nutrition Assistance Program (SNAP) and residing in a food desert. In 2020, 44% of SNAP participants were using food banks, and 29% were newly food insecure in 2020 but had not been food insecure in 2018 (Siddiqi et al. 2021).

As the pandemic dragged on, communities established food pantries to serve all groups, including middle-class and working-class people temporarily experiencing poverty and economic hardship. People in need, regardless of race, had similar experiences of adversity. Despite the commonality of hunger, racial groups remained separated socially, politically, and geographically.

Social Justice, Violence, and Black Lives Matter

With the pandemic as a backdrop, the fight for social justice emerged as a critical issue. This represented a retrogression to the challenges that the country faced in the 1970s, when Dr. Christmas gave her Solomon Carter Fuller speech. Social justice was a major issue at that time. Are we slipping back? In the aftermath of the killing of Black men or Black women by the police, white people and Black people march together again, carrying signs saying Black Lives Matter. At the same time, disruption of the political struggle is occurring because of increased violence from white nationalist groups. This violence perpetrated by white extremist groups is happening with greater frequency in America today, which is frightening for Black people, other people of color, and certain targeted religious groups. Superimposed on this is the violence by Black and brown people against members of their own communities, related in part to the blight, desperation, and hopelessness endemic in racially segregated urban areas.

A common thread in early childhood and adolescence among Black children and other children of color is that they have always experienced the police as a threatening force, even when they have not been involved in any wrongdoing. According to a study in the *Journal of Adolescent Health*,

> significant racial/ethnic disparities in feeling angry and unsafe during witnessed police stops emerged, with multiracial, Black, and Hispanic youth exhibiting the highest rates of these forms of emotional distress. In the case of Black and multiracial youth, officer intrusiveness and perceptions of procedural injustice collectively explain a large portion of disparities in emotional distress during witnessed stops. (Jackson et al. 2021, p. 250)

The study authors conclude that "youth of color are more likely to report emotional distress during witnessed police stops, largely due to the officer intrusiveness and perceived injustices that characterize these stops" (Jackson et al. 2021, p. 250).

Black people recognize the existence of differential treatment by law enforcement based on race. For example, the view of sympathetic legislators of the violent storming of the U.S. Capitol by whites on January 6, 2021, was of "tourists" expressing their First Amendment rights. If the attackers had been Black, they would have been in jail or killed. An order would have come to get rid of them. Knowing this affects the mental health of Black people (Shammas 2021).

In the South in the 1960s, police attacked people who were exercising their civil rights by protesting in a nonviolent way the unequal treatment of Black people under the law. Similarly, today, examples can be found of public officials using law enforcement to punish peaceful protesters. A case in point is the demonstrators who came out against the killing of George Floyd and other police killings. Black people are angry and are tired of this repetitive pattern of continued inequality and abuse in spite of the passage of civil rights legislation (Hawkins 2022).

Repeated trauma of Black people has taken its toll on their mental health. Research has found that highly public anti-Black violence is associated with poor mental health days for Black Americans. Curtis et al.

(2021) looked at data on 49 identified incidents of nationally publicized racial violence over a 5-year period. Using data from the Behavioral Risk Factor Surveillance System, they found that Black respondents indicated a significantly higher average of 0.31 more poor mental health days during weeks with two or more highly publicized racial incidents relative to weeks with none. Racial incidents did not predict average poor mental health days among white respondents. Further, a qualitative study using phenomenological interviews found that the "Black community can be traumatized by viewing graphic images or videos of police brutality. Interviewees reported a constant fear of dying, hyper alertness, and lack of coping mechanisms" (Hawkins 2022, p. 1120).

On a Saturday afternoon in 2022, an 18-year-old white supremacist killed 10 Black people, most of them older adults, in a supermarket in Buffalo, New York. The shooter was driven by racial hatred that was fueled by social media and powered with access to a semiautomatic weapon, and his terrorist attack unleashed trauma in a community historically beset with extreme segregation and systemic inequities (Closson 2022). In the immediate aftermath of this tragedy, residents of the Masten Park neighborhood in Buffalo's East Side were fearful of leaving their homes, and their community has become food insecure (B. Belim, personal communication, May 2022). The harm caused by this massacre extends beyond this Black neighborhood in western New York, affecting the mental health of Black people across the country. A nationwide poll conducted after the shooting reported that 75% of Black people in the United States worry that they or their loved ones will be a victim of a racial attack (Foster-Frau et al. 2022). The poll also found that the majority of Black Americans polled reported sadness and anger in association with the attack. Furthermore, only 1 in 10 surveyed believe that racism will improve during their lifetimes, whereas the majority think that racism will worsen.

Black communities also face racism from the law enforcement officers who are supposed to protect them. Dr. Christmas recounted a personal experience involving her 15-year-old son meeting a friend on West 96th Street and Central Park West in New York City (J. Christmas, personal communication, June 2021). A white police officer asked him what he was doing there, questioned him in a hostile manner, and told him to leave. Following this encounter, he wandered around afraid. In this context, Black police officers seek to prove themselves by identifying with the dominant group in law enforcement. When Eric Adams was a child, he and his brother were detained and beaten by police for stealing. Eventually, he served as a police officer and won election as mayor of New York City in 2021. The question is: do you work from within the "system," or do you work from without? Mental health professionals are partnering with police departments in communities around the country to implement a coresponder model that promotes a more appropriate response from the criminal justice system when alleged perpetrators have unmet mental health needs (Krider et al. 2020).

Reflecting on her upbringing in a racially mixed neighborhood in Cambridge, Massachusetts, in the 1920s, Dr. Christmas recalled that homes rented to Black people were located on clay pits, which would eventually sink, leading to their foundations becoming unstable (J. Christmas, personal communication, June 2021). This is an example of environmental racism involving the relegation of Black people to live in undesirable and segregated areas. Social injustice of this nature is common across the United States in areas of urban decay and deterioration. The water crisis in Flint, Michigan, is an ongoing disaster with long-term consequences affecting health, education, and the futures of generations of children (Seghal 2018).

COVID-19 and Mental Health in Black Communities

At the beginning of the COVID-19 pandemic, people commonly minimized the disease because they did not have a frame of reference to understand the lethality and devastation of such an infectious disease. Many people, including people of color, thought of COVID-19 as a bad case of the flu and said not to worry about it. Initially, public health officials noted that people with preexisting health conditions, such as heart disease and asthma, would be most at risk. The problem was that most Black people did not consider themselves to be medically vulnerable, even if they had hypertension, diabetes, and obesity. These were not conditions that would justify them, especially if they were essential workers, staying home and not going to work because their families were dependent on their financial support. This is another aspect of racism that puts people in subordinate positions because multigenerational limitations in educational and economic opportunities are difficult to escape.

When people began dying from COVID-19, it was frightening, but people continued going to work until the pandemic reached a crisis point in which hospitals were at capacity and medication and medical equipment were in short supply. Historically, some hospitals in New York City have been identified by Black communities as not wanting Black people as patients. When it was difficult to get into these hospitals during the pandemic, Black people were able to understand this exclusion through the lens of discrimination to which they were accustomed.

The issue of the COVID-19 vaccine for Black people is complex. The experience of Black people involved in research efforts without their permission and their sense of receiving lower-quality care are barriers to them accepting the vaccine easily. Frequently, even listening to trusted physicians describe the safety and efficacy of the vaccine cannot overcome these obstacles (Bogart et al. 2022). In actuality, it is common for people in Black communities to not have a primary care physician with whom they can discuss vaccination or even insurance coverage. As mentioned earlier, the states, especially in the South, that decided against Medicaid expansion left large numbers of Black people with limited or no insurance.

Shim and Starks (2021) characterized the complicated interplay of the COVID-19 pandemic, structural racism, and mental health inequities that has led to an array of disastrous health, economic, and social consequences. The interactions of these conditions is known as a *syndemic*, in which the synergies of the co-occurring epidemics, COVID-19 and racism, wreak havoc on society and create challenges in the realm of policy. However, these twin crises also provide an opportunity to address these challenges in an integrated and comprehensive way in order to achieve meaningful advances in finding solutions for the most vexing problems in our society.

Summary and Takeaways

Over the past three decades, the conditions in which Black people live have not changed much. Racial segregation in education continues in urban areas, and schools are significantly underresourced, resulting in lower academic achievement and lack of preparation for employment or higher education. Lack of affordable housing remains a critical issue across the country, especially for Black people. The destruction of public housing in areas such as New York City and Chicago has led to gentrification, which has built up these vacant spaces by replacing them with expensive luxury housing designed for affluent white people.

During the early 1960s, communities in New York City held town hall meetings to mandate planning under the Mental Health Act (J. Christmas, personal communication, June 2022). These meetings were effective for a while, and psychiatrists such as Dr. Christmas received plaques of appreciation for their involvement in program planning for people needing services for mental health and developmental disabilities. However, mental health budgets became strained, and funding, including from the federal government, is now limited, and as a result, prioritizing comprehensive mental health planning is no longer sustainable.

It is important to encourage young psychiatrists to pursue public service and go into government work with people in underserved communities, the Black community, and other communities of color. However, these young professionals may become frustrated with the slow pace of change. The change that a professional can foster in communities has a multigenerational impact from the prenatal period to early childhood and throughout the life span. Facilitating change in communities can be satisfying, but at times it can be discouraging. It also can be a mode of gaining insight into oneself and one's professional accomplishments. This is a call to service in which the practitioner should focus professional pursuits on fostering change in social conditions, with the goal of improving mental health and overall well-being in these communities.

References

Baumgartner JC, Collins SR, Radley DC, Hayes SL: How the Affordable Care Act has narrowed racial and ethnic disparities in access to health care. New York, Commonwealth Fund, 2020. Available at: www.commonwealthfund.org/publications/2020/jan/how-ACA-narrowed-racial-ethnic-disparities-access. Accessed May 1, 2022.

Bogart LM, Dong L, Gandhi P, et al: COVID-19 vaccine intentions and mistrust in a national sample of Black Americans. J Natl Med Assoc 113(6):599–611, 2022 34158171

Borno HT, Zhang S, Gomez S: COVID-19 disparities: an urgent call for race reporting and representation in clinical research. Contemp Clin Trials Commun 19:100630, 2020 32789282

Brennan Center for Justice: Voting laws roundup: October 2021. New York, Brennan Center for Justice, 2021. Available at: www.brennancenter.org/our-work/research-reports/voting-laws-roundup-october-2021. Accessed May 1, 2022.

Buchmueller TC, Levy HG: The ACA's impact on racial and ethnic disparities in health insurance coverage and access to care. Health Aff (Millwood) 39(3):395–402, 2020 32119625

Cefalu WT, Dawes DE, Gavlak G, et al: Insulin Access and Affordability Working Group: conclusions and recommendations. Diabetes Care 42(6):1299–1311, 2018 29739814

Centers for Disease Control and Prevention: Racism and health: racism is a serious threat to the public's health. Atlanta, GA, Centers for Disease Control and Prevention, November 2021. Available at: www.cdc.gov/minority-health/racism-disparities/index.html. Accessed May 1, 2022.

Christmas JJ: June Jackson Christmas papers, ScMG787. New York, Schomburg Center for Research in Black Culture, Manuscripts, Archives and Rare Books Division, New York Public Library, 1925–2008. Available at: https://archives.nypl.org/scm/22974. Accessed November 6, 2022.

Christmas JJ: Can psychiatry serve tomorrow's Black families: challenges for a profession in transition. Solomon Carter Fuller Award Lecture, American Psychiatric Association Annual Meeting, Miami, FL, June 1995

Closson T: Nobody cares about us here: anguish and anger on Buffalo's east side. New York Times, May 15, 2022. Available at: www.nytimes.com/2022/05/15/nyregion/east-side-buffalo-neighborhood.html. Accessed June 1, 2022.

Coalition for the Homeless: Basic facts about homelessness: New York City. Washington, DC, Coalition for the Homeless, 2021. Available at: www.coalitionforthehomeless.org/basic-facts-about-homelessness-new-york-city. Accessed May 1, 2022.

Commonwealth Fund: Status of Medicaid expansion. New York, Commonwealth Fund, September 22, 2021. Available at: www.commonwealth-fund.org/publications/maps-and-interactives/2021/jul/status-medicaid-expansion-and-work-requirement-waivers. Accessed May 1, 2022.

Cross-Call J: Medicaid expansion has helped narrow racial disparities in health coverage and access to care. Washington, DC, Center on Budget and Policy Priorities, 2020. Available at: www.cbpp.org/research/health/medicaid-expansion-has-helped-narrow-racial-disparities-in-health-coverage-and. Accessed May 1, 2022.

Curtis DS, Washburn T, Lee H, et al: Highly public anti-Black violence is associated with poor mental health days for Black Americans. Proc Natl Acad Sci USA 118(17):e2019624118, 2021 33875593

Czeisler MÉ, Marynak K, Clarke KE, et al: Delay or avoidance of medical care because of COVID-19-related concerns—United States, June 2020. MMWR Morb Mortal Wkly Rep 69(36):1250–1257, 2020 32915166

Dawes D: The Political Determinants of Health. Baltimore, MD, Johns Hopkins University Press, 2020.

Domonoske C: "Father of gynecology," who experimented on slaves, no longer on pedestal in NYC. Washington, DC, The Two-Way, National Public Radio, April 17, 2018. Available at: www.npr.org/sections/I-way/2018/04/17/603163394/-father-of-gynecology-who-experimented-on-slaves-no-longer-on-pedestal-in-nyc. Accessed May 1, 2022.

Duque RB: Black health matters too…especially in the era of Covid-19: how poverty and race converge to reduce access to quality housing, safe neighborhoods, and health and wellness services and increase the risk of co-morbidities associated with global pandemics. J Racial Ethn Health Disparities 8(4):1012–1025, 2021 32946069

Foster-Frau S, Hernandez AR, Clement S, Guskin E: Poll: Black Americans fear more racist attacks after Buffalo shooting. Washington Post, May 21, 2022. Available at: www.washingtonpost.com/nation/2022/05/21/post-poll-black-americans. Accessed June 1, 2022.

Frontline: Deinstitutionalization: a psychiatric "Titanic." Boston, MA, Public Broadcasting System, May 10, 2005. Available at: www.pbs.org/wgbh/pages/frontline/shows/asylums/special/excerpt.html. Accessed May 1, 2022.

Fryar CD, Ostchega Y, Hales CM, et al: Hypertension prevalence and control among adults: United States, 2015–2016. NCHS Data Brief No 289, October 2017. Atlanta, GA, Centers for Disease Control and Prevention. Available at: www.cdc.gov/nchs/products/databriefs/db289.htm. Accessed May 1, 2022.

Hawkins DS: "After Philando, I had to take a sick day to recover": psychological distress, trauma and police brutality in the Black community. Health Commun 37(9):1113–1122, 2022 33902344

Hawryluk M: Not pandemic-proof: insulin copay caps fall short, fueling underground exchanges. Kaiser Health News, October 5, 2020. Available at: https://khn.org/news/not-pandemic-proof-insulin-copay-caps-fall-short-fueling-underground-exchanges. Accessed May 1, 2022.

Jackson DB, Del Toro J, Semenza DC, et al: Unpacking racial/ethnic disparities in emotional distress among adolescents during witnessed police stops. J Adolesc Health 69(2):248–254, 2021 33814280

Jackson JS, Brown TN, Williams DR, et al: Racism and the physical and mental health status of African Americans: a thirteen-year national panel study. Ethn Dis 6(1–2):132–147, 1996 8882842

Kaiser Family Foundation: Status of state Medicaid expansion decisions: interactive map. San Francisco, CA, Kaiser Family Foundation, April 26, 2022. Available at: www.kff.org/medicaid/issue-brief/status-of-state-medicaid-expansion-decisions-interactive-map Accessed May 1, 2022.

Krider A, Huerter H, Gaherty K, Moore A: Responding to individuals in behavioral health crisis via co-responder models: the role of cities, counties, law enforcement, and providers. Policy Research Associates and National League of Cities Report, Delmar, NY, Policy Research Associates, 2020. Available at: www.prainc.com/resources/coresponder-models. Accessed May 1, 2022.

Lerner BH: Scholars argue over legacy of surgeon who was lionized, then vilified. New York Times, October 28, 2003. Available at: www.nytimes.com/2003/10/28/health/scholars-argue-over-legacy-of-surgeon-who-was-lionized-then-vilified.html. Accessed May 1, 2022.

Levitt AJ, Culhane DP, DeGenova J, et al: Health and social characteristics of homeless adults in Manhattan who were chronically or not chronically unsheltered. Psychiatr Serv 60(7):978–981, 2009 19564231

McGregor B, Li C, Baltrus P, et al: Racial and ethnic disparities in treatment and treatment type for depression in a national sample of Medicaid recipients. Psychiatr Serv 71(7):664–669, 2020 32237981

Meghani SH, Byun E, Gallagher RM: Time to take stock: a meta-analysis and systematic review of analgesic treatment disparities for pain in the United States. Pain Med 13(2):150–174, 2012 22239747

Reinert M, Fritze D, Nguyen T: The state of mental health in America 2022. Alexandria VA, Mental Health America, October 2021. Available at: https://mhanational.org/sites/default/files/2022%20State%20of%20Mental%20Health%20in%20America.pdf. Accessed May 1, 2022.

Robinson-Lane SG, Sutton NR, Chubb H, et al: Race, ethnicity, and 60-day outcomes after hospitalization with COVID-19. J Am Med Dir Assoc 22(11):2245–2250, 2021 34716006

Seghal P: Toxic history, poisoned water: the story of Flint. New York Times, July 3, 2018. Available at: www.nytimes.com/2018/07/03/books/review-poisoned-city-anna-clark-what-eyes-dont-see-mona-hanna-attisha-flint-water-crisis.html. Accessed May 1, 2022.

Shammas B: A GOP congressman compared Capitol rioters to tourists. Photos show him barricading a door. Washington Post, May 18, 2021. Available at: www.washingtonpost.com/politics/2021/05/18/clyde-tourist-capitol-riot-photos. Accessed May 1, 2022.

Shim RS, Starks SM: COVID-19, structural racism, and mental health inequities: policy implications for an emerging syndemic. Psychiatr Serv 72(10):1193–1198, 2021 33622042

Siddiqi SM, Cantor J, Dastidar MG, et al: SNAP participants and high levels of food insecurity in the early stages of the COVID-19 pandemic. Public Health Rep 136(4):457–465, 2021 33789530

Taylor J: Racism, inequality, and health care for African Americans. New York, The Century Fund, 2019. Available at: https://tcf.org/content/report/racism-inequality-health-care-african-americans. Accessed May 1, 2022.

Treatment Advocacy Center: Serious mental illness and homelessness. Arlington, VA, Treatment Advocacy Center, 2016. Available at: www.treatmentadvocacycenter.org/evidence-and-research/learn-more-about/3629-serious-mental-illness-and-homelessness. Accessed May 1, 2022.

U.S. Department of Health and Human Services: Improving data collection to reduce health disparities. Washington, DC, U.S. Department of Health and Human Services, 2012. Available at https://minorityhealth.hhs.gov/assets/pdf/checked/1/Fact_Sheet_Section_4302.pdf. Accessed May 1, 2022

Williams DR, Lawrence JA, Davis BA: Racism and health: evidence and needed research. Annu Rev Public Health 40:105–125, 2019 30601726

The Highs and Lows of Public Health Practice

David Satcher, M.D., Ph.D.

The history of public health practice is a history of highs and lows. Even now as we deal with COVID-19, we are experiencing high and low development that we will remember for years to come. If we look back to the last great pandemic 100 years ago, we see that there were also high points and low points. In fact, the Public Health Service (PHS) was born out of one of our most challenging public health experiences more than 200 years ago (Foege 2011).

One of my first experiences as I left my job as Director of the Centers for Disease Control and Prevention (CDC) to become the U.S. surgeon general was to revisit the yellow fever pandemic that took place in Philadelphia, Pennsylvania, in 1796—a pandemic that led to the death of more than 10% of the population of Philadelphia and led many survivors to abandon that city (Foege 2020). The 200th anniversary of the Philadelphia pandemic occurred just as I was beginning my job as the surgeon general.

Like many other outbreaks during that period, this yellow fever outbreak was related to a virus spread by soldiers returning from the war front. In time, President John Adams, while in the White House (the U.S. Capitol was still located in Philadelphia), would establish the PHS in Philadelphia. In 1998, as I started my tenure as surgeon general, I visited Philadelphia—the birthplace of the PHS going back to 1798—as well as cities such as Boston where hospitals were set up to quarantine and treat soldiers returning from the war front.

Most people would agree that one of the highest points in the history of public health was the eradication of smallpox disease. The two leading organizations in smallpox eradication were the CDC and the World Health Organization (WHO). The eradication of a disease means that it no longer exists anywhere in the world. The last case of smallpox was documented in India in 1978, but the disease was officially declared eradicated by the WHO in 1980 (World Health Organization 2020). In short, a disease is not eradicated until the WHO declares that it is eradicated. To date, no other disease has been declared eradicated.

The world is close to eliminating polio, which has been eliminated in most places except Afghanistan and Pakistan. When I was director of the CDC, we came close to eradicating polio. But because of the fighting in those countries, we could not get vaccinations to the children there. In short, politics can interfere with the eradication of a disease. Although most countries have now eliminated polio, the disease is not yet eradicated despite our ability to immunize against it in more than 99% of countries. It was indeed a momentous day when Africa was declared free of wild polio, but polio was not eradicated. Until every country has eliminated polio, it will not be globally eliminated.

But virtually in the same year that WHO declared smallpox eradicated, we began experiencing the rise of a new viral disease: HIV/AIDS. The rise in the prevalence of HIV/AIDS began in the early 1980s. In those early years, highly active retrovirus was seen in many gay men, which led to the misconception and labeling of AIDS as a gay-related disease. Like many other disparities in health, this was misunderstood and led to a delay in progress in controlling the disease. Between 1981 and early 2000, we saw a dramatic decline in AIDS prevalence and deaths in the United States (Centers for Disease Control and Prevention 2001a). Later, because of pre-exposure prophylaxis with tenofovir/emtricitabine, there was an overall drop in HIV infections from 2012 to 2016 and a decrease in AIDS, but in the absence of a vaccine our progress was to be limited. Until we can prevent a disease in addition to using drugs for diagnosis and treatment, progress is limited. Again, smallpox and polio are examples. Usually, prevention is brought about through drug development and use of vaccines, but other variables also have an impact on success in treatment. These variables can include politics and economics.

After serving for 5 years as director of the CDC, I took on many of our public health problems that were not due to infectious diseases, including many examples of disparities in health. Foremost among these were smoking and health and overweight and obesity.

Smoking and Health

In 1964, Dr. Luther Terry released the first official surgeon general's report to the American people, *Smoking and Health* (Centers for Disease Control and Prevention 2021b; Surgeon General's Advisory Committee on Smoking and Health 1964). In many ways, Dr. Terry's report was successful in that it dramatically decreased the number of persons who were developing as new smokers. It clearly demonstrated that smokers were not hopeless because many persons were able to quit smoking and many others made the decision to not begin smoking. Luther Terry's report was released on a Saturday morning, in part because it was not prime time for the news media. On the way to release the report, Dr. Terry was smoking more than usual. His assistant asked him if he was concerned that he might be asked about his own smoking. Dr. Terry replied, "Why would they ask me a question like that?" His assistant said, "Well, OK, Dr. Terry, we'll see." After Dr. Terry had finished announcing the release of the report, the first question from the media was, "Dr. Terry, do you smoke?" Dr. Terry replied, "No, no, I don't." The media person asking the question then asked, "When did you quit smoking?" Dr. Terry replied, "I quit 30 minutes ago." Dr. Terry never smoked again. In fact, according to Dr. Terry's son Michael, whom I got to know, Dr. Terry walked around the rest of his life with a lapel pin that said "Thank You for Not Smoking."

Overweight and Obesity

Just as the interventions dealing with smallpox disease proved to be successful and certainly one of the high points in the history of public health, we must admit that the high prevalence of overweight and obesity represents a low point in the history of public health. In "The Surgeon General's Call to Action to Prevent and Decrease Overweight and Obesity 2001," an estimated 61% of U.S. adults were overweight or obese and 13% of children and adolescents were overweight (Centers for Disease Control and Prevention 2001b). This is a struggle that continues today. Although we have made dramatic progress over the past few decades in achieving so many of our health goals, the statistics on overweight and obesity have steadily headed in the wrong direction. If this situation is not reversed, it could wipe out the gains that we have made in areas such as heart disease, diabetes, several forms of cancer, and other chronic health problems. Unfortunately, excessive weight for height is a risk factor for all of these conditions.

Many people believe that dealing with overweight and obesity is a personal responsibility, and they are right, but just as with COVID-19 and the use of vaccines, it is also a community responsibility. Overweight and obesity must be approached as preventable and treatable problems, with realistic and exciting opportunities to improve health and save lives. The challenge is to create a multifaceted public health approach capable of delivering long-term reductions in the prevalence of overweight and obesity. This approach should focus on health rather than appearance, and it should empower both individuals and communities to address barriers, reduce stigmatization, and move forward in addressing overweight and obesity in a positive and proactive fashion.

Several events have drawn attention to overweight and obesity as public health problems. In 1998, the National Heart, Lung, and Blood Institute, with the cooperation of the National Institute of Diabetes and Digestive and Kidney Diseases of the National Institutes of Health, released "Clinical Guidelines on the Identification, Evaluation, and Treatment of Obesity in Adults" (National Institutes of Health 1998). This report was the result of a thorough scientific review of the evidence related to the risk and treatment of overweight and obesity and provided evidence-based treatment guidelines for health care providers. In early 2000, Healthy People 2010 was released. This agenda identified overweight and obesity as major public health problems and set national objectives for reduction of their prevalence (Centers for Disease Control and Prevention 2010). The National Nutrition Summit in May 2000 illuminated the impact of dietary and physical activity habits on achieving healthy body weight and thus began a national dialogue on strategies for the prevention of overweight and obesity (Stockmyer et al. 2001). Finally, a surgeon general's listening session, held in late 2000, and a related public comment period generated many useful ideas for prevention and treatment strategies and helped forge and reinforce an important coalition of stakeholders. Participants in these events considered many prevention and treatment strategies, including such national priorities as ensuring daily physical education in schools, increasing research on the behavioral and environmental causes of obesity, and promoting breastfeeding.

Diabetes and Native Americans

I served as director of the CDC from October 1993 to October 1998. During this period, the CDC increasingly articulated a concern for disparities in health among different social and ethnic groups. We were concerned that of all the groups, Native Americans have a greater chance of having diabetes than any other racial group (Centers for Disease Control and Prevention 2017a). Diabetes is the leading cause of kidney failure, a costly condition that requires dialysis or kidney transplant for survival. Kidney failure, however, can be delayed or prevented by controlling blood pressure and blood sugar and by taking medicines that protect the kidneys. Good diabetes care includes regular kidney testing and education of the population about kidney disease and treatment.

Kidney failure from diabetes among Native Americans was the highest of any race. However, with the CDC's intervention, kidney failure has declined the fastest since the Indian Health Service began using population health and team-based approaches to diabetes and kidney care (Centers for Disease Control and Prevention 2017b). This is a potential model for other populations. It should be pointed out that even though this intervention for diabetes in Native Americans started in the mid-1990s, it was not until 2013 that other studies showed these benefits, including the fact that kidney failure dropped by 54% in Native Americans between 1996 and 2013. These interventions can be summarized under three health care system findings (Centers for Disease Control and Prevention 2017a):

1. Use population health approaches to diabetes care.
2. Develop a coordinated team approach to diabetes care.
3. Integrate kidney disease prevention and education into routine diabetes care.

Native American adults have more diabetes than any other race or ethnicity, and team-based and population approaches reduce kidney failure from diabetes in this population. Between 1996 and 2013, kidney failure from diabetes in Native Americans dropped more than for any other race or ethnicity. Figures 2–1 and 2–2 describe the intervention and the outcome of this particularly important study (Centers for Disease Control and Prevention 2017b).

In summarizing the outcome of the interventions that were implemented almost 10 years earlier, the CDC in 2013 made the following observations regarding outcomes:

1. Native Americans are twice as likely as whites to have diabetes.
2. In about two out of three Native Americans with kidney failure, diabetes is the cause.

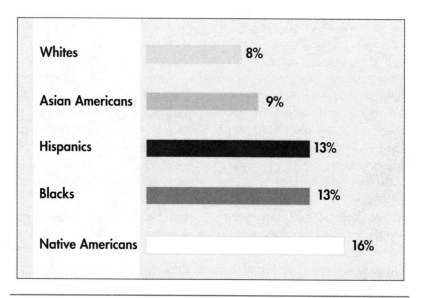

Figure 2-1.   Rates of diabetes by race/ethnicity, 2010–2012.
Source.   Centers for Disease Control and Prevention 2017b.

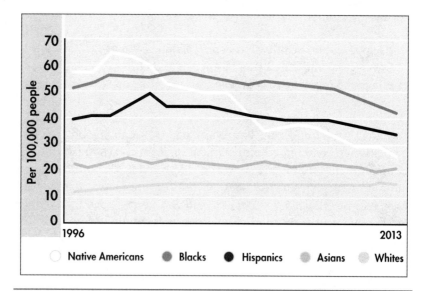

Figure 2-2.   Decline in kidney failure from diabetes in adults 18 and older, 1996–2013.
Source.   Centers for Disease Control and Prevention 2017b.

3. Kidney failure from diabetes dropped by 54% in Native Americans between 1996 and 2013 because of the health care system approach implemented in the mid-1990s described earlier.

A commitment to educate, motivate, and mobilize patients toward healthy lifestyles made the difference, and it can for others. As the former director of the CDC who implemented this intervention for Native Americans, I am grateful for the work of the chronic disease personnel who led this initiative at the CDC, and I am also grateful to former Speaker of the House Newt Gingrich and to Congress for providing the resources that allowed us to implement this intervention.

COVID-19

If the eradication of smallpox was an example of a high point in public health, then the current pandemic of COVID-19 must be examined as a low point in the history of public health. Advances in public health have built on the science that led to the eradication of smallpox disease. Three similarities stand out when comparing smallpox and COVID-19. First, scientists have developed a vaccine to reduce and prevent the spread of the virus. Second, conducting testing for presence of the virus permits intervention with strategies to significantly curtail the spread of the virus from person to person. And increasingly, we can treat persons with COVID-19 disease and thus reduce the magnitude of the illness, as was done with smallpox.

Some would argue that the COVID-19 outbreak and our experience with it is more likely to be remembered as a nadir in public health history. Despite the rapid development of a vaccine for COVID-19, less than 70% of Americans in 2020 said they would get the vaccine. For political and other reasons, many persons in the United States have refused the vaccine, and more than 1.1 million Americans have died from COVID-19. The virus continues to mutate and spread from person to person, with original development of variants that may not be sensitive to existing vaccines.

Of great concern is the fact that there are major disparities in the sensitivity to and impact of the COVID-19 virus. This means that disparities in health among different racial and ethnic groups in public health outcome measures may be increasing, especially among people of color. Because public health is driven by the collective efforts of a society to create the conditions in which people can be healthy, the disproportionate impact of COVID-19 on African Americans and other people of color tends to widen the public health gap that currently exists in our society—and, to a great extent, the world.

In short, disparities in health lead to disproportionate impact on different populations. The public health impact of new viruses on society depends on the susceptibility of populations. Disparities in access to vaccines lead to disparities in our ability to control the spread of the disease and is one of the ways of increasing the public health gaps among and/or between populations. It is imperative to develop a novel approach to public health that targets the population as a whole, with the goal of elevating the public health system.

What if We Had Eliminated Disparities in the Past Century?

In 2005, while Dr. George Rust and I were working toward the goal of eliminating disparities in health, we decided to examine the impact on public health if we had achieved such a goal in the past century. The results of our study were published in the journal *Ethnicity and Disease* (Satcher and Rust 2006). Our findings included the following: There would have been 83,500 fewer Black deaths in the year 2000 alone. This number would have included 24,000 fewer deaths from heart disease, 7,000 fewer deaths from HIV/AIDS, 4,700 fewer infant deaths, 22,000 fewer deaths from diabetes, and 2,000 fewer women dying from breast cancer. In addition to preventing these deaths, there would have been a major difference in the segment of the population covered by health insurance. This would have included 2.5 million more Black people, of which 620,000 would have been children.

When these data were graphed as standardized mortality ratios for Black people and white people by gender, a few messages were clear (Satcher and Rust 2006). Between 1980 and 1990 there was a major change for African American males and females. The mortality risk for Black males increased dramatically, whereas these ratios for Black females continued to decline. Although it is difficult to accurately pinpoint the causes of these changes, they are associated with two major factors in Black communities: 1) the incarceration of Black males due to drug intervention and 2) the resulting breakup of Black families.

Health equity is the equal opportunity to be healthy. The McKinlay model of health promotion (Figure 2–3) divides these opportunities into three levels: upstream, midstream, and downstream (McKinlay 1995). Upstream opportunities are related to policies that are made by legisla-

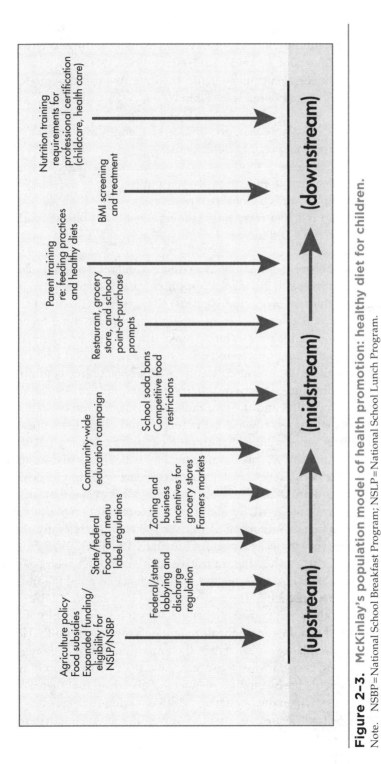

Figure 2–3. McKinlay's population model of health promotion: healthy diet for children.

Note.   NSBP=National School Breakfast Program; NSLP=National School Lunch Program.

Source.   Adapted from Glanz 1999; McKinlay 1995.

tors, midstream opportunities are created in the community, and downstream opportunities include motivation to eat healthy and to be physically active (Douglas et al. 2019; Glanz 1999).

At the Satcher Health Leadership Institute, we use this model to help teach six lessons about leadership:

1. Leadership responds to opportunities, challenges, and crises.
2. Leadership is not position dependent.
3. Leadership is a team sport.
4. Effective leadership transforms communities.
5. Leadership requires a global perspective.
6. Leadership is like a relay race: leaders must build on the work of those who preceded them.

It must be borne in mind that the reduction and ultimate elimination of disparities in health is a job for our public health system, and eliminating disparities involves more than just changes to health care. For example, as with the eradication of smallpox, we must come together around an agenda for prevention to make dramatic progress in reducing smoking and lung cancer and other diseases associated with it. We need to provide education and incentives for prevention to continue to reduce smoking and enhance health. Health care must be seen as a key part of public health, and the two must work together so we can continue to make progress toward the reduction and ultimate elimination of smoking as a major public health problem in America.

Just as important as encouraging healthy behavior is discouraging harmful behaviors. For example, along with encouraging physical activity on a regular basis, we should discourage behaviors that require little or no physical activity. Similarly, regular consumption of fruits and vegetables is just as important as the avoidance of excess fatty foods and sweets. This was clearly shown in the CDC study of the early twenty-first century showing a positive relationship between healthy behaviors in Native Americans and the avoidance of renal failure and heart disease (Centers for Disease Control and Prevention 2017b).

Throughout recent periods, where records are kept, healthy living has promoted health, and nonhealthy living has led to ill health. However, there are still gray areas where the impact on health of a range of styles of living is not always clear (e.g., how the consumption of milk harms or benefits the health of consumers). This means that there is still a need for research on the impact on health of various living habits and lifestyles. We must keep an open mind as well as keeping our eyes open to the latest information about health and how best to promote it.

Mental Health

In order to practice public health successfully in the future, we must do a better job of incorporating mental health. In "Mental Health: A Report of the Surgeon General," mental health is defined as the successful performance of mental function resulting in productive activity, fulfilling relationships with others, and the ability to adapt to change and successfully cope with adversity (Center for Mental Health Services 1999). On the other hand, mental illness or mental disorders are characterized by abnormalities in cognition, emotion, and mood or the highest integrative aspects of behavior, such as the ability to be productive or to manage relationships with others. Risk factors for mental illness include 1) prenatal damage through exposure to alcohol, illegal drugs, or tobacco; 2) low birth weight; 3) difficult temperament or predisposition to mental disorders; 4) external risk factors (e.g., poverty, deprivation, abuse, neglect); 5) unsatisfactory relationships; 6) parental mental health disorders; and 7) exposure to traumatic events.

In the surgeon general's report on mental health, mental health is defined as "the successful performance of mental function, resulting in productive activities, fulfilling relationships with others, and the ability to adapt to change and to successfully cope with adversity" (Center for Mental Health Services 1999, p. 36). The mental health matrix in the report highlighted "productive activities, the ability to adapt to change, fulfilling relationships and to successfully cope with adversity" (p. 37). Although this first surgeon general's report on mental health reflected noteworthy progress in our understanding and appreciation of mental health, there is still much to understand and learn about the brain and the mind-body relationship and how it is molded at various stages of development. This will also improve our understanding of mental illness.

In the surgeon general's report, mental disorders are described as abnormalities in cognition, emotion, or mood or the highest integrative aspects of behavior such as the ability to be productive or to manage relationships with others at various stages of life. It is important to understand what a mentally healthy child is and that such a child must have opportunities to enjoy a positive quality of life. The following are aspects of mental health in children:

- The child functions well at home, in school, and in their community and family.
- The child is free of disabling symptoms of psychopathology.

The surgeon general's report on mental health (Center for Mental Health Services 1999) included the following key messages:

- Mental health is fundamental to overall health and well-being.
- Mental disorders are real.
- Mental disorders are common.

Each year, one in five Americans will experience a mental illness (Centers for Disease Control and Prevention 2021a). Mental disorders are as disabling as cancer or heart disease in terms of premature death and lost productivity. In fact, the global burden of mental disorders is so great that in 2019, more than 970 million people were living with a mental illness worldwide (World Health Organization 2022). Globally, mental health problems are the leading cause of disability (Pan American Health Organization 2019). Among the major disabilities are

- Depression
- Anxiety
- Dementia
- Alcohol use disorder

The good news is that mental disorders are treatable (American Psychiatric Association 2022). Unfortunately, fewer than half (47.2%) of adults receive help for their mental health needs (National Institute of Mental Health 2023). In particular, depression in African Americans is often undiagnosed and undertreated. Additionally, among African American patients, schizophrenia is often misdiagnosed or overdiagnosed. One of the major barriers to treatment is stigma, which impedes treatment on three levels:

- Individual—keeps people who are experiencing a problem from acknowledging it
- Family/community/society—keeps people from acknowledging problems among family and friends or recommending help
- Policy—keeps government and the private sector from addressing problems

Another mental health crisis area is suicide, which is a significant public health problem:

- The majority of suicides are related to psychiatric illnesses, with depression, substance use disorders, and psychotic illnesses carrying the greatest risk (Brådvik 2018).

- Suicide was the twelfth leading cause of death in 2020 (National Institute of Mental Health 2023).
- Each day, approximately 130 Americans die of suicide (American Foundation for Suicide Prevention 2023).
- In 2020, more than 1 million people attempted suicide (Centers for Disease Control and Prevention 2022).

Mental illness is a problem throughout the life span. When left untreated, mental illness can result in the following:

- Lost productivity
- Unsuccessful relationships
- Significant distress and dysfunction
- Adverse impact on childcare

Disability due to mental illness in people older than 65 will become a major public health problem as a result of the aging of the nation and the high percentage of older adults. Continued intellectual, social, and physical activity throughout the life cycle are important for mental health. It should be noted that the prevalence of depression in chronic diseases ranges from 30% to 40% in Parkinson's disease (Frisina et al. 2008), from 8% to 24% in cancer patients (Krebber et al. 2014), from 11% to 31% in diabetes (Katon 2008), and up to 50% in Alzheimer's disease (Chi et al. 2014). These depression and chronic disease comorbidities underscore the importance of primary care providing screening, diagnosis, treatment, and referral of individuals, especially older adults with depression.

One of the greatest gaps in our health care system is in mental health. This gap is in our attitudes, our diagnosis, our treatment, and our research. It is time to close that gap. We continue to pay a tremendous price for it. We pay for crimes that would not be committed if we were active in educating about mental illness. We know how to punish individuals for crimes, and we disproportionately punish those who do not know how to control their own behavior. We pay for the injuries that victims of these behaviors receive from others. We also pay for injuries to each other, including loved ones. We pay to intervene to prevent the violence and injuries that occur when we fail to help people deal with behaviors that would be otherwise controllable and preventable. Although individuals in the criminal justice system provide a valuable service, we will not be able to punish our way out of our current crisis of crime and punishment and more crime and punishment. It is time for us to find a way to prevent the crime that is so damaging to our families and communities.

Our attitude and behavior are based on the philosophy that violent behavior is not controllable. But we can do better. We can develop more positive relationships with each other. We can better control ourselves and our behaviors toward each other. It is also time for us to invest more time and resources in understanding mental health so that we will be able to better diagnose often undiagnosed individuals.

We must continue to remind ourselves that just as things go wrong with the heart and lungs, the kidneys and liver, things go wrong with the brain. They always have and they always will. The question is how will we as individuals and families respond? How will our health system respond, and will we care enough about each other? Are we willing to invest in those who are caught up in a system of hopelessness and who often strike out at the rest of society? Yes, we must care for all of them, including the least of them.

Alzheimer's Disease

Of all the major causes of death, Alzheimer's disease stands out in several ways. First, the odds of developing Alzheimer's disease double every 5 years. In that sense, Alzheimer's can be considered a disease of aging. The national Alzheimer's strategy or plan has been limited by the long-standing belief that the course of the disease is more dependent on genetics and cannot be altered. In recent years, it has become increasingly clear that the onset and the advancement of Alzheimer's disease is, in fact, related to lifestyle, including nutrition, education, physical activity, and related factors. As such, the determinants of health that we developed during my first year as surgeon general are just as applicable to the development of Alzheimer's disease as they are to other illnesses.

The Lancet Commission recently reported that up to 40% of the risks for Alzheimer's disease are modifiable risks, including education, physical activity, nutrition, and related factors (Livingston et al. 2020). This finding represents both good news and unwelcome news. First, it is good news that, increasingly, we may be able to alter the risk of individuals for acquiring Alzheimer's disease. The risk of Alzheimer's is not equally distributed in our society but varies by socioeconomic factors that include poverty, race, and even discrimination among individuals and groups. Thus, the risk factors for Alzheimer's disease vary not only by age but also by race and socioeconomic status. The gap in the occurrence of Alzheimer's disease will continue until we are able to close the socioeconomic and related gaps in our society. This also implies that the cost to payment systems such as Medicaid and Medicare may vary by as much as threefold, more or less. People who are dependent on public insurance are vulnerable to receiving limited care for Alzheimer's disease depending on the state in which they reside and that state's health policies.

The prevalence of Alzheimer's disease from the year 2000 to 2050 will increase from 5.8 million to 13.8 million. Likewise, we can project that Medicare and Medicaid spending for people with Alzheimer's disease will grow from $206 billion in 2020 to $777 billion in 2050 (Alzheimer's Impact Movement 2020).

Research in Alzheimer's disease shows that keeping up with the growth of the disease could have prohibitive costs to society. There are, however, encouraging signs with regard to public health and Alzheimer's disease that indicate advancement in the right direction. For example, studies show that children who receive proper nutrition and physical activity are at lower risk for Alzheimer's disease.

Need for New Partnerships

The greatest advancement in health care over the past 25 years has been the development of new partnerships. These new partnerships have often resulted in the development of not only new relationships but new professions such as physician assistants and nurse practitioners. It is agreed that these new professions have added to the quality and quantity of care provided. For example, in addition to investing heavily in enriching patient care at the top of the chain, we now see the advantage of investing in the care team for the control of chronic diseases such as hypertension.

The team approach to care of hypertension has led to better control of blood pressure and other chronic diseases. This approach allows more patients to be followed more effectively. Better use of a well-trained team has made an enormous difference in the control of some of the most dangerous of chronic diseases and will be expanded in the future.

References

Alzheimer's Impact Movement: Costs of Alzheimer's to Medicare and Medicaid. Alzheimer's Association Fact Sheet, Chicago, IL, Alzheimer's Association, March 2020. Available at: https://act.alz.org/site/DocServer/2012_Costs_Fact_Sheet_version_2.pdf?docID=7161. Accessed July 12, 2022.

American Foundation for Suicide Prevention: Suicide statistics. New York, American Foundation for Suicide Prevention, 2023. Available at: https://afsp.org/suicide-statistics. Accessed March 28, 2023.

American Psychiatric Association: What is mental illness? Washington, DC, American Psychiatric Association, November 2022. Available at: www.psychiatry.org/patients-families/what-is-mental-illness. Accessed March 28, 2023.

Brådvik L: Suicide risk and mental disorders. Int J Environ Res Public Health 15(9):2028, 2018 30227658

Center for Mental Health Services: Mental Health: A Report of the Surgeon General. Bethesda, MD, National Institute of Mental Health, 1999

Centers for Disease Control and Prevention (CDC): HIV and AIDS—United States, 1981–2000. MMWR Morb Mortal Wkly Rep 50(21):430–434, 2001a 11475378

Centers for Disease Control and Prevention: The Surgeon General's Call to Action to Prevent and Decrease Overweight and Obesity 2001. Rockville, MD, Office of Disease Prevention and Health Promotion, 2001b. Available at: www.cdc.gov/nccdphp/dnpa/pdf/CalltoAction.pdf. Accessed July 12, 2022.

Centers for Disease Control and Prevention: Healthy People 2010: nutrition and overweight. Atlanta, GA, Centers for Disease Control and Prevention, 2010. Available at: www.cdc.gov/nchs/data/hpdata2010/hp2010_final_review_focus_area_19.pdf. Accessed July 12, 2022.

Centers for Disease Control and Prevention: Remarkable progress made reducing kidney failure from diabetes in Native American populations. Atlanta, GA, Centers for Disease Control and Prevention, 2017a. Available at: www.cdc.gov/media/releases/2017/p0110-diabetes-native-americans.html. Accessed July 12, 2022.

Centers for Disease Control and Prevention: Vital Signs: Native Americans with diabetes: better diabetes care can decrease kidney failure. Atlanta, GA, Centers for Disease Control and Prevention, January 10, 2017b. Available at: www.cdc.gov/vitalsigns/aian-diabetes/infographic.html. Accessed July 11, 2022.

Centers for Disease Control and Prevention: About mental health. Atlanta, GA, Centers for Disease Control and Prevention, June 28, 2021a. Available at: www.cdc.gov/mentalhealth/learn. Accessed March 28, 2023

Centers for Disease Control and Prevention: Smoking and tobacco use: a brief history. Atlanta, GA, Centers for Disease Control and Prevention, October 19, 2021b. Available at: www.cdc.gov/tobacco/sgr/history/index.htm. Accessed July 12, 2022.

Centers for Disease Control and Prevention: Facts about suicide. Atlanta, GA, Centers for Disease Control and Prevention, October 24, 2022. Available at: www.cdc.gov/suicide/facts/index.html. Accessed, March 28, 2023.

Chi S, Yu J-T, Tan M-S, Tan L: Depression in Alzheimer's disease: epidemiology, mechanisms, and management. J Alzheimers Dis 42(3):739–755 2014 24946876

Douglas MD, Willock RB, Respress E, et al: Applying a health equity lens to evaluate and inform policy. Ethn Dis 29(suppl 2):329–342, 2019 31308601

Foege B: Opinion: Lessons of smallpox eradication and COVID-19. Atlanta Journal Constitution, May 16, 2020

Foege WH: House on Fire: The Fight to Eradicate Smallpox. Berkeley, University of California Berkeley Press, 2011

Frisina PG, Borod JC, Foli NS, Tenenbaum HR: Depression in Parkinson's disease: health risks, etiology, and treatment options. Neuropsychiatr Dis Treat 4(1):81–91, 2008 18728814

Glanz K: Progress in dietary behavior change. Am J Health Promot 14(2):112–117, 1999 10724722

Katon WJ: The comorbidity of diabetes mellitus and depression. Am J Med 121(11 suppl):S8–S15, 2008 18954592

Krebber AMH, Buffart LM, Kleijn G, et al: Prevalence of depression in cancer patients: a meta-analysis of diagnostic interviews and self-report instruments. Psychooncology 23(2):121–130, 2014 24105788

Livingston G, Huntley J, Sommerlad A, et al: Dementia prevention, intervention, and care: 2020 report of the Lancet Commission. Lancet 396(10248):413–446, 2020 32738937

McKinlay JB: Preparation for aging, in The New Public Health Approach to Improving Physical Activity and Autonomy in Aging Populations. Edited by Heikinen E, Kuusinen J, Ruppila I. New York, Plenum, 1995, pp 87–103

National Institute of Mental Health: Mental illness. Bethesda, MD, National Institute of Mental Health, March 2023. Available at: www.nimh.nih.gov/health/statistics/mental-illness#:~:text=In%202021%2C%20among%20the%2057.8,services%20in%20the%20past%20year. Accessed March 28, 2023.

National Institutes of Health: Clinical guidelines on the identification, evaluation, and treatment of overweight and obesity. Rep No 98-4083. Bethesda, MD, National Heart, Lung, and Blood Institute, 1998. Available at: www.ncbi.nlm.nih.gov/books/NBK2003. Accessed July 12, 2022.

Pan American Health Organization: Mental health problems are the leading cause of disability worldwide, say experts at PAHO Directing Council side event. Washington, DC, Pan American Health Organization, 2019. Available at: www3.paho.org/hq/index.php?option=com_content&view=article&id=15481:mental-health-problems-are-the-leading-cause-of-disability-worldwide-say-experts-at-paho-directing-council-side-event&Itemid=0&lang=en#gsc.tab=0. Accessed March 28, 2023.

Satcher D, Rust G: Achieving health equity in America. Ethn Dis 16(2 suppl 3):8–13, 2006 16774018

Stockmyer C, Kuester S, Ramsey D, Dietz WH: National Nutrition Summit, May 30, 2000: results of the obesity discussion groups. Obes Res 9(4):41S–52S, 2001 11393160

Surgeon General's Advisory Committee on Smoking and Health: Smoking and health: report of the Advisory Committee to the Surgeon General of the Public Health Service. Washington, DC, Office of the Surgeon General, 1964. Available at: https://profiles.nlm.nih.gov/spotlight/nn/feature/smoking. Accessed March 29, 2023.

World Health Organization: Commemorating smallpox eradication—a legacy of hope, for COVID-19 and other diseases. Geneva, Switzerland, World Health Organization, May 8, 2020. Available at: www.who.int/news/item/08-05-2020-commemorating-smallpox-eradication-a-legacy-of-hope-for-covid-19-and-other-diseases. Accessed July 12, 2022.

World Health Organization: Mental disorders. Geneva, Switzerland, World Health Organization, June 9, 2022. Available at: www.who.int/news-room/fact-sheets/detail/mental-disorders. Accessed March 28, 2023

3

Why Economic Disparities Matter in Mental Health

Hassell H. McClellan, M.B.A.

The purpose of this chapter is to examine mental health through a lens that acknowledges and assesses the links between economic disparities and mental health. Greater understanding of these links is imperative considering the disproportionate impacts mental well-being and increased disparities have on the economy and society, particularly for African Americans, who make up approximately 12% of the U.S. population (McKnight-Eily et al. 2021; U.S. Census Bureau 2021). Although awareness of the correlations between economic factors and mental health is not a new phenomenon, increasing economic volatility and increasing disparities correlated with race and other factors make the links more salient (Broady and Romer 2021; Little 2021; Tham et al. 2021). This salience has been highlighted in a variety of socioeconomic assessments. One observer, for example, has noted that "...mental distress increased for some and varied widely across geography, race and ethnicity, age, education, income and gender in 2020" (Myshko 2021).

To examine the implications of an increasing relationship between economic disparities and mental health, I will focus on *economic disparities* simply in the sense of absolute differences rather than equitableness or unfairness, which are embodied in the more complicated notion of *inequities*. The fundamental premise is that economic disparities not only matter but are highly consequential for understanding and addressing mental health challenges in society in general and in selected populations specifically. Given this premise, this chapter will have three primary areas of focus:

1. Examination of the links between economic factors and mental health through the lens of economic disparities
2. Detailed examination of the impactful role that one highly salient economic factor and stressor, financial stress, plays in affecting mental health
3. Consideration of the link between economic factors and mental health metrics for African Americans compared with other subgroups of the population

Motivation for these areas of focus is twofold. First, mental health is an increasingly impactful issue for society and the economy (National Alliance on Mental Illness 2022). Data on mental health in the United States suggest that mental health concerns will continue to require significant attention from public policy makers, corporate leaders, and medical and health practitioners over the near future (see Table 3–1).

As Table 3–1 illustrates, 21% of adults—more than 52 million Americans—experienced a mental illness in 2020. A simple extrapolation of this number in terms of potential lost work time, lessened productivity, and cost of treatment easily adds up to an economic drain of billions of dollars each year from the U.S. economy. The exponentially growing economic costs of failing to more appropriately address mental health challenges related to economic disparities have the potential to become an economic "tsunami."

Table 3–1. State of mental health in America

21% of U.S. adults (52 million) experienced a mental illness in 2020

55% of adults with a mental illness (28 million) reported receiving no treatment in 2020

60% of youth with major depression reported not getting needed treatment

11% of Americans with a mental illness were uninsured in 2020

115 million people live in designated mental health professional shortage areas

Serious mental illness causes $193.2 billion in lost earnings annually

Source. National Alliance on Mental Illness 2022; Reinert et al. 2022.

A second motivation is that continuing evidence of correlations between mental health and economic disparities, particularly among African Americans, suggests that there is much to be gained by increased understanding of 1) the relationship of disparities reflected in economic factors and mental health outcomes and 2) the impact of economic factors, particularly financial stress, on perceived and actual behavioral and mental health. That behavior, the result of mental processes, has intertwined economic and societal links is not a new revelation, but it continues to be inadequately understood by policy makers and practitioners. As early as the 1930s, a prominent British economist, Lionel Robbins, commented on the link between mental processes and economic factors. In simple terms, he defined economics as "the science which studies human behavior as a relationship between ends and scarce means which have alternative uses" (Robbins 1932, p. 15). Notably, his observation was made during the Great Depression in the United States, a period of one of the greatest displays of the impact of economic factors on human behavior in history. It might be inferred from Robbins's observation that this linkage is inherent in the term *socioeconomic*. Numerous health and socioeconomic studies have indeed examined and confirmed how differences in *economic resources* (*means*) and financial exigencies (scarce resources) may affect individual and collective behavior (mental health) (Macintyre et al. 2018; Marmot 2005; Melita et al. 2021).

In examining economic disparities, a particular emphasis will be placed on access to economic resources and education. Income is a core determinant and metric of access to resources and socioeconomic status. It is often perceived as a means of protection against the many stresses that accompany lack of access to resources such as desirable housing, sufficient food, necessary education, adequate clothing, and upward social mobility. Notably, income and wealth, fundamental to resource access, tend to vary across race, gender, and geography (Peter G. Peterson Foundation 2021). Educational attainment is also spotlighted because it generally is highly correlated with higher income and higher levels of health, including mental well-being. Considerable research has also parsed out the reality that differences or disparities in economic factors often illuminate differences in health and mental well-being across various subgroups of populations (Carratala and Maxwell 2020). Thus, in both the economic and health professions, it should be a foregone conclusion that economics do matter in behavioral and mental health outcomes. The implications are particularly significant for practitioners and policy makers striving to address mental well-being as a growing social conundrum. Continuing to highlight that disparities do matter is beneficial because gaps remain in practitioners' and policy makers' appreciation of the contribution of economic disparities to mental well-being and physical manifestations of mental health issues.

Clarifying Disparities Versus Inequities

Nowhere in the field of health and well-being is the distinction between disparities and inequities more informative than the link between variances in economic factors and observed or perceived mental health outcomes. To put the discussion in context, let us first consider how disparities differ from inequities. When discussing differences in manifestations and measures in health and mental well-being, we have an unfortunate tendency to conflate economic disparities with economic inequalities, which often devolves into quagmires of political, moral, and ethical debates. Distinguishing between the two definitions is important; as noted by Meghani and Gallagher (2008),

> "Disparity" and "inequity" are two interdependent, yet distinct concepts. In the literal sense, disparity merely implies a "difference" or a "lack of parity" of some kind. Inequity, on the other hand, implies "a state of being unfair." In the context of health care, these two concepts may have distinct implications for practice and policy. (pp. 613–614)

This delineation parallels in some way the articulated distinction between *positive economics*, which is generally limited to analysis of cause and effect, and *normative economics*, whose focus is on fairness or what should be. For purposes of this chapter, the focus, or "what matters," is disparities, in particular the link between disparities in economic factors and mental health across specific populations. A fundamental principle is that economic disparities do matter and should matter to policy makers and practitioners. Having a broad positive economics perspective on the extent to which economic disparities exist and are relevant is key for understanding and addressing mental health challenges in our society.

A central premise of this chapter is that disparities in and of themselves are manifestations of underlying root issues. In that sense, I would point out that observed disparities are not necessarily the intrinsic cause of mental health issues, although perceived economic disparities may contribute to internalized emotional responses that lead to mental health challenges such as stress, low self-esteem, and depression (Wilkinson and Pickett 2017). I would also note that the size of a given disparity may be consequential in the propensity for selected stressors to become problematic by causing dysfunctional behavior and/or actual physical harm. There may be threshold levels of disparities where the resultant stressor becomes negatively catalytic of mental health issues (Knapp and Wong 2020; Pickett et al. 2006). For example, financial stress is most commonly associated with a negative gap between required expenditures and resources or income necessary to meet expenses (Richardson et al. 2013; Satter 2016). However, the disparity between annual incomes of $200,000 and $100,000 is far less impactful as a stressor than a threshold income disparity that is below the poverty line.

To illustrate the existence of economic disparities in general, Table 3–2 presents information on select social and economic characteristics of U.S. households. As Table 3–2 illustrates, disparities exist across several survey characteristics and can exist across multiple demographics, as can be seen in the differences in income by gender and race.

Economic Disparities and Mental Health: An Undeniable Link

Considerable evidence has suggested that the links between economic factors, economic disparities, and mental health issues are quite strong (Wilkinson and Pickett 2017; Wolla and Sullivan 2017). One study published in 2005 examined a database of more than 34,000 patients with two or more psychiatric hospitalizations during 1994–2000 (Hudson 2005). Hudson suggested three important and relevant conclusions:

1. The poorer one's socioeconomic conditions are, the higher the risk is for mental disability and psychiatric hospitalization.
2. The correlation between these factors was found regardless of the person's economic hardship or type of mental illness.
3. Strong evidence exists that socioeconomic conditions affect the development of mental illness directly, as well as indirectly through the association between mental health and adverse economic stressful conditions among lower-income groups.

Others have found that significant differences in income or income inequality have a causal effect on general health, life span, and mental illness: "The effect of income on health is arguably most consequential in its role in extending life, and there is strong evidence for negative, nonlinear association between income and mortality in the United States" (Avanceña et al. 2021, pp. 1404–1408).

Table 3–2. Income summary measures by selected characteristics

Characteristic	2019		2020	
	Number (thousands)	Estimated median income (dollars)	Number (thousands)	Estimated median income (dollars)
All households	128,451	69,560	129,931	67,521
Type of household				
Family households	83,677	89,249	83,907	86,372
Married couple	62,342	103,585	61,454	101,517
Female householder, no spouse present	14,832	48,698	15,490	49,214
Male householder, no spouse present	6,503	70,108	6,963	67,304
Nonfamily households	44,774	41,747	46,024	40,464
Female householder	23,470	35,044	24,244	35,574
Male householder	21,304	49,101	21,781	47,259
Race and Hispanic origin of householder				
White	100,568	73,105	101,582	71,231
White, not Hispanic	84,868	77,007	85,336	74,912
Black	17,054	46,005	17,358	45,870
Asian	6,853	99,400	6,987	94,903
Hispanic (any race)	17,667	56,814	18,349	55,321

Table 3–2. Income summary measures by selected characteristics *(continued)*

Characteristic	2019 Number (thousands)	2019 Estimated median income (dollars)	2020 Number (thousands)	2020 Estimated median income (dollars)
Age of householder				
Younger than 65 years	93,524	78,845	94,243	76,800
15–24 years	5,406	48,532	5,485	46,886
25–34 years	20,424	71,161	20,654	71,566
35–44 years	21,432	89,968	22,105	85,694
45–54 years	21,659	93,372	21,663	90,359
55–64 years	24,603	76,631	24,336	74,270
65 years and older	34,927	47,949	35,688	46,360
Region				
Northeast	22,031	77,172	22,082	75,211
Midwest	27,757	69,208	27,865	66,968
South	49,486	62,657	50,385	61,243
West	29,177	76,714	29,600	74,951

Table 3–2. Income summary measures by selected characteristics (*continued*)

Characteristic	2019		2020	
	Number (thousands)	Estimated median income (dollars)	Number (thousands)	Estimated median income (dollars)
Educational attainment of householder				
Total, age 25 and older	123,045	71,186	124,446	69,228
No high school diploma	10,310	31,347	10,052	29,547
High school, no college	31,071	49,316	31,647	47,405
Some college	33,852	65,510	33,646	63,653
Bachelor's degree or higher	47,812	110,002	49,102	106,936

Note. Income in 2020 dollars, adjusted using the Consumer Price Index for All Urban Consumers Retroactive Series. Households are listed as of March of the following year. Information on confidentiality protection, sampling error, nonsampling error, and definitions is available at www2.census.gov/programs-surveys/cps/techdocs/cpsmar21.pdf. Inflation-adjusted estimates may differ slightly from other published data because of rounding.
Source. Shrider et al. 2021.

That income is an important factor in the mental health universe is not a surprise. As data and research indicate, income influences and/or is a determinant of a number of health care outcomes, including access to care, awareness of treatments, access to insurance that covers mental health issues, and, in many cases, quality of care. Notably, having access to resources such as insurance is not always correlated with accessing treatment for mental health problems. Some data have shown that 86% of adults who did not receive mental health treatment were covered by health insurance (United Health Foundation 2021a). It would be invaluable to know more about how much socioeconomic issues (e.g., race and ethnicity, level of education, perception of cost of treatment, ability to take time for treatment, perceived risk, stigmas associated with getting treatment for various income levels, lack of awareness of coverage) play into individuals not availing themselves of the benefit of health insurance coverage.

Disparities in income and resultant differences in manifestation of mental health challenges have also been observed across states as shown in Tables 3–3 and 3–4. As can be seen, median income in selected states tends to have a fairly consistent correlation with health and behavioral challenges. The data in Table 3–4, for example, highlight that states with higher median income (Connecticut, New Jersey, Massachusetts, Maryland) tend to have higher rankings on behavioral health, depression, and health outcomes. The states ranked lowest on median household income tend also to be ranked low on all of the same factors, including economic resources. As the data suggest, states in the South tend to have lower incomes and health ratings. Because more than 50% of African Americans live in the South, a significant portion of African Americans as a group are challenged by availability of mental health resources related to governmental polices in areas where they reside.

Notably, the effects of the COVID-19 pandemic on the economy only served to underscore the impact of economic disparities on mental health and has had a catalytic impact on mental health issues (Gaetano 2020). Economic effects of the pandemic have included job losses and increased insecurity, and people were unable to move out of cities because dramatic increases in suburban home prices affected their ability to acquire a second home or purchase a home in a mentally appealing environment. On the other hand, individuals with higher socioeconomic attributes benefited from great increases in wealth and income portfolios as a result of having resources to capitalize on investment opportunities in the stock market (Kent and Ricketts 2021). Thus, the disparity in income and resources and the availability of and access to mental health resources increased dramatically during the pandemic. As discussed in

Table 3–3. U.S. real per capita income by selected states

State	Rank	Real per capital personal income[a]
Connecticut	1	$68,533
New Jersey	6	$59,584
Massachusetts	2	$65,893
Maryland	12	$56,578
Alabama	46	$46,963
Arkansas	42	$47,765
West Virginia	47	$46,130
Mississippi	50	$43,284

[a]Real personal income per capita based on the Bureau of Economic Analysis definition: income per person adjusted for state price level differences and national inflation.
Source.   DePietro A: U.S. per capita income by state in 2021. Forbes, December 28, 2021. Available at: www.forbes.com/sites/andrewdepietro/2021/12/28/us-per-capita-income-by-state-in-2021. Accessed May 6, 2022.

this chapter, disparities in insulation from stress-inducing economic and financial circumstances play an outsize role in mental health and well-being.

Disparities in income and socioeconomic status also tend to be highly correlated with levels of educational attainment. As shown in Tables 3–3 and 3–4, higher income tends to be correlated with better health outcomes. Table 3–5 data for 2020 illustrate that disparities in income and unemployment may accrue as a result of educational attainment levels (Torpey 2021). Given that ability to access health care may be affected by economic resources, income does matter with regard to mental health treatment and access. Again, this portends ominously because economic data from the pandemic show a dramatic increase in disparity on the basis of income. Individuals most susceptible to loss of employment because they were not able to work from home remotely tended to be those at the lower end of the economic spectrum. The uncertainty and potential loss of economic sustainability that comes with loss of employment create conditions that are ripe for one of the most powerful contributors to a decline in mental well-being: stress. Robinson and Smith 2022 succinctly captured the essence of the power of economically based stress: "While we all know deep down there are many more important things in life than money, when you're struggling financially fear and stress can take over your world."

Table 3–4. America's health rankings 2021 for selected states

State	Median household income	Rank					
		Poverty	Economic resources	Behavioral health	Depression	Multiple chronic health problems	Health outcomes
Connecticut	$70,098	13	34	5	18	6	3
New Jersey	$69,160	7	17	15	5	5	7
Massachusetts	$71,919	12	14	10	20	13	1
Maryland	$73,971	2	6	3	7	6	10
Alabama	$42,830	44	46	35	45	48	49
Arkansas	$41,262	46	44	42	45	46	46
West Virginia	$41,059	47	47	37		48	48
Mississippi	$39,680	49	49	14	31	44	48

Source. United Health Foundation 2021b.

Table 3–5. Unemployment rate by level of education and income, 2020

Level of education	Median usual weekly earning	Unemployment rate, %
Doctoral degree	$1,885	2.5
Professional degree	$11,893	3.1
Master's degree	$1,545	4.1
Bachelor's degree	$1,305	5.5
Associate degree	$938	7.1
Some college, no degree	$877	8.3
High school diploma	$781	9.0
Less than high school diploma	$619	11.7

Source.   Torpey 2021.

Economic Disparities, Financial Stress, and Mental Health

With the onset of the COVID-19 pandemic in 2020, the pervasive sense of higher levels of stress and anxiety across all segments of the U.S. population has been palpable. Without question, the very real threat of severe illness, dramatic increase in mortality rates, isolation-induced social distancing, and decline in economic activity all have contributed to a high level of stress in the environment. One observer indicated that more than 70% of Americans ranked their finances as the most significant source of stress in their life (Gaetano 2020). Increasingly, researchers are pointing out the impactful role of economic and financial stress in mental health and alludes to the role of economic disparities. Common themes in their conclusions are that 1) mental health and economic issues are linked, 2) financial stressors are one of the highest sources of stress, and 3) stress is a major contributor to a variety of financial challenges and affects mental well-being (Connolly and Slade 2018; Davis and Mantler 2004; Macintyre et al. 2018).

1.   Mental health and financial and economic issues are linked.
2.   Financial stress is one of the highest stressors.

3. Stress is a contributor to many financial challenges and mental health issues.
4. Stress affects mental health, which, in turn, affects financial well-being.
5. Access to mental health care is negatively affected by lower economic resources.

However, stress as a major influencer of mental health has been problematic since long before the pandemic. Of the various types of stress that affect mental health, financial stress has consistently emerged as being particularly pernicious and as a particularly salient issue in mental health and well-being. In research reported in *Everyday Health*, 52% of respondents indicated that financial stress issues regularly stressed them out, a number that was considerably higher than the next most common stressor, jobs and careers (35%) (Connolly and Slade 2018). Connolly and Slade also noted that "prolonged or unremitting stress exacts a stunningly toxic toll on the body, brain, mind, and soul" and that worries about finances were the number one source of stress.

In a 2004 study, "The Consequences of Financial Stress for Individuals, Families, and Society," Christopher G. Davis and Janet Mantler conducted research that focused on the emotional, cognitive, and behavioral changes that are linked to stress (Davis and Mantler 2004). They concluded that financial stress is associated with both mental health issues and physical and emotional well-being. One of their views is particularly beneficial for assessing the role of stress appropriately in mental health contexts: They noted that although economic hardship is a key stressor, it should be distinguished from financial stress. In their view, financial stress is a subjective feeling, which may or may not be based on objective data and assessment of one's financial situation, whereas economic hardship refers to the objective circumstances that give rise to feelings of financial stress. The link between economic hardship and financial pressure is complex and should not be viewed in a linear manner—some people without economic hardship feel financial pressure, whereas other people experiencing economic hardships do not feel pressure. Additionally, it is useful to note that perceived financial stress can be as negatively impactful as actual stress. The data of Davis and Mantler and other researchers have led to conclusions on a number of topics that matter for mental health practitioners and society in general:

1. Financial stress is linked to lowered self-esteem, an increasingly pessimistic outlook on life, and reduced mental health.
2. Financial stress is linked to an increase in depression and hostility.

3. Financial stress is linked to suicide and alcohol consumption, which are directly related to increased levels of depression.
4. Financial stress is associated with declining physical health, including headaches, stomachaches, and insomnia.
5. Financial stress has a direct and often causal link to marital discord and dissolution of marriages.
6. Financial stress is linked to parents being less responsive to children's needs, less nurturing, and less consistent in their discipline.
7. Behaviors induced by financial stress in parents are linked to increased risk of socioemotional problems in children, including low self-esteem, depression, impulsive behavior, health problems, poor academic performance, deviant behavior, drug and alcohol use, withdrawal from relationships, and reduced aspirations and expectations.

Table 3–6 summarizes some of the critical economic implications that the psychological and physical manifestations of financial stress may have on individuals.

Table 3-6. Impact and economic consequences of financial stress

	Manifestation	Consequences	Economic implications
Psychological effects	• Depression • Anxiety • Mood changes • Memory loss	• Workplace absenteeism • Poor workplace culture • Substance abuse • Employee turnover	• Lower productivity • Higher health care costs • Higher public funding costs • Higher cost for treatments • Higher unemployment
Physical effects	• Cardiovascular disease • Increase in mortality • Hypertension • Increase in suicide rates	• Workplace disruption • Loss of experienced talent • Poor workplace performance	• Higher health care costs • Lower workplace productivity • Higher unemployment • Higher sick leave costs

It is also notable that financial stress has no respect for age or generation. In 2021, Best Money Moves identified four key financial stress statistics that reflect a growing problem for the American workforce across generational groups:

1. As a whole, the American workforce is stressed out about money, even more so than about the pandemic; 73% of Americans ranked their finances as the most significant source of stress in their lives.
2. Gen Z and millennial employees were feeling the crunch the most; 82% of Gen Z respondents and 81% of millennial respondents indicated that their finances were at least somewhat stressful.
3. The cost of medical care is a major concern.
4. Most people (e.g., 62% of Gen Z respondents) are unprepared for financial emergencies (Konstantino 2021).

Disparities, Stress, and African Americans

As has been suggested, stress affects all demographic groups, regardless of race, gender, ethnicity, or age (Adler and Ostrove 1999; Davis and Mantler 2004). However, because of economic disparities, differences are often reflected in both the impact of stress and responses to it, particularly for African Americans. Notably, because of unequal access to education, historical discrimination in employment, and bias in promotion to higher-compensated jobs, race and ethnicity have generally been acknowledged as frequent correlated and explanatory factors in economic disparities and determining perceived socioeconomic status (Ajilore 2020; Kent and Ricketts 2020, 2022; Strauss 2017).

Consequently, significant economic and socioeconomic disparities are often reflected in metrics regarding African Americans (Bhutta et al. 2020). Many of these socioeconomic metrics show significant disparities in income, wealth, and education compared with other groups such as Non-Hispanic whites and Asians (Bhutta et al. 2020; Kent and Ricketts 2020, 2022). These disparities are often rooted in years of historical discrimination, which resulted in a lack of opportunities for African Americans to accumulate wealth, obtain higher-paying employment, and access financial resources to acquire homes, the latter of which is a major source of wealth accumulation in the United States (Strauss 2017; Wilson 2020). Equally important has been the lack of access to information on investing and the lack of generational transmission of financial information and wealth on a wide scale (Torpey 2021; Wolla and Sullivan 2017).

As a result, data for African Americans as a group tend to show significant disparities in economic resources and demographics when compared with other groups (Adler and Ostrove 1999; Ajilore 2020; Bhutta et al. 2020). Having comparatively fewer resources to navigate financial situations, African Americans are notably more vulnerable to financial stress. And the disparity in impact is great (McKnight-Eily et al. 2021).

Equally as significant, disparities in economic resources appear to contribute to financial stress in African Americans in ways that have serious consequences for major physical health problems. The differences in income between African Americans and other groups are very divergent, and therefore the burden born by African Americans and other groups for mental health challenges and stress is considerably greater (Choi 2009; Davis and Mantler 2004). Cheryl Clark, a hospitalist and researcher at Brigham and Women's Hospital, made the following observation on the basis of the Jackson Heart Study, a longitudinal study of more than 2,200 participants: "Stress is known to contribute to heart disease, but the data from our study suggest a possible relationship between financial stress and heart disease that clinicians should be aware of as we research and develop intervention to address social determinants of health disparities" (St. Peter 2019). Clark also concluded that "[a]s we think about policies to prevent heart disease, we need to know a lot more about how economic volatility and financial stress may be connected to heart disease" (St. Peter 2019). The Jackson Heart Study found that African American men and women who experienced moderate to high financial stress had almost three times greater risk of a heart disease event than did individuals who did not experience financial stress (National Heart, Lung, and Blood Institute 2019). Individuals with mild financial stress appeared to have nearly two times the risk (Moran et al. 2019; St. Peter 2019).

That economic disparities and access to financial resources have a major impact on access to mental health services, as well as on finding ways to mitigate the impact of stress, should not be surprising (Baumgartner et al. 2021; Carratala and Maxwell 2020). African Americans, who have comparatively few economic resources as a group, would appear to access mental health services at significantly lower rates than do whites (Table 3–7).

It is also noteworthy that some studies have shown that African Americans with mental health challenges are treated differently by practitioners when they do seek mental health services. The American

Table 3–7. Access to health care for Black vs. white adults, 2019

	Non-Hispanic Black adults age 18 and over	Non-Hispanic white adults age 18 and over
Percentage who received mental health services in the past year	9.8	16.6

Source. Substance Abuse and Mental Health Services Administration: National Survey on Drug Use and Health 2019. NSDUH-2019-DS0001. Rockville, MD, Substance Abuse and Mental Health Services Administration, 2020. Available at: www.datafiles.samhsa.gov/dataset/national-survey-drug-use-and-health-2019-nsduh-2019-ds0001. Accessed March 29, 2023.

Psychiatric Association has noted that although rates of mental illnesses in African Americans are similar to those in the general population, disparities exist in treatment and access to mental health care services (Baumgartner et al. 2021; Young 2020). African Americans also frequently receive poor quality of care and less access to culturally competent care. This disparity also contributes to unwillingness to access treatment for mental illness even when care is available via insurance.

Health insurance coverage is widely regarded as an important factor in healthcare and propensity for individuals to seek treatment for both mental and physical health issues. Data on type of health insurance coverage by various demographic groups are shown in Table 3–8. As reflected in the data, African Americans tend to lag all other demographic groups, except Hispanics, in access to any health insurance as well as private insurance categories. Notably, African Americans tend to have relatively higher coverage through public health mechanisms, which frequently provide care that is less comprehensive and is perceived as being of lower quality. For individuals with mental health challenges, lack of insurance can be a particularly onerous obstacle to seeking and obtaining treatment. Given the link between insurance coverage and cost, the implications of disparities in income, education, and employment for addressing mental health challenges in specific demographic populations cannot be overlooked (Young 2020).

Conclusion

On the basis of the emerging evidence and data discussed in this chapter, there should not be any question that economic disparities both matter and are frequently correlated with disparities in occurrence of,

Table 3–8. Selected characteristics of individuals by health insurance coverage status, 2021[a]

	Number in thousands	Any health insurance, %	Private health insurance, %	Public health insurance, %	Uninsured, %
Total	328,074	91.7	66.0	34.5	8.3
Race and Hispanic origin					
White	248,776	91.8	67.8	35.0	8.2
White, not Hispanic	194,186	94.8	73.2	34.6	5.2
Black	43,963	91.0	55.1	42.7	9.0
Asian	20,681	93.8	72.4	27.4	6.2
Hispanic (any race)	61,915	81.7	48.8	37.0	18.3
Region					
Northeast	56,045	94.7	68.1	38.8	5.3
Midwest	67,933	94.5	71.0	35.3	5.5
South	125,144	88.6	63.3	34.0	11.4
West	77,933	92.1	64.4	37.0	7.9

[a]Population as of March of the following year.
Source.   U.S. Census Bureau: 2020 Annual Economic Supplement (CPS ASEC). Suitland, MD, U.S. Census Bureau, 2020.

access to, and treatment of mental health challenges. For Black and African Americans, the data and metrics resoundingly suggest that mental health issues are even more acute than they are in other populations and are highly linked to disparities in resources and access to appropriate treatment (Williams 2018). A number of conclusions have important implications for many stakeholders, including the mental health profession, policy makers, the business community, and the African American community. Key among the conclusions are the following:

- Economic factors are critical in understanding the sources of mental health issues.
- Disparities in income and education are highly correlated with disparities in access to and treatment of mental health issues.
- Where you live is a significant factor in access to mental health treatment and care.
- Financial stress is one of the most impactful stressors that contribute to mental health challenges in general and to the African American community in particular in light of significant disparities in income, access to resources, and education.
- Recent economic upheavals and the COVID-19 pandemic have increased the conditions that make a rise in stress and resultant mental health challenges more likely.

For the future, it is reasonable to conclude that mental health and well-being will continue to challenge policy makers, health care professionals, and private sector decision-makers to develop solutions that mitigate the impact of mental health problems in the U.S. population in general and among groups that may be more susceptible to economically induced stress. As emphasis on efficiency, automation, and use of technology continues to increase, greater substitution of technology for labor is likely to occur. A result may be great uncertainty in employment in many economic sectors, which will create a fertile ground for greater financial stress and thereby increase the need for greater provision of mental health services.

For the African American community, it is imperative to develop great awareness of both the symptoms of stress and the harm that untreated stress can have on physical and mental well-being. Efforts to reduce the stigma associated with acknowledging mental health concerns within the African American community will be particularly helpful and can help promote more proactive responses to stress, such as seeking out mental health services.

At a more fundamental level, it would be appropriate to conclude that ongoing efforts to reduce economic disparities will pay significant dividends in mitigating financial stress and, in turn, incidences of mental and physical health problems (Keisler-Starkey and Bunch 2020). Economic disparities are a clear and present danger to mental well-being in the United States, and greater focus on helping individuals cope with financial stress will be beneficial.

References

Adler NE, Ostrove JM: Socioeconomic status and health: what we know and what we don't. Ann N Y Acad Sci 896(1):3–15, 1999 10681884

Ajilore O: The persistent Black-white unemployment gap is built into the labor market. Washington, DC, Center for American Progress, September 28, 2020. Available at: www.americanprogress.org/article/persistent-black-white-unemployment-gap-built-labor-market. Accessed May 6, 2022.

American Psychological Association: Stress in America 2020: a national mental health crisis. Washington, DC, American Psychological Association, October 2020. Available at: www.apa.org/news/press/releases/stress/2020/report-october. Accessed May 6, 2022.

Avanceña ALV, DeLuca EK, Iott B, et al: Income and income inequality are a matter of life and death. What can policymakers do about it? Am J Public Health 111(8):1404–1408, 2021 34464177

Baumgartner JC, Collins SR, Radley DC: Racial and ethnic inequities in health care coverage and access, 2013–2019. New York, Commonwealth Fund, June 9, 2021. Available at: www.commonwealthfund.org/publications/issue-briefs/2021/jun/racial-ethnic-inequities-health-care-coverage-access-2013-2019. Accessed May 6, 2022.

Bhutta N, Chang AC, Dettling LJ, Hsu JW: Disparities in wealth by race and ethnicity in the 2019 Survey of Consumer Finances. Washington, DC, Board of Governors of the Federal Reserve System, September 28, 2020. Available at: www.federalreserve.gov/econres/notes/feds-notes/disparities-in-wealth-by-race-and-ethnicity-in-the-2019-survey-of-consumer-finances-20200928.htm. Accessed May 6, 2022.

Broady K, Romer C: Despite June's positive jobs numbers, Black workers continue to face high unemployment. Washington, DC, Brookings Institution, July 2, 2021. Available at: www.brookings.edu/blog/the-avenue/2021/07/02/despite-junes-positive-jobs-numbers-black-workers-continue-to-face-high-unemployment. Accessed May 7, 2022.

Carratala S, Maxwell C: Health disparities by race and ethnicity. Washington, DC, Center for American Progress, May 7, 2020. Available at: www.americanprogress.org/article/health-disparities-race-ethnicity. Accessed May 6, 2022.

Choi L: Financial stress and its physical effects on individuals and communities. Community Development Investment Review 5(3):120–122, 2009

Connolly M, Slade M: The United States of stress 2019. Everyday Health, October 23, 2018. Available at: www.everydayhealth.com/wellness/united-states-of-stress. Accessed May 6, 2022.

Davis CG, Mantler J: The Consequences of Financial Stress for Individuals, Families, and Society. Ottawa, Doyle Salewski, 2004

Gaetano C: Survey: 77% of Americans stressed over finances. New York State Society of Certified Public Accountants, January 28, 2020. Available at: www.nysscpa.org/most-popular-content/survey-77-percent-of-americans-stressed-over-finances-012820#sthash.M4UNh13o.dpbs. Accessed May 6, 2022.

Hudson CG: Socioeconomic status and mental illness: tests of the social causation and selection hypotheses. Am J Orthopsychiatry 75(1):3–18, 2005 15709846

Keisler-Starkey K, Bunch LN: Health insurance coverage in the United States: 2019. Suitland, MD, U.S. Census Bureau, September 15, 2020. Available at: www.census.gov/library/publications/2020/demo/p60-271.html. Accessed May 6, 2022.

Kent AH, Ricketts LR: Has wealth inequality in America changed over time? Here are key statistics. St. Louis, MO, Federal Reserve Bank of St. Louis, December 2020. Available at: www.stlouisfed.org/open-vault/2020/december/has-wealth-inequality-changed-over-time-key-statistics?print=true. Accessed May 7, 2022.

Kent AH, Ricketts LR: Wealth gaps between white, Black and Hispanic families in 2019. St. Louis, MO, Federal Reserve Bank of St. Louis, January 5, 2021. Available at: www.stlouisfed.org/on-the-economy/2021/january/wealth-gaps-white-black-hispanic-families-2019. Accessed May 7, 2022.

Kent AH, Ricketts LR: Racial and ethnic household wealth trends and wealth inequality. St. Louis, MO, Federal Reserve Bank of St. Louis, November 29, 2022. Available at: www.stlouisfed.org/institute-for-economic-equity/the-real-state-of-family-wealth/racial-and-ethnic-household-wealth. Accessed March 20, 2023.

Knapp M, Wong G: Economics and mental health: the current scenario. World Psychiatry 19(1):3–14, 2020 31922693

Konstantino D: 5 financial stress statistics for 2021. Best Money Moves, February 3, 2021. Available at: https://bestmoneymoves.com/blog/2021/02/03/5-financial-stress-statistics-for-2021. Accessed May 6, 2022.

Little K: Americans are just as anxious about money as they were one year ago: here is how to manage the stress. NextAdvisor, August 5, 2021. Available at: https://time.com/nextadvisor/in-the-news/survey-americans-anxious-about-money-post-covid. Accessed May 7, 2022.

Macintyre A, Ferris D, Gonçalves B, Quinn N: What has economics got to do with it? The impact of socioeconomic factors on mental health and the case for collective action. Palgrave Commun 4(1): doi.org/10.1057/s41599-018-0063-2, 2018

Marmot M: Social determinants of health inequalities. Lancet 365(9464):1099–1104, 2005 15781105

McKnight-Eily LR, Okoro CA, Strine TW, et al: Racial and ethnic disparities in the prevalence of stress and worry, mental health conditions, and increased substance use among adults during the COVID-19 pandemic—United States, April and May 2020. MMWR Morb Mortal Wkly Rep 70(5):162–166, 2021 33539336

Meghani SH, Gallagher RM: Disparity vs inequity: toward reconceptualization of pain treatment disparities. Pain Med 9(5):613–623, 2008 18777609

Melita D, Willis GB, Rodríguez-Bailón R: Economic inequality increases status anxiety through perceived contextual competitiveness. Front Psychol 12:637365, 2021

Moran KE, Ommerborn MJ, Blackshear CT, et al: Financial stress and risk of coronary heart disease in the Jackson Heart Study. Am J Prev Med 56(2):224–231, 2019 30661571

Myshko D: Americans' health during the COVID-19 pandemic. Managed Healthcare Executive, December 7, 2021. Available at: www.managedealth careexecutive.com/view/americans-health-during-the-covid-19-pandemic. Accessed March 19, 2023.

National Alliance on Mental Illness: Mental Health by the Numbers. Arlington, VA, National Alliance on Mental Illness, February 2022. www.nami.org/mhstats. Accessed May 7, 2022.

National Heart, Lung, and Blood Institute: Stress, financial or otherwise, increases heart risks for African Americans. Bethesda, MD, National Heart, Lung, and Blood Institute, May 2, 2019. Available at: www.nhlbi.nih.gov/news/2019/stress-financial-or-otherwise-increases-heart-risks-african-americans. Accessed May 7, 2022.

Peter G. Peterson Foundation: Income and wealth in the United States: an overview of recent data. New York, Peter G. Peterson Foundation, November 17, 2021. Available at: www.pgpf.org/blog/2021/11/income-and-wealth-in-the-united-states-an-overview-of-data. Accessed May 7, 2022.

Pickett KE, James OW, Wilkinson RG: Income inequality and the prevalence of mental illness: a preliminary international analysis. J Epidemiol Community Health 60(7):646–647, 2006 16790839

Reinert M, Fritze D, Nguyen T: The State of Mental Health in America. Alexandria, VA, Mental Health America, October 2022. Available at: https://mhanational.org/sites/default/files/2023-State-of-Mental-Health-in-America-Report.pdf. Accessed March 20, 2023.

Richardson T, Elliott P, Roberts R: The relationship between personal unsecured debt and mental and physical health: a systematic review and meta-analysis. Clin Psychol Rev 33(8):1148–1162, 2013 24121465

Robbins LR: An Essay on the Nature and Significance of Economic Science. London, Macmillan, 1932

Robinson L, Smith M: Coping with financial stress. Santa Monica, CA, Helpguide, August 30, 2022. Available at: www.helpguide.org/articles/stress/coping-with-financial-stress.htm. Accessed March 20, 2023.

Satter MY: Top 7 causes of financial stress. BenefitsPRO, August 26, 2016. Available at: www.benefitspro.com/2016/08/26/top-7-causes-of-financial-stress/?slreturn=20220406210450. Accessed May 7, 2022.

Shrider EA, Kollar M, Chen F, Semega J: Income and poverty in the United States: 2020. Current Population Rep P60-273. Washington, DC, U.S. Government Publishing Office, 2021

St. Peter E: Financial stress linked to heart disease risk among African-Americans. Harvard Gazette, January 17, 2019. Available at: https://news.harvard.edu/gazette/story/2019/01/financial-stress-linked-to-heart-disease-risk-among-african-americans. Accessed May 7, 2022.

Strauss S: The connection between education, income inequality, and unemployment. December 6, 2017. Available at: www.huffpost.com/entry/the-connection-between-ed_b_1066401. Accessed May 7, 2022.

Tham WW, Sojli E, Bryant R, McAleer M: Common mental disorders and economic uncertainty: evidence from the COVID-19 pandemic in the U.S. PLoS One 16(12):e0260726, 2021 34855850

Torpey E: Education pays, 2020. Washington, DC, Career Outlook, U.S. Bureau of Labor Statistics, June 2021. Available at: www.bls.gov/careeroutlook/2021/data-on-display/education-pays.htm Accessed March 20, 2023.

United Health Foundation: America's Health Rankings Annual Report 2021. Minneapolis, MN, UnitedHealth Group, 2021a. Available at: www.americashealthrankings.org/learn/reports/2021-annual-report. Accessed May 7, 2022.

United Health Foundation: America's Health Rankings Health Disparities Report 2021. Minneapolis, MN, UnitedHealth Group, 2021b. Available at: www.americashealthrankings.org. Accessed May 6, 2022.

U.S. Census Bureau: Racial and ethnic diversity in the United States: 2010 Census and 2020 Census. Suitland, MD, U.S. Census Bureau, August 12, 2021. Available at: www.census.gov/library/visualizations/interactive/racial-and-ethnic-diversity-in-the-united-states-2010-and-2020-census.html. Accessed May 7, 2022.

Wilkinson R, Pickett K: How inequality endangers our mental health. Washington, DC, Institute for Policy Studies, June 4, 2017. Available at: https://inequality.org/research/inequality-endangers-mental-health. Accessed May 7, 2022.

Williams DR: Stress and the mental health of populations of color: advancing our understanding of race-related stressors. J Health Soc Behav 59(4):466–485, 2018 30484715

Wilson V: Racial disparities in income and poverty remain largely unchanged amid strong income growth in 2019. Washington, DC, Economic Policy Institute, September 16, 2020. Available at: www.epi.org/blog/racial-disparities-in-income-and-poverty-remain-largely-unchanged-amid-strong-income-growth-in-2019. Accessed May 7, 2022.

Wolla SA, Sullivan J: Education, income, and wealth. St. Louis, MO, Federal Reserve Bank of St. Louis, January 2017. Available at: https://research.stlouisfed.org/publications/page1-econ/2017/01/03/education-income-and-wealth. Accessed May 7, 2022.

Young CL: There are clear, race-based inequalities in health insurance and health outcomes. Washington, DC, Brookings Institution, February 19, 2020. Available at: www.brookings.edu/blog/usc-brookings-schaeffer-on-health-policy/2020/02/19/there-are-clear-race-based-inequalities-in-health-insurance-and-health-outcomes. Accessed March 20, 2023.

4

African Americans and Substance Use

H. Westley Clark, M.D., J.D., M.P.H.

Historical Context

The adverse impact of slavery and the ongoing subjugation of Black people during Reconstruction and the Jim Crow era should be obvious. What may not be quite as obvious and is often missing from the discussion of race in this country is the impact of racism on the health of Black America and on access to health care services in general and substance use disorder (SUD) services in particular. This racism includes naive beliefs going back to the early days of the United States, such as Dr. Benjamin Rush's belief that Blacks were immune to yellow fever.

The experience of Black people with the indifference of the medical establishment to their well-being was not just with Dr. Rush's dangerous belief or the infamous Tuskegee syphilis experiment. Dr. James Marion Sims, often lauded as the father of modern gynecology, conducted research on enslaved Black women without anesthesia during the mid-1840s. Given that Dr. Sims was a slaveholder, it is possible that he felt that his property was not due any more than "it" received. As recently as 2006, some people have rushed to defend Dr. Sims, essentially arguing that he was a man of his times who was providing a needed medical service to the benefit of his enslaved patients (Wall 2006). In defending Sims, some argue that his intervention was one of last resort and that the slave women in his charge "clamored" for the operation, which often failed.

In considering the historical Black experience, we are not dealing simply with a preoccupation with antebellum history. As recently as 1989, the Medical University of South Carolina (MUSC) adopted a policy that singled out for drug testing indigent Black women who had sought prenatal care and childbirth services (Paul-Emile 1999). Black women who tested positive were arrested, incarcerated, and prosecuted (American Civil Liberties Union 2021). These women were concerned enough to present for medical care despite their substance use, and when they were most vulnerable, the medical establishment turned on them and handed them over to the police and prosecutors. In reality, the records of MUSC indicated that Black patients used drugs at about the same rate as white patients; however, of the 30 women arrested, 29 were Black. This amounted to neither appropriate care nor equal justice. How are Black people supposed to trust the health care delivery system?

These historical events are not lost on the Black community. Black people are reluctant to engage with the medical establishment given the historical memory of no health care, poor health care, medical experimentation, the legacy of slavery and Jim Crow, police brutality, and intergenerational trauma that results from persistent experiences with the microaggressions of a perceived hostile environment. A discussion of health disparities in general is too broad for this chapter, but it is sufficient to state that racism, separate but unequal social policies, and the corresponding lack of access to health care are inextricably tied to the overall health and well-being of Black Americans today.

The multigenerational experience of slavery, segregation, racism, prejudice, and discrimination contributes to the historical trauma, predisposing Blacks to high rates of alcoholism, domestic violence, child abuse, drug use, and physiological and psychological problems (Williams-Washington and Mills 2018). Compounding historical trauma, of course, is the use of the criminal justice system to contain and control Black Americans. Two streams of social and political events are relevant to this chapter: 1) alcohol and Prohibition and 2) the drug wars. Both phenomena set the stage for the conflating of substance use with criminal sanctions, and both resulted in the felonization of African Americans.

Alcohol, Prohibition, and African Americans

Alcohol use and misuse in America cannot be constructed solely as a "Black" problem. Alcohol consumption and the people who use alcohol, however, are influenced by the intersections of class, economic status, race, gender, sexual orientation, and other factors. When chronicling his experiences as a slave, Black abolitionist and civil rights leader Frederick Douglass wrote in 1845 that slave owners would get their slaves drunk to keep them divided, disorganized, and dominated (Douglass 1846). Alcohol, from his perspective, was an effective tool for slave owners to subdue their slaves' inclinations toward insurrection. Consistent with his efforts to gain freedom for Black people, Douglass advocated for temperance and women's suffrage in addition to the abolition of slavery.

Prohibition notwithstanding, it is important to look at the prevalence of alcohol use from the perspective of dysfunctional consumption. As Figure 4–1 reveals, the past month prevalence of binge alcohol use (defined as five or more drinks on a single occasion in the past 30 days) hovers around 25% of whites, Blacks, Hispanics, and American Indians/Alaska Natives. For Asians the prevalence of binge drinking is below 15%.

Despite the similarity in prevalence rates for binge alcohol use among people of various races/ethnicities, numerically, the overwhelming number of past month binge drinkers ages 18 years or older in 2021 were white, with 36.9 million whites admitting to binge drinking, compared with 11.2 million Hispanics, fewer than 7.4 million Blacks, 1.75 million Asians, and 370,000 American Indians/Alaska Natives, according to data from the Substance Abuse and Mental Health Services Administration (2021).

Prohibition became the progenitor of the war on drugs and a justification for social control. The repeal of Prohibition in 1933 left in place a bureaucratic apparatus that had nothing to do. It chose to go after drugs.

Drug Laws and Oppression of Black People

Unlike Prohibition, which evolved from the concerns about the adverse effects of alcohol on the family, the drug wars were launched by a different agenda, an agenda that was manifestly based on race and ethnicity. In this section, I focus on three drug classes to highlight my points: 1) opioids, 2) cocaine, and 3) marijuana. These three drugs are symbolic

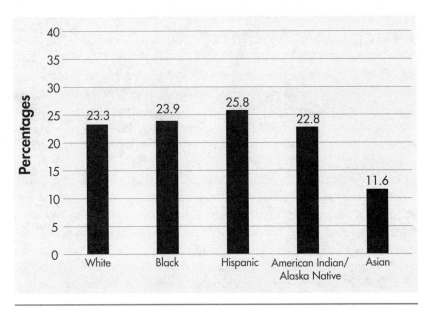

Figure 4-1. **Binge alcohol use in the past month among persons 18 years or older by race/ethnicity, 2021.**
Source. Substance Abuse and Mental Health Services Administration (2021).

of the experience of Asians, Hispanics, and African Americans in America; all three drugs have been used to justify racist and exclusionary policies directed against people of color. Because of economic goals and xenophobia, people of color have been demonized and mischaracterized—attitudes and beliefs that must be considered when addressing the medical aspects of mental health.

The issues of Black crime and Black violence were promoted as justification for the need to legislate both opioids and cocaine (Courtwright 1983). In the early twentieth century, the image of the Negro as a cocaine fiend was promoted in a *New York Times* article by Dr. Edward H. Williams, who succumbed to the tendency to stereotype and vilify African Americans (New York Times 1913; Williams 1914). Although this infamous article is often discussed and decried (Netherland and Hansen 2016), what is often missing from the discussion is the fact that Dr. Williams was an early addiction medicine specialist and anti-Prohibitionist. Courtwright (1983) argued that Dr. Williams may have been implying that alcohol was the lesser of two evils in suggesting that when denied alcohol, Blacks turned to cocaine; however, even if this were true, it only shows that Black people were regarded as throwaway objects in the service of some other policy agenda. That an addiction medicine specialist would do so points to the problem with racism and the dehumanization of Blacks as a means to an end.

There is more to the story of Edward H. Williams. He refused to bow down to the anti-addict posture of Harry Anslinger, commissioner of the Federal Bureau of Narcotics, and continued to treat persons with opioid use disorders (OUDs). One day, an informant entered Williams's clinic in withdrawal; Dr. Williams treated that informant with a narcotic and was arrested. Dr. Williams was subsequently incarcerated for his belief that persons with OUDs should be treated (Hari 2015). Here was a man who was so dedicated to treating persons with OUDs that he went to jail in support of his beliefs, but despite his heroics, his 1914 article in the *New York Times* captured his underlying racism and willingness to sacrifice Black people in the service of his agenda.

An unusual aspect of Dr. Williams's story is that his brother subsequently cowrote *Drug Addicts Are Human Beings: The Story of Our Billion-Dollar Racket, How We Created It and How We Can Wipe It Out*, a book that advocates for the treatment of people with SUDs (Williams and Smith 1938). However, in the 287-page book, the word "Negro" appears only three times, two of which involve Blacks murdering someone, and one of which involves a Black patient in Portland, Oregon, who, on hearing that the narcotic clinic was closed, "hurled himself on the concrete floor with such violence as to knock himself out completely" (Williams 1938, p. 37).

It is important to look at the invidious and pernicious effects of racism within the character of physicians like Dr. Williams. The unwillingness to see Black people as equals within community creates a visible distance between non-Black practitioners and Black patients. The core issue is race.

Opioids

The issue of iatrogenic SUD is a part of the historical matrix under discussion. Iatrogenic substance use has been a part of the warp and woof of American history since before its founding, and physicians have been major vectors of opioid use. Of course, until recently, Black patients had less to fear about iatrogenic opioid use because systemic bias resulted in Black patients being less likely to receive adequate pain management for either acute or chronic pain; this included Black patients who presented to emergency departments for acute injuries incurred, for example, in motor vehicle accidents (Morales and Yong 2021). In fact, Hoffman et al. (2016) found that many medical students and medical residents hold false biological beliefs about the thickness of Black skin and the sensitivity of nerve endings of Black people, justifying in their minds prescribing fewer pain medications.

OPIOID USE AND OPIOID USE DISORDER

Drug laws pursued by individuals with a criminal justice perspective ignore the epidemiology of drug use in America. Data from the federal government's Substance Abuse and Mental Health Services Administration (SAMHSA) reveal only slight variations by race or ethnicity in the prevalence rates for illegal drug use in America. Figure 4–2 shows that the past month drug use prevalence rate among the following racial and ethnic groups is about equal: the prevalence rate for past month marijuana use in 2021 was 15.5% for whites, 17.5% for Blacks, 12.9% for Hispanics, and 29.3% for American Indians/Alaska Natives (Substance Abuse and Mental Health Services Administration 2021). Furthermore, the prevalence of opioid use hovers around 1% across whites, Blacks, and Hispanics and 1.8% for American Indians/Alaska Natives. There are variations in cocaine and methamphetamine use, with slight elevations for cocaine use for Blacks and methamphetamine use for whites and American Indians/Alaska Natives.

SAMHSA data for 2019 revealed that the past month prevalence of the misuse of pain relievers for persons 18 or older was 0.9% for whites (or 1.4 million people) and 1.1% for Blacks (or 329,000 people) (Substance Abuse and Mental Health Services Administration 2021). The paradox here is that race played a role for access to pain medications, with Black people often denied therapeutic and clinically indicated pain medications because of bias and discrimination (Hoffman et al. 2016).

Prevalence rates tell one story, but the actual numbers of users tell an additional story. Whereas fewer than 6 million Blacks or Hispanics used illicit drugs in the past month in 2021, 24.5 million whites used illicit drugs. In addition, whereas about 5 million Blacks and Hispanics used marijuana in the past month in 2021, an estimated 22 million whites used marijuana (Substance Abuse and Mental Health Services Administration 2021). If the object of drug laws is to curtail the use of illicit drugs, then the criminal justice focus on Blacks and Hispanics is clearly misplaced. Numerically, whites have the highest incidence of illicit drug use, so why does law enforcement focus on people of color as the highest priority?

The CDC reports that nearly 841,000 people have died from a drug overdose between 1999 and 2020 (Craft et al. 2022). More than 70% of drug overdose deaths in 2019 involved an opioid, and more than 70% of the opioids were synthetic opioids, such as fentanyl (Mattson et al. 2021). The number of drug overdose deaths involving fentanyl more

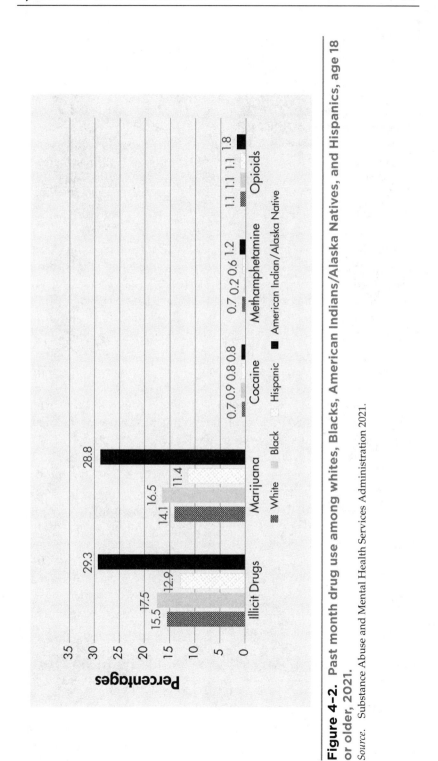

Figure 4–2. Past month drug use among whites, Blacks, American Indians/Alaska Natives, and Hispanics, age 18 or older, 2021.

Source. Substance Abuse and Mental Health Services Administration 2021.

than doubled, from 1,905 deaths to 4,200 deaths, in a single year (2013–2014; Warner et al. 2016). It was thought that the opioid overdose issues were about whites (Hansen and Netherland 2016), but research funded by the National Institute on Drug Abuse found an opioid overdose death rate in 2019 of 41 per 100,000 for non-Hispanic whites and 43.2 per 100,000 for non-Hispanic Blacks (Larochelle et al. 2021). The rates of drug overdose deaths involving fentanyl for non-Hispanic white persons ranged from 0.7 to 0.8 per 100,000 from 2011 through 2013, then increased by 108.8% from 2013 through 2016 (Spencer et al. 2019). Non-Hispanic Black persons had the largest annual percentage increase in fentanyl overdose death rates from 2011 through 2016 (140.6% per year), followed by Hispanic persons (118.3% per year) (Spencer et al. 2019).

An added complication to the opioid overdose crisis is the COVID-19 pandemic. Increases in opioid overdose deaths among Blacks during the pandemic have been reported in Alabama, Virginia, and Pennsylvania. Public health measures such as masking, social distancing, and social isolation coupled with historical social inequities and health disparities may predispose Black people to heightened vulnerability to opioid use and opioid overdose deaths; both social distancing and social isolation are associated with relapse for people in recovery from substance use (Patel et al. 2021)

As we look at the issue of overdose deaths, we need to keep in mind that Black families had been dealing with this problem years before the issues of prescription drugs and fentanyl. As with stimulants (discussed in the section "Cocaine"), the response of authorities and the medical community was to stigmatize Black victims. Once the epidemiology made it clear that white lives were also endangered by the disease of opioid misuse and that white people were dying from the very same drugs that were killing Black people, a public health emergency was declared (Haffajee and Frank 2018). In addition, substantial funding was made available to address the issue (Hansen and Netherland 2016). This funding was not for more arrests and more prosecution but for harm reduction, prevention, treatment, and recovery, something that was missing from the government's response to crack cocaine, which was considered to affect mostly Black people.

RACIAL DISPARITIES AND MEDICATION FOR OPIOID USE DISORDERS

In addition to making more money available to address the opioid epidemic, the federal government changed the law to permit prescription of buprenorphine, a Schedule III drug, to treat OUDs. By 2002, buprenorphine, which was previously used for postsurgical analgesia, was brought to market for the treatment of OUDs. Until the availability of buprenorphine to treat OUD, individuals who needed opioid medication for withdrawal or maintenance had to be treated in a network of 1,611 federally regulated and licensed clinics that dotted the country and that used the full opioid agonist methadone, approved in 1972 for this purpose (Institute of Medicine (US) Committee on Federal Regulation of Methadone Treatment 1995).

Methadone clinics gained a negative reputation in communities and among law enforcement because of their location in marginal neighborhoods, long lines of clients, and concerns about drug dealing and irregular activities in and around the clinics. Black patients dependent on opioids were disproportionately represented in opioid treatment programs that used methadone. Because federal regulations used a highly structured approach to treatment, such as prescribed supervised dosing, limits on take-home medications, and stipulated urine drug screenings, some patients viewed methadone negatively.

Andraka-Christou (2021) contends that not only is methadone associated with racial discrimination in health care settings, the political image of methadone treatment is that it is for poor Black and Hispanic patients. I do not agree with this assessment of methadone treatment. Keep in mind that for 50 years, the only legally acceptable maintenance medication was methadone, and the industry around its use grew up within an atmosphere of restrictive covenants, "not in my backyard" local resistance, and the Controlled Substances Act (and its predecessor, the Harrison Narcotics Tax Act); these two acts made it illegal to treat opioid use disorders with an opioid. At the very least, the advent of methadone signaled a shift in political attitudes toward the individuals experiencing an OUD, even if that shift still retained elements of inconvenience and social control. Blaming the medication instead of policies and social attitudes is an error in judgment.

A third medication, extended-release naltrexone, an opioid antagonist, was approved in 2010. With the advent of buprenorphine and, subsequently, extended-release naltrexone, the clinical issue should be patient choice. However, this is where the issue of disparities surfaces. Because of systemic issues, the options for Black and Hispanic patients have been compromised. Research has shown that buprenorphine is being used disproportionately by white patients and those with private insurance or who can self-pay out of pocket (Lagisetty et al. 2019). Two key barriers limit patient access to buprenorphine: 1) where to get it and 2) how to pay for it. Given that there are more than 1 million physicians in the United States and that all a physician has to do to prescribe buprenorphine for OUD is to complete 8 hours of training to get a special registration (X-waiver), many physicians should be available to treat OUDs. However, that is not the case. Only a minority of physicians have registered to prescribe buprenorphine. The same two questions apply to extended-release naltrexone, but no 8-hour training or special registration is required.

As a result of only a minority of physicians being willing to prescribe buprenorphine, federal legislation was changed to permit physician assistants, nurse practitioners, and other advanced practice nurses to prescribe buprenorphine in their practices. However, if those buprenorphine prescribing providers are not located in areas to which Black patients have access, the increased number of buprenorphine prescribers will only further skew the disparity issue.

Pharmacies are another bottleneck in accessing buprenorphine. Once the prescriber writes the prescription, a pharmacy generally must dispense the buprenorphine. First, there needs to be a pharmacy; then, the pharmacy must carry the buprenorphine. Research shows that Black and Hispanic neighborhoods have fewer pharmacies compared with white neighborhoods; in addition, such neighborhoods are more likely to experience pharmacy closures (Guadamuz et al. 2021). This lack of pharmacies, known as *pharmacy deserts*, adversely affects access to buprenorphine and to other prescription medications and over-the-counter medications as well (Qato et al. 2014). Prescribers should be aware of whether pharmacies within their service areas carry buprenorphine. One study showed that one in five pharmacies in counties with high overdose mortality rates do not dispense buprenorphine and that this limitation is more common in Southern states and among independent pharmacies (Kazerouni et al. 2021). Pharmacy deserts also affect the availability and price of naloxone for opioid overdose reversals, further dramatizing the issue of racial and economic disparity facing the Black community (Gilbert et al. 2021).

Once a prescriber and a pharmacy have been identified, the next issue is how to pay for the prescriber visit and the buprenorphine. Lagisetty et al. (2017) addressed income and racial disparities, noting that approximately 40% of buprenorphine visits are self-pay, whereas only 4.5% of visits without buprenorphine are self-pay. However, they did not ask why this is the case. I believe that the issue of stigma associated with being in treatment is important across the board. Under the self-pay rule in the Health Insurance Portability and Accountability Act, patients have greater discretion to limit access to the information in their medical records if they pay for the entire transaction out of pocket (Gellman and Dixon 2014). However, it is not clear who is deciding the issue of paying out of pocket; if it is the prescriber, then this creates an extra barrier for the patient; if it is the patient, then this empowers the patient to control information about their OUD.

If the patient does not have the resources to pay out of pocket or does not have private insurance to cover the cost of either buprenorphine or extended-release naltrexone, then the patient must rely on either Medicaid or subsidized care. As of this writing, 12 states have not adopted Medicaid expansion: Alabama, Florida, Georgia, Kansas, Mississippi, North Carolina, South Carolina, South Dakota, Tennessee, Texas, Wisconsin, and Wyoming. Many of these states have large Black populations. For instance, 38% of Mississippi's population, 33% of Georgia's population, 27% of Alabama's population, 27% of South Carolina's population, 22% of North Carolina's population, 17% of Florida's population, 17% of Tennessee's population, and 13% of Texas's population identify as being Black (U.S. Census 2021). Black patients in those jurisdictions who cannot access Medicaid cannot use this funding mechanism to pay for medications for OUD treatment. All states receive some block grant funding from SAMHSA for SUD treatment, and patients in non–Medicaid expansion states are dependent on the rules and regulations of those states. One final note on the issue of Medicaid: physicians are less likely to take new Medicaid patients than patients who are on Medicare or have private insurance (MACPAC 2021). Strategies must be developed to address the administrative hurdles that discourage practitioners from accepting new Medicaid patients.

Barbara Andraka-Christou (2021) made the following policy recommendations to enhance access to medications for OUDs: 1) expand Medicaid in all states, 2) provide grants to expand buprenorphine treatment, 3) expand access to practitioners in communities of color, 4) make methadone treatment more flexible and convenient, and 5) cover ancillary services to increase retention in treatment. Fulfilling these five policy proposals would help reduce the barriers to medications for OUDs for Black people, other people of color, and people living in poverty.

Cocaine

As mentioned in the section "Drug Laws and Oppression of Black People," the exaggerated relationship between cocaine and African Americans became a tool for a racist narrative, reinforcing attitudes against Blacks and serving to foster the evolving foundation of law that has carried over into the twenty-first century and threatens to persist well beyond. However, as with opioids, the issue is not just about cocaine. It is about race and the views about the constitution of Black people, views that diminish the autonomy of Black people and damage both their health and their liberty. Prejudicial attitudes from even the most well-meaning practitioners in medicine and law who simply saw Black people as different set the stage across centuries for the continued oppression of Black people by the field of medicine itself.

Evidence of the lasting effects of the prejudice associated with that exaggerated narrative can be found later in the twentieth century when, in 1986, President Ronald Reagan signed into law the Anti-Drug Abuse Act, which created large disparities between the mandatory sentencing for crack cocaine and powdered cocaine (P.L. 99-570 1986). Under this law, the mandatory sentence for 5 g of crack cocaine was the same as for 500 g of cocaine hydrochloride (powdered cocaine). This 100:1 ratio meant that the law fell disproportionately on Black people, who were more likely to use crack cocaine because of its lower cost. The law required mandatory sentencing of at least 5 years.

The interesting thing about the 1986 law was that it was launched by the death of Black basketball player Len Bias. Bias died from an overdose of cocaine hydrochloride, but it was assumed that because he was Black, he had died of an overdose of crack cocaine. The antidrug bill was introduced in the House of Representatives on September 8, passed the U.S. Senate on October 17, and was signed into law on October 27. Given what it did, whom it would affect, and how much it cost to implement, this criminal legislation passed with lightning speed.

Following the passage of stiffer penalties for crack cocaine and other drugs, the Black incarceration rate in America exploded from about 600 per 100,000 people in 1970 to 1,808 per 100,000 in 2000. It is also interesting that several prominent Black members of Congress were cosigners of this bill. These Black members of Congress joined a gallery of moderate to liberal white politicians in getting this rapid-fire legislation passed. When I looked for hearings on this legislation, I could find none that demonstrated a reliance on the science. No one seemed to ask about the epidemiology of crack cocaine use or what it was about the difference between crack cocaine and cocaine hydrochloride that would warrant a 100:1 disparity in criminal penalties. Had there been a serious inquiry into the science of cocaine use, legislators would have discovered that there was no justification for the disparate treatment (Hatsukami and Fischman 1996).

What is clear is that the low cost of crack cocaine made this form of cocaine accessible to low- to middle-income people, including Black people, and because it affected Black people, harsher sentences could be countenanced. Despite this, Black politicians were willing to sign on. It was the lack of knowledge of the epidemiology and science that marked the decision-making about crack cocaine. As with Benjamin Rush, Edward Williams, and then the U.S. Congress, assumptions about Black people—not science—drove decision-making.

When looking at cocaine use in America in 2021, for non-Hispanic whites, the past year prevalence for those 18 years or older was 1.8% or an estimated 2.9 million people (Substance Abuse and Mental Health Services Administration 2021). For non-Hispanic Blacks, the prevalence rate for those 18 years old or older was 1.9% or an estimated 594,000 people. Looking at crack cocaine use by non-Hispanic whites, the past year prevalence rate was 0.3% for those 18 years or older or an estimated 535,000. For non-Hispanic Blacks, the prevalence rate for those 18 years or older was 1.0% or an estimated 300,000. Yet crack cocaine is seen as a Black drug, even though more whites than Blacks use it.

As Figure 4–3 shows, when looking at use of cocaine and crack cocaine in 2021, the rates for past month use by Blacks were 0.9% and 0.5%, respectively, and the rates for use by whites and Hispanics were 0.8% for cocaine and 0.1% for crack cocaine (Substance Abuse and Mental Health Services Administration 2021). However, when looking at actual numbers of users of cocaine and crack cocaine, Figure 4–4 reveals a different story. Whites make up the largest single group of both cocaine and crack cocaine users.

In contrast to the harsh sentencing laws for crack cocaine, the federal government has taken a very different approach to the other major stimulant of interest, methamphetamine. The past year prevalence of use of methamphetamines in 2021 among whites 18 years or older was 1.2% or 1,855,000 people (Substance Abuse and Mental Health Services Administration 2021). Among Blacks 18 years or older, the prevalence of methamphetamine use was 0.5% or 142,000 people. In short, methamphetamine was more clearly a "white" drug, and despite the problems associated with its use, Congress did not rush to pass any laws with outrageous sentencing associated with this drug. The data from 2021 represent only the second wave of methamphetamine use in recent years. When the first wave occurred in the 1990s and early 2000s, the reaction of Congress was not to increase sentencing but to pass the Combat Methamphetamine Epidemic Act of 2005 (H.R. 3199 2005) to regulate over-the-counter sales of ephedrine and pseudoephedrine.

In addition to the issue of substance use, there is the issue of individuals with SUDs, that is, those who use alcohol or drugs to the point of having clinically significant impairment of function. As Figure 4–5 shows, the prevalence of SUDs among whites, Blacks, and Hispanics ranges from 16.8% to 18.3%, with a lower rate for Asian Americans and a higher rate for American Indians/Alaska Natives (Substance Abuse

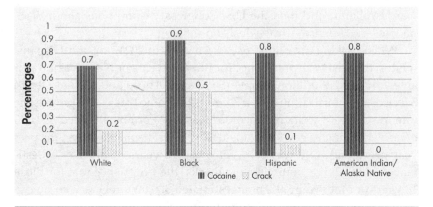

Figure 4-3. **Past month cocaine and crack cocaine use (percentage) among whites, Blacks, Hispanics, and American Indians/ Alaska Natives age 18 or older, 2021.**
Source. Substance Abuse and Mental Health Services Administration 2021.

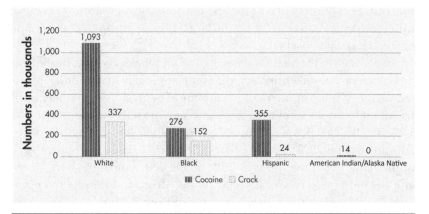

Figure 4-4. **Past month cocaine and crack cocaine use (in thousands) among whites, Blacks, Hispanics, and American Indians/ Alaska Natives age 18 or older, 2021.**
Source. Substance Abuse and Mental Health Services Administration 2021.

and Mental Health Services Administration 2021). In addition to similar prevalence rates for SUDs, the prevalence rates for the receipt of substance use treatment for the past year among persons 18 or older by race/ethnicity can be seen in Figure 4–6. These data show that there was no important difference between whites, Blacks, or Hispanics in terms of SUDs and general SUD treatment. Thus, policies that disparage people of color for substance use are inherently discriminatory.

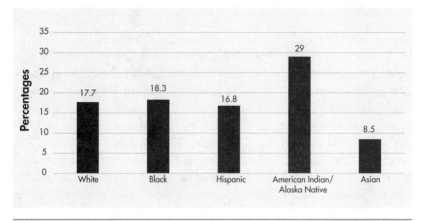

Figure 4-5. Substance use disorder in the past year among persons 18 or older by race/ethnicity, 2021.
Source. Substance Abuse and Mental Health Services Administration 2021.

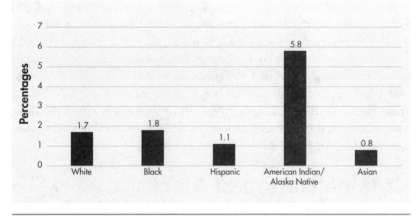

Figure 4-6. Substance use treatment received in the past year among persons 18 or older by race/ethnicity, 2021.
Source. Substance Abuse and Mental Health Services Administration 2021.

The issues of substance use, SUDs, and substance use treatment cut across all populations in the United States. The targeting of African Americans and Hispanics through use of the criminal justice system as an intervention reflects a systemic inequity in society. As mentioned in the section "Opioids," the meta-message to all those thousands of Black men and women who were incarcerated for either marijuana or cocaine offenses and their families is that Black lives do not matter.

Marijuana

The issue of marijuana from a sociomedical perspective is heavily weighed down by racial and ethnic factors. Marijuana was made illegal by a number of states in the early 1900s and at the federal level by the Marijuana Tax Act of 1937. The Boggs Act of 1951 imposed a mandatory minimum sentence of 2–10 years for a first-offense conviction for marijuana possession (P.L. 82-255 1951). Marijuana was subsequently classified as a schedule I drug in 1970 under the Controlled Substances Act. (P.L. 91-513 1970). In addition to federal laws, states created their own laws. All of these laws created criminal sanctions for those who violated them. King and Mauer (2006) pointed out that during the 1990s, 30% of marijuana arrests were of Black people, although Blacks made up only 14% of the population. There were 8.2 million marijuana arrests between 2001 and 2010, and the American Civil Liberties Union (2013) noted that Blacks were 3.73 times more likely to be arrested for marijuana possession than whites; in fact, Black arrest rates went from 537 per 100,00 in 201 to 716 per 100,000 in 2010. The difference between white marijuana use and Black marijuana use (see Figure 4–2) does not justify the disparity in arrest. Furthermore, although marijuana reform began in California in 1996 with the legalization of medical marijuana and expanded by 2023, with 38 other states joining California, Blacks have continued to be arrested for marijuana-related violations. In addition, in 2012, Colorado and Washington State made adult use of marijuana legal; by 2023, 21 states had legalized some form of recreational marijuana. Nevertheless, the racial disparity between Black and white arrests of marijuana possession persists (American Civil Liberties Union 2020).

Criminalization of Blacks

I focus on the 1986 Anti-Drug Abuse Act because the core issue there is substance use, but Elizabeth Hinton (2016) has argued that the drive toward mass incarceration in America predated the 1986 Anti-Drug Abuse Act. She dates the push toward mass incarceration to the administration of President Lyndon Johnson, noting that it was he who called for a "war on crime." Hinton contends that Johnson's antipoverty policies focused more on fighting the effects of inequality than on inequality itself. Johnson's administration adopted the view that Black pathology, not social injustice, unemployment, and racism, was at the root of Black poverty. As a result, the war on crime and the war on poverty merged, yielding what Hinton calls "the carceral state" that targeted Black people.

Much has been written about the impact of the 1986 Anti-Drug Abuse Act and its 100:1 crack cocaine versus powder cocaine provision. Within 9 years of the passage of this act, the U.S. Sentencing Commission concluded, "While some aspects of crack cocaine use and distribution suggest that a higher penalty for crack offenses compared to powder cocaine offenses is appropriate, the present 100-to-1 quantity ratio is too great." The Commission also concluded, "Among other problems, the 100-to-1 quantity ratio creates anomalous results by potentially punishing low-level (retail) crack dealers far more severely than their high-level (wholesale) suppliers of powder cocaine that served as the product for conversion into crack" (U.S. Sentencing Commission 1995, p. i).

For public health in general, and behavioral health in particular, the issue of using the criminal justice system both for exploiting labor and for culling young Black people, especially men, from the community is a substantial problem. The Bureau of Justice Statistics revealed a steady rise in Black imprisonment from 1986 to about 2009, the apparent peak year of Black incarceration. In 2009, the Black imprisonment rate was 2,134 per 100,000, compared with 308 per 100,000 for whites. Although the imprisonment rate for Blacks has since dropped to 1,446 per 100,000, that number is still substantially higher than the 263 per 100,000 for whites (Carson 2020).

From a behavioral health perspective, we must think about the impact of antidrug legislation on the cultural environment for Blacks. With mass incarceration comes the rotation of young men and women, but particularly young men, in and out of the criminal justice system. Mandatory minimum sentences guarantee that those incarcerated for 5 years or more are out of their family for a sustained period. This leads to a normalization of incarceration. Once young Blacks start to expect that they will go to jail or prison, incarceration becomes a rite of passage. I believe that this normalization of incarceration leads to adaptive behaviors that adversely influence the values and expectations of Black Americans, further isolating them from the socioeconomic mainstream. In addition, the institutional morality that young people acquire in the penal system poorly equips them for appropriate roles in civil society.

The deaths of George Floyd, Breonna Taylor, Philando Castile, and others at the hands of police officers involved drugs. Reactions to George Floyd's death were complicated by the issue of his being under the influence at the time. Breonna Taylor was killed while she was asleep when police entered her apartment searching for drugs, which were not found there. The police officer who shot Philando Castile stated that he feared for his own life because of alleged marijuana use by individuals in

Castile's car. The cases go on. Police-related drug-involved shootings of Black people have become so common that they are expected (NewsOne 2023). However, they are only part of the larger issue of police-involved shootings of African Americans. The paradox of public safety and police brutality makes it difficult for Black people to rely on the police, especially when the usual outcome is that the police are not held accountable for their misdeeds. The attitudes that presume that Black people, especially Black men, are coked-up fiends indifferent to bullets create a society that is unsafe for Black people. Drugs simply become another rationalization for the summary shooting of Blacks. However, Black people suffering mental health crises have also been the victims of unwarranted police shootings (King 2019).

An adversarial relationship between law enforcement and the Black community creates an adversarial relationship between the Black community and laws. The net effect contributes substantially to the normalization of incarceration. An example of the normalization of incarceration can be found in an unusual case in Baltimore in which 13 female guards were indicted for smuggling drugs and phones into the city jail and 4 of the guards were impregnated by the same inmate, the alleged leader of a jailhouse gang (CBS News Baltimore 2013). The women in this case were tried for corruption. One commentator asked if the women guards were predators or prey and concluded that they were predators (Dvorak 2013). Although it is clear that criminal laws were violated in this case, another issue that should be entertained from a clinical perspective is normalization of incarceration. I believe that with so many young Blacks, especially Black men, rotating in and out of incarceration, incarceration becomes normalized and destigmatized. Although the Baltimore example may be an outlier and unusual in its dimensions, it does capture the theme of how Black people can respond to an environment that marginalizes them. This, then, spills over into the clinical context, in which the norms of the clinician are at loggerheads with the norms of the patient because the worldview of the patient is at loggerheads with the worldview of the clinician.

Although the poverty rate for Black families declined from 31.3% in 1993 to 16.8% in 2020, unemployment and underemployment for formerly incarcerated people can reach 35%, leaving them to fend for themselves or their families in the alternative marketplaces of income (Sawyer 2020). To make matters worse, unemployment is not the only risk factor derived from the war on drugs. Tolani Britton (2019) points out that incarceration made people ineligible for both federal Pell grants and student loans while in prison, limited young adults' ability to receive student aid from the government after release, and had a dampening effect on the education of youth. Given the discrimination against formerly incarcerated persons, being asked about imprisonment serves as a deterrent in applying for financial aid and college.

When incarceration is normalized and a living wage is denied, social inequities are perpetuated. With that comes a healthy suspicion of the motives of that society. Then along came the COVID-19 pandemic, which highlighted not only those inequities but also the lack of trust that Black people have in the medical community. In a systematic review, Yasmin et al. (2021) found a high level of vaccine hesitancy in 2020 among Blacks. In addition to vaccine hesitancy, Yasmin et al. invoked the Tuskegee syphilis study as an explanation for the suspicion about the health care delivery system; preexisting health care delivery system disparities were also discussed as a contributing factor.

The recognition that professional associations have been complicit in the perpetuation of stigmatizing and discriminatory practices against Black Americans has been slow in coming. Still, the American Psychiatric Association (APA) in 2021 apologized for the history of racism, declaring the following:

> Since APA's inception, practitioners have at times subjected persons of African descent and Indigenous people who suffered from mental illness to abusive treatment, experimentation, victimization in the name of "scientific evidence," along with racialized theories that attempted to confirm their deficit status. Similar race-based discrepancies in care also exist in medical practice today as evidenced by the variations in schizophrenia diagnosis between white and BIPOC [Black, Indigenous, and People of Color] patients, for instance. (American Psychiatric Association 2021)

Ten months after the medical APA issued its apology, the American Psychological Association adopted a resolution that apologized to people of color for its role in promoting, perpetuating, and failing to challenge racism, racial discrimination, and human hierarchy in the United States (American Psychological Association 2021).

The two APAs were not the only organizations to address the issue of racial justice. The American Society of Addiction Medicine (ASAM) also acknowledged that racism in addiction medicine was a reality:

> ASAM recognizes the racism and discrimination that BIPOC patients, their families, and addiction medicine professionals consistently face in their personal and professional lives. Every day, addiction medicine professionals confront the tragic consequences of racial injustice among the patients and communities we serve — from the disproportionate incarceration of BIPOC with the disease of addiction, to treatment barriers for many BIPOC, to rising overdose deaths and ongoing discrimination. ASAM denounces and commits to challenging racial injustice by work-

ing toward solutions to the addiction crisis that recognize the role of systemic racism in creating and reinforcing health inequities.

Drug policy has supported systemic racism. Drug controls arose from a mix of motives, some of which were laudable, but many of which were based in racist ideology. Racial bias has emerged in policies as written and applied. (American Society of Addiction Medicine 2021)

National Association for Alcoholism and Drug Abuse Counselors (2021) promulgated a code of ethics that addressed the issue of working in a culturally diverse world, stressing respect, cultural humility, and confidentiality and privacy. Other organizations, such as Mental Health America (2021) and the National Council for Mental Wellbeing (2021), have issued statements on racism as well.

The COVID-19 pandemic has created an awareness among those in public health about the inequities in American society. That progressive organizations are touting their public policy statements is encouraging. However, the Black community has witnessed progressive statements of interest that have then dissipated, often within a short period of time. Historically, the Reconstruction period is a good starting example. The war on poverty from the 1960s is another good example. The commitment of behavioral health organizations to addressing social inequities, including addressing the social determinants of health, will need to be met with performance metrics that can be evaluated and verified. Otherwise, the many apologies and policy statements that evolved from the observations from the COVID-19 pandemic will be only exercises in sophistry.

Veterans

The U.S. Department of Veterans Affairs (VA) health care system is the largest integrated health care system in the United States, with more than 9 million veterans enrolled, and it is also the largest provider of SUD care. The VA health care system is less dependent on income and other socioeconomic factors and more dependent on service-connected disability and other eligibility criteria. Data from the VA indicate that in 2019, 28.9% of active-duty women were Black and 16.9% of active-duty men were Black (Patten and Parker 2011). Despite the fact that Blacks make up such a large proportion of the men and women in arms, of the 41 most senior commanders in the military (with four-star rank), only two are Black (Cooper 2020). Black soldiers who served in the armed forces in World War II, Korea, and Vietnam faced hatred and racism both in the military and on their return home. The prevailing attitudes about Black soldiers were not restricted to life after the military but affected how they were treated in the military.

Racism in the military and in military medicine over the many periods of military action in which America has participated has been documented as limiting the type of medical care to which Black soldiers had access. Attitudes and beliefs about pain in Black patients appear to have continued over into the care that Black veterans receive in the VA health system. For example, opioids have a place for treatment of soldiers, especially those suffering from physical trauma from wounds or diarrhea from lack of combat arena sanitation. However, Black soldiers have had substantial lack of access to opioids for medical treatment, including pain from severe war-related wounds. In a retrospective cohort study of almost 100,000 veterans in 2006, it was found that Black veterans with moderate to high pain levels were less likely than whites to receive opioids (Burgess et al. 2014). This disparity leads to one of two conclusions: poorly treated veterans are left to cope as best they can, or they end up seeking access to opioids from the street (e.g., illegal prescriptions, heroin, fentanyl). Adding PTSD to the calculus results in an obviously complicated picture.

Data show that black Vietnam veterans have greater rates of PTSD, as well as more persistent effects, than do white veterans. An additional contextual note is that in a general population sample, the lifetime prevalence of PTSD for Blacks as determined by the National Epidemiologic Survey on Alcohol and Related Conditions was 8.7%, a rate higher than the 7.4% prevalence rate for whites, with higher risk of witnessing domestic violence as a child and higher rates of war-related events (Roberts et al. 2011). It has been shown that Black veterans receive less intensive treatment for PTSD, are more likely to receive a minimal trial of treatment, and are less likely to be service connected (i.e., to receive disability payments) for PTSD. In fact, Black veterans are more likely than white veterans to be denied PTSD status as well as PTSD service connection by the VA disability assessment process (Marx et al. 2017).

It is well established that PTSD commonly co-occurs with SUDs, each complicating the course of the other disorder. Nevertheless, PTSD trials have consistently excluded patients with SUDs, both in the past and currently (Najavits et al. 2020). In short, Black veterans with SUDs and PTSD may find it difficult to receive adequate care from VA facilities. It also should be stressed that SUDs alone do not make a veteran eligible for service-connected disability; thus, a compensation and pension examination that deems substance use to be primary will result in the denial of service-connected disability (Jankowski et al. 2019). Naturally, where bias and discrimination exist within the VA compensation and pension system, Blacks and Hispanics will be disadvantaged.

On reentering society, Black military veterans who developed OUDs during American war efforts in the 1970s found opioid treatment limited.

Although the VA officially expanded its capacity to provide opioid agonist therapy to veterans presenting with OUD, it apparently could not move beyond the issue of disparities in how Black and white veterans receive this therapy. The choice between receiving methadone from a federally regulated clinic or buprenorphine from an office-based practice should be driven by medical or psychiatric comorbidities, service use characteristics, and patient choice. Office-based buprenorphine offers greater flexibility in dosing, fewer administrative restrictions, and less stigma than does clinic-based methadone. However, a national study of veterans suffering from OUD found differences in access to buprenorphine based on race and urban versus rural residence rather than clinical conditions. In short, Black veterans were three times more likely to receive methadone rather than buprenorphine, and this could not be explained by medical or psychiatric comorbidities or service use characteristics (Manhapra et al. 2016).

The circumstances of Black women veterans, specifically, must be addressed. Women, including Black women, make up about 9% of veterans; that means about 1.7 million women (Vespa 2020). Women veterans made up 3.7% of Vietnam War era veterans, but they make up 14.6% of Gulf War veterans and 16.8% of post-9/11 veterans (Vespa 2020). Black women make up 29% of active duty enlisted women and 19% of women veterans (Office of Data Governance and Analytics 2017).

The lifetime prevalence of PTSD is higher among female veterans than male veterans. In addition, using data compiled from the National Survey on Drug Use and Health, Hoggatt et al. (2017) estimated that the prevalence of past-month heavy episodic drinking is about 19% for women veterans overall; the prevalence of past-year illicit drug use for women is about 11%. The overall prevalence of past-year prescription drug misuse among female veterans is 5%.

Finally, the issues of military sexual trauma PTSD and premilitary trauma-related PTSD need to be mentioned here for both female veterans in general and Black female veterans in particular (Lehavot and Simpson 2014; Relyea et al. 2020). The trauma experiences of heterosexual and lesbian or bisexual Black female veterans should be considered as a part of a clinical workup for substance use, anxiety, depression, or other psychiatric conditions.

Conclusion

In this chapter, I have attempted to scan a few critical issues associated with substance use among Black Americans. I have attempted to show that social beliefs and political biases contribute to systemic issues that are critical contributors to health disparities. Through policy and practice, authorities have viewed Black people as inferior to whites intellectually, morally, and physically, and this diffuses into the practice of health, whether public health, mental health, or general health. Blaming Black people through microaggressions or systemic features of public policy reinforces the disparities that disadvantage the Black community and American society in general.

Thus, viewing the current state of race relations from an evolutionary perspective is essential because each epoch—colonial, Revolutionary, Civil War, Reconstruction, Jim Crow, post–World War II, and modern—carried with it an undercurrent of social and psychological attitudes about Black people, and those attitudes were carried forward by clergy, politicians, medical personnel, researchers, and average white people in all parts of the United States. The perceived threat of Blacks and the willingness to disregard the welfare of Black people have controlled public policy. This is not a matter of a progressive or conservative agenda. It is a matter of race. Even in comprehensive health care systems such as the VA health system, disparities are found time and again. In short, if we are to change things, concerned Black Americans must have greater participation in the institutions that function as the bulwark of the American enterprise.

In the academic year 2018–2019, only 6.2% of medical school graduates, or 1,238 individuals, identified as Black (Association of American Medical Colleges 2019). In addition, of full-time medical school faculty in the United States, only 3.6%, or 6,288 individuals, identified as Black. If medical schools, with almost 185,000 individuals in them, have so few Black graduates or Black faculty, then neither the general medical school student body nor the faculty are in a position to benefit from challenges to their beliefs about Black people (Association of American Medical Colleges 2020). These biases, stereotypes, and racial tropes linger in the consciousness of non-Blacks. Whatever non-Blacks learned from their parents, schools, and social environments is what they bring to the laboratory, the clinic, and the operating room.

The issue of systemic factors is not limited to medical schools and physicians. All institutions that make policy, formulate regulations, and deliver services follow a similar vein. As a civil servant, I found that Black people in positions of authority were often treated more negatively than white people in authority. The priorities germane to the Black community often took a back seat to the vision of non-Blacks. That must change.

If changes are going to occur, the following things must happen:

1. We need more Black people in positions of authority in federal and state bureaucracies.

2. We need more Black scholars and researchers funded by the National Institutes of Health and its component institutes and involving the National Science Foundation and the Departments of Justice, Education, Labor, Agriculture, and Housing.
3. We need appropriate training of medical students, nursing students, dental students, and public health students.
4. We need a commitment from society to allow Black people to acquire their fair share of the American dream, which means eliminating many of the artificial barriers to training, education, and employment.
5. We need to recognize that health disparities manifest not only in physical and mental health but also in housing, food security, and income security.
6. We need to promote access to health care for all Americans.
7. We need an action agenda that is long range and long term.
8. We need to promote better science about the various substances of misuse to inform harm reduction, prevention, treatment, and recovery strategies.

The changes that are required to allow Black people full participation in American society will be perceived by some as encroaching on the economic interests of non-Blacks; this attitude will generate pushback and a digging in of heels to preserve the status quo. In addition to economic interests, some people simply believe that Black people are less than non-Blacks and are thus undeserving; this attitude is a recurrent theme in American consciousness. As a society, we must address both attitudes.

References

American Civil Liberties Union: The war on marijuana in Black and white. New York, American Civil Liberties Union, June 2013. Available at: www.aclu.org/report/report-war-marijuana-black-and-white. Accessed March 15, 2023.

American Civil Liberties Union: A tale of two countries: racially targeted arrests in the era of marijuana reform, 2020. Available at: www.aclu.org/report/tale-two-countries-racially-targeted-arrests-era-marijuana-reform. Accessed March 15, 2023.

American Civil Liberties Union: Ferguson v City of Charleston: social and legal contexts. New York, American Civil Liberties Union, 2021. Available at: www.aclu.org/other/ferguson-v-city-charleston-social-and-legal-contexts. Accessed October 29, 2021.

American Psychiatric Association: APA Board issues apology for history of racism. Washington, DC, American Psychiatric Association, February 3, 2021. Available at: https://psychnews.psychiatryonline.org/doi/full/10.1176/appi.pn.2021.2.45. Accessed October 31, 2021.

American Psychological Association: Apology to people of color for APA's role in promoting, perpetuating, and failing to challenge racism, racial discrimination, and human hierarchy in U.S. Washington, DC, American Psychological Association, October 29, 2021. Available at: https://www.apa.org/about/policy/racism-apology. Accessed October 31, 2021.

American Society of Addiction Medicine: Public policy statement on advancing racial justice in addiction medicine, February 25, 2021. Available at: www.asam.org/advocacy/public-policy-statements/details/public-policy-statements/2021/02/25/public-policy-statement-on-advancing-racial-justice-in-addiction-medicine. Accessed May 6, 2022.

Andraka-Christou B: Addressing racial and ethnic disparities in the use of medications for opioid use disorder. Health Aff (Millwood) 40(6):920–927, 2021 34097509

Association of American Medical Colleges: Diversity in medicine: facts and figures 2019. Washington, DC, Association of American Medical Colleges, 2019. Available at: www.aamc.org/data-reports/workforce/interactive-data/figure-13-percentage-us-medical-school-graduates-race/ethnicity-alone-academic-year-2018-2019. Accessed December 23, 2021.

Association of American Medical Colleges: Faculty roster: U.S. medical school faculty. Washington, DC, Association of American Medical Colleges, 2020. Available at: www.aamc.org/data-reports/faculty-institutions/report/faculty-roster-us-medical-school-faculty. Accessed December 23, 2021.

Britton T: Does locked up mean locked out? The effects of the anti-drug act of 1986 on Black male students' college enrollment. Working Paper 101-19. Berkeley, CA, Institute for Research on Labor and Employment, April 2019. Available at: http://irle.berkeley.edu/files/2019/04/Does-Locked-Up-Mean-Locked-Out.pdf. Accessed May 6, 2022.

Burgess D, Nelson D, Gravely A, et al: Racial differences in prescription of opioid analgesics for chronic noncancer pain in a national sample of veterans. J Pain 15(4)447–455, 2014 24440840

Carson EA: Prisoners in 2019. Bureau of Justice Statistics Bull NCJ255115. Washington, DC, Bureau of Justice Statistics, 2020

CBS News Baltimore: Jailhouse soap opera: 13 female guards indicted for smuggling drugs and phones; 4 impregnated by same inmate. Baltimore, MD, CBS News, April 30, 2013. Available at: https://baltimore.cbslocal.com/2013/04/23/25-correctional-officers-inmates-indicted-for-gang-activity-in-baltimore-jails. Accessed October 28, 2021.

Cooper H: African-Americans are highly visible in the military, but almost invisible at the top. New York Times, May 25, 2020. Available at: www.nytimes.com/2020/05/25/us/politics/military-minorities-leadership.html. Accessed October 18, 2021.

Courtwright DT: The hidden epidemic: opiate addiction and cocaine use in the South, 1860–1920. J South Hist 49(1):57–72, 1983 11614816

Craft WH, Tegge AN, Keith DR, et al: Recovery from opioid use disorder: a 4-year post-clinical trial outcomes study. Drug Alcohol Depend 234:109389, 2022 35287034 [Erratum Drug Alcohol Depend 241:109687, 2022 36334989]

Douglass F: Temperance and anti-slavery. Address delivered at Paisley Scotland, March 30, 1846. Renfrewshire Advertiser, April 11, 1846

Dvorak P: Were the female guards indicted in Baltimore prison scheme predators or prey? Washington Post, April 25, 2013. Available at: www.washington post.com/local/were-the-female-guards-indicted-in-baltimore-prison-scheme-predators-or-prey/2013/04/25/d75fa3fe-adbc-11e2-8bf6-e70cb6 ae066e_story.html. Accessed May 6, 2022.

Gellman R, Dixon P: Paying out of pocket to protect health privacy: a new but complicated HIPAA option. Lake Oswego, OR, World Privacy Forum, 2014. Available at: www.worldprivacyforum.org/2014/01/wpf-report-paying-out-of-pocket-to-protect-health-privacy. Accessed December 23, 2021.

Gilbert L, Elliott J, Beasley L, et al: Naloxone availability in independent community pharmacies in Georgia, 2019. Subst Abuse Treat Prev Policy 16(1):63, 2021 34419089

Guadamuz JS, Wilder JR, Mouslim MC, et al: Fewer pharmacies in black and Hispanic/Latino neighborhoods compared with white or diverse neighborhoods, 2007–15. Health Aff (Millwood) 40(5):802–811, 2021 33939507

Haffajee RL, Frank RG: Making the opioid public health emergency effective. JAMA Psychiatry 75(8):767–768, 2018 29710123

Hansen H, Netherland J: Is the prescription opioid epidemic a white problem? Am J Public Health 106(12):2127–2129, 2016 27831792

Hari J: Chasing the Scream. New York, Bloomsbury, 2015

Hatsukami DK, Fischman MW: Crack cocaine and cocaine hydrochloride: are the differences myth or reality? JAMA 276(19):1580–1588, 1996 8918856

Hinton E: From the War on Poverty to the War on Crime. Cambridge, MA, Harvard University Press, 2016

Hoffman KM, Trawalter S, Axt JR, Oliver MN: Racial bias in pain assessment and treatment recommendations, and false beliefs about biological differences between blacks and whites. Proc Natl Acad Sci USA 113(16):4296–4301, 2016 27044069

Hoggatt KJ, Lehavot K, Krenek M, et al: Prevalence of substance misuse among US veterans in the general population. Am J Addict 26(4):357–365, 2017 28370701

H.R. 3199, USA Patriot Improvement Act of 2005, Title VII

Institute of Medicine (US) Committee on Federal Regulation of Methadone Treatment: Federal Regulation of Methadone Treatment. Edited by Rettig RA, Yarmolinsky A. Washington, DC, National Academies Press, 1995. Available at: www.ncbi.nlm.nih.gov/books/NBK232105. Accessed May 6, 2022.

Jankowski RL, Black AC, Lazar CM, et al: Consideration of substance use in compensation and pension examinations of veterans filing PTSD claims. PLoS One 14(2):e0210938, 2019 30726261

Kazerouni NJ, Irwin AN, Levander XA, et al: Pharmacy-related buprenorphine access barriers: an audit of pharmacies in counties with a high opioid overdose burden. Drug Alcohol Depend 224:108729, 2021 33932744

King RS, Mauer M: The war on marijuana: the transformation of the war on drugs in the 1990s. Harm Reduct J 3:6, 2006 16469094

King S: If you are Black and in a mental health crisis, 911 can be a death sentence. The Intercept, 2019. Available at: https://theintercept.com/2019/09/29/police-shootings-mental-health. Accessed October 31, 2021.

Lagisetty P, Klasa K, Bush C, et al: Primary care models for treating opioid use disorders: what actually works? A systematic review. PLoS One 12(10):e0186315, 2017 29040331

Lagisetty P, Ross R, Bohnert A, et al: Buprenorphine treatment divide by race/ethnicity and payment. JAMA Psychiatry 76(9):979–981, 2019 31066881

Larochelle MR, Slavova S, Root ED, et al: Disparities in opioid overdose death trends by race/ethnicity, 2018–2019, from the HEALing Communities Study. Am J Public Health 111(10):1851–1854, 2021 34499540

Lehavot K, Simpson TL: Trauma, posttraumatic stress disorder, and depression among sexual minority and heterosexual women veterans. J Couns Psychol 61(3):392–403, 2014 25019543

MACPAC: Physician acceptance of new Medicaid patients: findings from the National Electronic Health Records Survey. Fact sheet. Washington, DC, Medicaid and CHIP Payment and Access Commission, June 2021. Available at: www.macpac.gov/wp-content/uploads/2021/06/Physician-Acceptance-of-New-Medicaid-Patients-Findings-from-the-National-Electronic-Health-Records-Survey.pdf. Accessed December 23, 2021.

Manhapra A, Quinones L, Rosenheck R: Characteristics of veterans receiving buprenorphine vs. methadone for opioid use disorder nationally in the Veterans Health Administration. Drug Alcohol Depend 160:82–89, 2016 26804898

Marx BP, Engel-Rebitzer E, Bovin MJ, et al: The influence of veteran race and psychometric testing on Veterans Affairs posttraumatic stress disorder (PTSD) disability exam outcomes. Psychol Assess 29(6):710–719, 2017 28594214

Mattson CL, Tanz LJ, Quinn K, et al: Trends and geographic patterns in drug and synthetic opioid overdose deaths: United States, 2013–2019. MMWR Morb Mortal Wkly Rep 70(6):202–207, 2021 33571180

Mental Health America: Racism and Mental Health. Alexandria, VA, Mental Health America, 2021. Available at: www.mhanational.org/racism-and-mental-health. Accessed October 31, 2021.

Morales ME, Yong RJ: Racial and ethnic disparities in the treatment of chronic pain. Pain Med 22(1):75–90, 2021 33367911

Najavits LM, Clark HW, DiClemente CC, et al: PTSD/substance use disorder comorbidity: treatment options and public health needs. Curr Treat Options Psychiatry 7(4):544–558, 2020 35444925

National Association for Alcoholism and Drug Abuse Counselors: Introduction to NAADAC/NCC AP Ethical Standards. Alexandria, VA, National Association for Alcoholism and Drug Abuse Counselors, January 1, 2021. Available at: www.naadac.org/code-of-ethics. Accessed October 31, 2021.

National Council for Mental Wellbeing: Statement from executive leadership team of the National Council for Mental Wellbeing on the death of George Floyd. Washington, DC, National Council for Mental Wellbeing, 2021. Available at: www.thenationalcouncil.org/news/statement-from-executive-leadership-team-of-the-national-council-for-mental-wellbeing-on-the-death-of-george-floyd. Accessed March 15, 2023.

Netherland J, Hansen HB: The war on drugs that wasn't: wasted whiteness, "dirty doctors," and race in media coverage of prescription opioid misuse. Cult Med Psychiatry 40(4):664–686, 2016 27272904

NewsOne: 144 Black men and boys killed by police. NewsOne, March 3, 2023. Available at: https://newsone.com/playlist/black-men-boys-who-were-killed-by-police/item/1. Accessed March 15, 2023.

New York Times: 10 dead, 20 hurt in a race riot; drug-crazed Negroes start a reign of terror and defy whole Mississippi town. New York Times, September 29, 1913

Office of Data Governance and Analytics: Women veterans report. Washington, DC, National Center for Veterans Analysis and Statistics, Department of Veterans Affairs, 2017

Patel I, Walter LA, Li L: Opioid overdose crises during the COVID-19 pandemic: implication of health disparities. Harm Reduct J 18(1):89, 2021 34399771

Patten E, Parker K: Women in the U.S. military: growing share, distinctive profile. Washington, DC, Pew Research Center, December 2011. Available at: www.pewresearch.org/social-trends/2011/12/22/women-in-the-u-s-military-growing-share-distinctive-profile. Accessed March 11, 2023.

Paul-Emile K: The Charleston policy: substance or abuse. Mich J Race Law 4:325–387, 1999

P.L. 82-255, 82nd Congress, 1951

P.L. 91-513, 91st Congress, 1970

P.L. 99-570, 99th Congress, 1986

Qato DM, Daviglus ML, Wilder J, et al: "Pharmacy deserts" are prevalent in Chicago's predominantly minority communities, raising medication access concerns. Health Aff (Millwood) 33(11):1958–1965, 2014 25367990

Relyea MR, Portnoy GA, Combellick JL, et al: Military sexual trauma and intimate partner violence: subtypes, associations, and gender differences. J Fam Violence 35(4):349–360, 2020

Roberts AL, Gilman SE, Breslau J, et al: Race/ethnic differences in exposure to traumatic events, development of post-traumatic stress disorder, and treatment-seeking for post-traumatic stress disorder in the United States. Psychol Med 41(1):71–83, 2011 20346193

Sawyer W: Visualizing the racial disparities in mass incarceration. Northampton, MA, Prison Policy Initiative, July 27, 2020. Available at: www.prisonpolicy .org/blog/2020/07/27/disparities/?gclid=Cj0KCQjwlOmLBhCHARIs AGiJg7l5SN6l_u5IXEET2iowRd2mPOE-p6tRR6iqlBHl689fRsZb_HBY-isaAnEeEALw_wcB. Accessed October 29, 2021.

Spencer MR, Warner M, Bastian BA, et al: Drug overdose deaths involving fentanyl, 2011–2016. Natl Vital Stat Rep 68(3):1–19, 2019 31112123

Substance Abuse and Mental Health Services Administration: National Survey on Drug Use and Health 2018. Rockville, MD, Center for Behavioral Health Statistics and Quality, Substance Abuse and Mental Health Services Administration, 2018

Substance Abuse and Mental Health Services Administration: National Survey on Drug Use and Health 2021. Rockville, MD, Center for Behavioral Health Statistics and Quality, Substance Abuse and Mental Health Services Administration, 2021

U.S. Census: QuickFacts: Population Estimates, July 1, 2021. Available at: www.census.gov/quickfacts/fact/table/US/PST045221. Accessed December 23, 2021.

U.S. Sentencing Commission: 1995 Report to the Congress: Cocaine and Federal Sentencing Policy. Washington, DC, U.S. Sentencing Commission, 1995. Available at: www.ussc.gov/research/congressional-reports/1995-report-congress-cocaine-and-federal-sentencing-policy. Accessed March 14, 2023.

Vespa JE: Those who serve: America's veterans from World War II to the war on terror. Rep ACS-43. Suitland, MD, American Community Survey, June 2020

Wall LL: The medical ethics of Dr J Marion Sims: a fresh look at the historical record. J Med Ethics 32(6):346–350, 2006 16731734

Warner M, Trinidad JP, Bastian BA, et al: Drugs most frequently involved in drug overdose deaths: United States, 2010–2014. National Vital Statistics Rep Vol 65 No 10. Hyattsville, MD, National Center for Health Statistics, 2016

Williams EH: Negro cocaine "fiends" are a new Southern menace; murder and insanity increasing among lower class Blacks because they have taken to "sniffing" since deprived of whisky by prohibition. New York Times, February 8, 1914, Section M, p 12

Williams MD, Smith H: Drug Addicts Are Human Beings: The Story of Our Billion-Dollar Drug Racket, How We Created It and How We Can Wipe It Out. Washington, DC, Shaw, 1938

Williams-Washington KN, Mills CP: African American historical trauma: creating an inclusive measure. J Multicult Couns Devel 46:246–263, 2018

Yasmin F, Najeeb H, Moeed A, et al: COVID-19 vaccine hesitancy in the United States: a systematic review. Front Public Health 9:770985, 2021 34888288

Black Psychiatrists Responding to the Mental Health Impact of Natural and Human-Caused Disasters and Systemic Inequities

Annelle B. Primm, M.D., M.P.H., DLFAPA

Inaction in the face of need is the hallmark of structural racism.
Camara Phyllis Jones, M.D., M.P.H., Ph.D. (Jones 2021b)

In this chapter I describe the efforts of Black psychiatrists and community health advocates from a variety of disciplines and sectors who have focused on supporting Black communities and other historically marginalized populations in the aftermath of disasters of all types.

Any discussion of the involvement of Black psychiatrists in disasters should include the late Phyllis Harrison-Ross, M.D. (August 14, 1936 to January 16, 2017), a child psychiatrist and prominent figure who was instrumental in developing culturally aligned responses to disasters in communities of color, including 9/11 and the fallout of mass incarceration, on the well-being of families. Dr. Harrison-Ross was the author of *The Black Child*, a community activist and visionary, and one of the early presidents of the Black Psychiatrists of America (BPA). She was an academic psychiatrist and a major force in community mental health, serving in the role of chief of service for psychiatry at New York City's Metropolitan Hospital, overseeing mental health services in some of the city's most economically fragile communities. Many people for whom she provided care were experiencing mental illnesses and a plethora of other challenges, including substance use disorders, chronic diseases, physical disabilities, unstable housing, and high incarceration rates.

Dr. Harrison-Ross took immense pride in her ability to build teams of professionals to work within the framework of public psychiatry to address the needs of individuals with mental illnesses, multiple co-occurring health conditions, and adverse social circumstances. She was fully aware of the dysfunction and barriers inherent in urban mental health systems and the complexities individuals encounter navigating those systems. As a Black psychiatrist, she embraced these challenges despite the frustrations and was conscious of the responsibility of professionals who shared her racial identity to provide hope, help, and healing "in the face of the many problems confronting [Black] communities across America." She stated, "...it is our skills, our know-how, our understanding that can help Black women, men, children, and families navigate the rocky road towards both physical and mental health" (Harrison-Ross 2004, p. 3).

In the latter part of her career, Dr. Harrison-Ross was appointed commissioner of the Medical Review Board of the New York State Department of Corrections, where she advocated for major changes in that system to improve mental health care for incarcerated individuals—a disproportionate number of whom are members of Black communities and other marginalized racial identity groups. Dr. Harrison-Ross was also a pioneer in the use of telehealth for mental health services and televisiting to connect children with their incarcerated parents. This connection promotes bonding that helps protect children's mental health and facilitates eventual parental reentry into family life.

Another dimension of Dr. Harrison-Ross's contributions to society was her deep commitment to her faith community, the New York Society for Ethical Culture. As chair of its Social Services Review Board, she created and championed numerous community-focused initiatives addressing societal disasters such as housing for battered and displaced women, healing initiatives for people traumatized by 9/11, and outreach to socially isolated older adults. She was keenly aware of the impact of public policies on health, which drove her to establish a series of programs called Champions of Change to hold politicians accountable for the impact of their legislative decision-making on the well-being of communities.

Dr. Harrison-Ross was the American Psychiatric Association Solomon Carter Fuller awardee in 2004, and her lecture, "I Am a Fact, Not a Fiction," paid homage to Dr. Fuller (Harrison-Ross 2004). She said that Fuller was "a pioneer…a first…a trailblazer. It is because of him that the idea of a Black psychiatrist became a reality. And because of the reality that he created, I am a fact, not a fiction. I—and all Black psychiatrists—owe our existence to Dr. Fuller, who opened the door that we have been able to walk through" (Harrison-Ross 2004, p. 4).

Dr. Harrison-Ross focused on what Black and other marginalized communities need in order to be whole and experience mental health, well-being, and quality of life. She established as fact that

> as Black psychiatrists, we must practice well-informed, culturally balanced, and technologically pertinent psychiatry. We must do so in the face of restraints…constraints…and dwindling resources. Our existence as African Americans gives us insight into the particular needs of Black communities. When we leave the office, and work and live in the community, we reconnect with the universe of needs that our patients have and the impact of community on their physical and mental health. (Harrison-Ross 2004, pp. 5, 7)

Given Dr. Harrison-Ross's major contributions to social and community psychiatry, this chapter is a fitting tribute to an important aspect of her professional life. In it, I seek to provide a platform to amplify her work in the area of disasters of all types and their impact on Black and other historically marginalized communities. I also shed light on how her work evolved over time and has led to initiatives focused on natural and human-caused disasters, which are occurring with increasing frequency and with greater impacts in Black and other marginalized communities.

Formation of All Healers Mental Health Alliance

Hurricane Katrina, the catastrophic storm that hit New Orleans and the Gulf Coast in August 2005 and caused a devastating death toll of more than 1,800 people, was a game changer among disasters. Katrina exposed the reality that economically fragile communities are at a distinct disadvantage during and after disasters, which reinforce and intensify preexisting disparities and suffering. There was also a racial dynamic to the destruction of Hurricane Katrina. People of color relegated to low-lying areas vulnerable to flooding, a form of racial segregation combined with environmental racism, experienced the highest levels of mortality and displacement. Watching in horror on television the vast devastation and human suffering in the wake of Katrina and the disproportionate impact on economically distressed communities of color prompted me, along with Dr. Harrison-Ross and Dr. Lucille Norville Perez, former president of the National Medical Association, to act swiftly in response to the tragedy that unfolded post-Katrina. We immediately convened a group of health professionals, academics, faith leaders, first responders, and other community health advocates from various parts of the nation to focus on what could be done to facilitate culturally grounded responses to the mental health needs of communities directly affected by this unprecedented disaster.

Recognizing that it was neither possible nor prudent to drop everything and go rushing to the Gulf Coast to help communities harmed by Katrina, we began to meet weekly via telephone conference call in an effort to assist by coordinating actions to support affected communities from a distance. The group called itself All Healers Mental Health Alliance (AHMHA), which reflects an inclusive organization, multidisciplinary and multisectoral in nature, that was intent on developing comprehensive and strategic responses that incorporate a variety of perspectives, including public health, clinical care, social work, community organizing, and faith-based efforts.

Over time, AHMHA continued to convene forums for information exchange, resource sharing, and technical assistance for solving local problems rooted in gaps and unmet needs of marginalized communities following disasters. In addition, AHMHA partners have mobilized collaborations to promote healing and thriving and have coordinated support services for disaster-affected communities, caregivers, and first responders. During its history, AHMHA has engaged more than 50 leaders associated with large national Black organizations; academic institutions, including historically Black colleges and universities (HBCUs); faith communities; nonprofit organizations; and small businesses across the nation, including the U.S. Virgin Islands.

Necessity of Collaboration

As a result of climate change, natural disasters are occurring with increasing frequency. Communities of color are hit harder by disasters than other communities because of disproportionate, preexisting economic disparities and other inequities, including environmental racism (Millar 2021). These inequities and harsh circumstances place these social groups in harm's way in floodplains, which are vulnerable to climate-related disasters, and in areas exposed to other environmental calamities such as poor air quality and polluted water. These communities are typically neglected by and receive unequal treatment from emergency response efforts (Flavelle 2021).

There is a glaring lack of racial diversity in leadership among disaster and emergency management professionals, which is one of the drivers of disparities in disaster response to racially marginalized communities. Disaster organizations on the national and state levels typically take a one-size-fits-all approach, which is not helpful. Furthermore, the emergency management community holds stereotypes that Black organizations are not involved in disaster response (D. Gibson, personal communication, October 2021). This attitude is a result of historical patterns and economic disadvantage in Black communities and organizations, which serve as barriers to them mounting large-scale disaster responses.

Another dimension of this attitude is the *white savior complex*. This term describes the tendency of some white people to work from a perspective of superiority in which they assume they understand the needs of Black and other racially marginalized communities. They dismiss the legitimacy of leaders of color, whom they inappropriately deem to be lacking in the wherewithal and intellectual ability to serve their own communities after disasters (Raypole 2021). Black psychiatrists and other leaders have concluded that it is they who must conceive the solutions for their own communities because no one else may come to the rescue or fully understand their culture or the extent of their needs in the context of disasters.

Responding to Katrina and Beyond

The multidisciplinary team of psychiatrists, psychologists, social workers, nurses, faith leaders, first responders, academics, advocates, and activists who are partners of AHMHA worked together to engage frontline colleagues and caregivers to obtain a firsthand view of what was occurring on the ground in the Gulf Coast, including New Orleans. By supporting these practitioners, AHMHA partners were indirectly providing care for the caregiver and helping them to feel supported in a chaotic, highly stressful environment, which in some cases involved even their own displacement because of the disaster. AHMHA's focus was on schools, primary care settings, and churches, which are places where people gather and on which they rely for support before, during, and after a disaster.

AHMHA developed a collaboration with Morehouse School of Medicine, the HBCU medical school in Atlanta, and its Regional Coordinating Center for Hurricane Response, led by Dr. Dominic Mack. The collaboration supported mental health after Katrina by using videophones, a rudimentary precursor of videoconferencing that used fax lines (Mack et al. 2021). Use of this simple mechanism was spearheaded by Dr. Harrison-Ross, who was an early adopter of employing technology to provide mental health services to her geographically distant patients. Using this technology in the aftermath of a disaster such as Hurricane Katrina makes it possible for mental health professionals to provide counseling from afar to disaster-affected people located in areas where psychiatric services were scarce prior to a disaster and remain scarce afterward.

In addition, access to telehealth resources facilitates mental health professionals in providing consultation to primary care practitioners and faith leaders to assist people who come to them for counseling and emotional support. AHMHA leaders are aware that typically, few people come directly to psychiatrists when in distress, preferring primary care practitioners and the faith community. Furthermore, as with Katrina, psychiatric practitioners often are in short supply because the majority of the few available before the disaster have been displaced by the storm to other geographical areas themselves. People are more likely to engage gatekeepers, such as faith community leaders, who are trusted and less likely to raise the specter of stigma typically associated with specialty mental health help seeking, even in the aftermath of a disaster (U.S. Department of Health and Human Services 2022). Indeed, the psychological distress associated with disaster is not necessarily pathological but rather a natural response to the disequilibrium associated with displacement and disruption by lack of housing, food, and other essential comforts to which people are accustomed.

The weekly Sunday calls provided a supportive space in which leaders on the forefront of the fallout from the devastation left by Katrina could unload their burdens and AHMHA partners could care for the caregivers to help them keep going and continue their efforts. By working to keep up the spirits and rejuvenate the energy of these individuals who were often working long hours to assist disaster-affected communities, AHMHA helped increase the service capacity of first responders.

One of the concerns that arose in response to survivors of Hurricane Katrina was that the cultural dimensions of the needs of the people were in some instances disregarded. Volunteers from disaster relief organizations displaced survivors to parts of the country with unfamiliar cultures and few people of color. In some instances, this led to a cultural disconnect and social isolation. Examples of this cultural mismatch with the disaster-affected community include the absence of disaster relief workers who understood the local dialect and the undesirable foods that were served that were out of keeping with cultural norms.

After turning its attention to a spate of natural disasters, including Hurricane Katrina, AHMHA partners realized they needed to focus on both natural and human-caused disasters that have a disproportionately negative impact on Black and other historically marginalized communities. In both Katrina and the Deepwater Horizon oil spill, which devastated fishermen of color on the Gulf Coast, AHMHA found a way to assist. In the latter case, AHMHA hired a filmmaker to document the plight of the fishermen of Pointe à La Hache to call attention to the fishermen's inability to make a living in the aftermath of the destruction caused by the oil spill. After the national media moved on to other news topics, the affected community continued to languish. AHMHA did what it could to raise awareness, and, as a result, the community received donations that helped the fishermen move forward with a modicum of hope. Awareness of the existence of this type of racial disparity and its impact on mental health and economic well-being in the wake of even human-caused environmental disasters was a motivation for AHMHA to develop similar strategies for action going forward.

Racism Is the Ultimate Disaster

AHMHA discovered racism to be the ultimate disaster undergirding the disparately devastating impact of natural and human-caused disasters on historically marginalized communities. This devastation comes in many forms and shows up in all aspects of life through social determinants of physical health and mental health, including but not limited to exclusion, discrimination, segregation, substandard housing, underresourced educational systems, economic inequality and unemployment, food insecurity, toxic environments, and limited access to health care (Compton and Shim 2015). Racism is at the root of disparities in social determinants of health and mental health that plague racially marginalized communities and intensify the impact of disasters on communities of color. Racial discrimination is a main driver of the low-level, delayed, or completely absent response and recovery efforts. Racial disparities also underpin the fallout of displacement and resultant rending of social fabric among desperate families who are forced to leave their communities and relocate elsewhere after disasters, either temporarily or permanently (Fullilove 2016).

Racism is also a factor in climate change consequences, given the disproportionate effects on people of color. As victims of environmental racism, they are often relegated to living in segregated higher-risk areas prone to flooding and other undesirable climate-based impacts. Furthermore, people of color are more likely than their white counterparts to experience preexisting, multilayered adverse social determinants of physical health and mental health, which result in them having reduced access to resources to prepare for disasters and experiencing more difficult recoveries. All of these factors can precipitate or compound trauma, psychological distress, social isolation, depression, anxiety, loss, grief, and a sense of hopelessness.

Racism is an underlying cause of mundane *extreme environments*, in which racism and racially oppressive forces are continuous and omnipresent and abound in everyday occurrences. These racism-laden environments cause significant stress that piles up over time, having a negative and draining impact and taking a significant toll on the psychological and physical health status of Black individuals (Carroll 1998; Pierce 1981). The amalgam of the stress of racism superimposed on the stress of disasters is a double whammy on the Black community and other communities of color. In addition to destruction of their homes, these communities experience the additional stress and despair associated with loss of employment and income, loss of personal belongings, displacement, disenfranchisement, loss of property, and the destruction and ultimate gentrification of neighborhoods by predatory developers.

An example of the interplay of these factors is Black communities in Eastern North Carolina that were severely affected by a succession of natural disasters in the form of Hurricanes Matthew (2016) and Florence (2018). Black communities, including churches, had not recovered from Matthew before they were hit hard again with floods and destruction of their homes and churches caused by Hurricane Florence. These extreme conditions set the stage for toxic stress, weathering, and allostatic load of repeated exposures to highly stressful conditions (Geronimus et al. 2006) and associated shortened life spans among Black people regardless of socioeconomic status. This stress is multilayered with the intergenerational impact of more than 400 years of enslavement and its aftermath of Jim Crow and racial discrimination in all aspects of life. These historical forces undergird the Dred Scott decision that a Black man "has no rights which the white man is bound to respect" (Arenson 2015). In fact, members of the communities affected by the storms have been suffering because of their inability to afford insurance and to get federal aid to repair or rebuild. AHMHA has supported these communities when they were threatened by local officials and saw nooses in local newspapers intended to scare them off from asking for help, which local authorities equated with causing trouble (L. Dunston, personal communication, January 2019).

Attitudes borne by age-old policies and practices covertly drive the maldistribution of opportunity and promote racial disparities in deprivation and punishment. This is consistent with the words of Dr. Camara Phyllis Jones, a leading U.S. physician, epidemiologist, and antiracism activist, who has stated that "Black people tend to be on top of every bad list, and the bottom of every good list" (Jones 2021a). A common saying is that "When the white community catches a cold, the Black community catches pneumonia," and in many ways, communities of color represent a canary in the coal mine, foreshadowing the vulnerability of the people of our nation and the planet to disasters as a result of climate change, a crumbling national infrastructure in urban and rural environments, and numerous other perils (CDC 2022).

The AHMHA Approach to Helping Communities Postdisaster

The hazards described in this chapter do not spell doom for vulnerable communities given the work of AHMHA and other community-focused organizations who elect to emphasize the phrase "risk factors are not predictive factors because of protective factors." AHMHA highlights protective factors in the form of information exchange, resource sharing, thought leadership, brainstorming, and culturally consonant technical assistance for solving local problems associated with gaps in support to marginalized communities after disasters. One set of approaches that AHMHA follows is drawn from a meta-analysis of studies of factors that maximize mental health after a disaster. These factors include the promotion of calm, safety, collective and self-efficacy, social connectedness, and hope (Hobfoll et al. 2007). Many of these mediators of mental health align with psychological first aid, which is an approach used by the American Red Cross to support people through the early postdisaster stages (Brymer et al. 2006).

Best Practices, Lessons Learned, and Cases in Point

In this section, I describe in detail some of the key elements that Dr. Phyllis Harrison-Ross set in motion during the 12 years she was in a leadership role with AHMHA.

FOSTERING A MINISTRY OF PRESENCE

A critical aspect of addressing the loss of connection and social isolation that many marginalized communities experience in the aftermath of disasters is fostering a ministry of presence. When communities feel neglected and bypassed, this only adds to their stress and misery. Addressing this aspect has provided an essential role for AHMHA: to organize, facilitate, and mobilize culturally aligned responses to disaster-related needs of Black and other historically marginalized populations. In rural North Carolina, AHMHA connected with Black churches whose parishioners were reeling from floods and water-damaged homes caused by successive storms, including Hurricane Florence and Hurricane Matthew. Some residents of these rural areas had not been able to recover from previous storms. The Eastern North Carolina chapter of the National Association of Black Social Workers and members of the Department of Psychiatry at East Carolina University came to the rescue and provided psychological first aid and information on stress management techniques to the disaster-affected families. They also brought donations of food and items such as toiletries, bedding, linens, backpacks, and coloring books for children. Donations helped to support the provision of warm food of the familiar culturally based cuisine that was preferred by the disaster-affected people of this area. The totality of the components of disaster response in these rural areas was a village approach, which gave a strong signal to these communities that they had not been forgotten. AHMHA's partnership with faith communities, an important organizing force in Black communities, was highly effective in giving people hope and a sense of connection when hopelessness and isolation were lurking.

Another example of the ministry of presence occurred after Superstorm Sandy, when AHMHA convened healers from various mental health and human service professions for a disaster training at a New York City church. Groups of Black organizations from the New York metropolitan area "adopted" the hardest-hit communities of color in remote areas of New York City. They bore witness to hardships in these communities wrought by Sandy, reported to the Federal Emergency Management Agency (FEMA) on the needs of disaster-affected residents, and provided supportive and healing services. These approaches were important for guarding against the inequities in distribution of resources that occurred in some of these communities and the condescending attitudes with racial overtones among some of the volunteer relief workers from around the country, many of whom were not accustomed to interacting with people of color. In other disasters, people of color received threats that if they talked about what they did or did not receive and complained about disparities, they would be punished by not receiving additional services or losing their employment (D. B. Gibson, personal communication, October 2021).

PROVIDING ACCESS TO COLLECTIVE RESOURCES

Another aspect of AHMHA's postdisaster work focused on marginalized communities of color is providing access to collective resources. After Hurricane Harvey in the Houston area in 2017, AHMHA partners engaged scouts on the ground and connected community leaders in Port Arthur, Texas, to FEMA to ensure that neglected neighborhoods received disaster relief. In some ways counterintuitively, AHMHA's orchestration of delivery of truckloads of food and supplies in collaboration with Unity in Disasters, a Black-led disaster relief organization, had an impact on the mental health of disaster populations by restoring basic comforts that are so essential to a decent quality of life. Gathering and sending supplies and donations to hard-hit communities in need is an essential component of the work of AHMHA because it has an ameliorative impact on mental health by decreasing stress. Providing food and supplies was counterintuitive because one might assume that AHMHA's efforts would be focused directly on mental health supports rather than basic needs such as food and supplies (e.g., cleaning supplies, diapers, wipes) that may not be usually associated with mental health.

PROMOTING CULTURALLY GROUNDED RESPONSES TO DISASTERS

The failures of Katrina, when some communities of color were looked on and treated as refugees, became a clarion call for promoting culturally grounded responses to disasters and prompted AHMHA to contribute a section on culturally sensitive disaster mental health services to the American Red Cross Disaster Mental Health Handbook of 2012. AHMHA recommended that disaster workers use cultural brokers and *promotoras* (community members trained to provide health education) as translators and ambassadors to ensure that disaster-related services being provided to communities of color consider and accommodate their cultural beliefs and preferences in their preferred language.

Responding to mental health needs postdisaster is a critical component of the work of AHMHA, but this is not to suggest that people's mental health responses to disasters are considered pathological or that psychiatry was being practiced in the response to Katrina and other disasters. However, people with preexisting psychiatric disorders that are exacerbated in the wake of a disaster do need psychiatric care. AHMHA facilitated provision of telemental health services to people who needed mental illness care in New Orleans and remote Gulf Coast areas affected by Katrina. AHMHA also coordinated healing circles where survivors were taught relaxation techniques to help ameliorate the long-lasting effects of the trauma. In addition, for seniors displaced by Katrina from New Orleans to Houston, AHMHA convened support groups in a nursing facility to foster thriving.

USING MEDIA AND COMMUNICATION

Use of media and communication is a critical part of the work of AHMHA and serves as a mediator of mental health–related support to disaster-affected communities. Delivering online training to Disaster Distress Helpline crisis counselors is one component of this effort. The training helps to ensure that counselors have a working knowledge of some of the cultural factors at play in communities such as the U.S. Virgin Islands, which was devastated by Hurricanes Irma and Maria. Another dimension of the use of media is providing context for articles in the Black press and other socially conscious media to raise awareness of the plight of communities of color affected by disasters. Also, it is crucial to use radio, online resources, and social media to share culturally tailored disaster preparedness tools and tips on coping after disaster for families and children. In recent years, AHMHA has developed tip sheets on what items to have handy in case of a disaster requiring evacuation. These tip sheets are culturally customized and include images of a Black family to ensure that the resource will resonate with the intended audience. Another example of the use of culturally tailored media messaging is the public service announcements developed by AHMHA partners, which have been helpful in encouraging vaccination against COVID-19 in Black communities in Cleveland, Ohio.

PROVIDING CARE FOR THE CAREGIVER

AHMHA has created a forum for first responders and health care practitioners in which providing care for the caregiver is an essential feature. AHMHA meetings have become a sought-after safe space where leaders can unload their challenges and elevate their need for support for strategic direction. AHMHA convenings include trusted experts from a variety of fields and disciplines, which accrues to the benefit of communities and their leaders struggling to promote recovery in the wake of disasters. Self-care and tools for physical, mental, and spiritual health are shared on a regular basis to encourage community leaders on the front line to rejuvenate. Investing in individual wellness is paramount in ensuring that people providing assistance to their communities can continue to do so.

HOLDING CELEBRATORY EVENTS

Celebratory events give people the chance to tell their stories and be praised publicly for their sacrifices for and contributions to the healing of displaced people and devastated communities. These Heroes of Healing celebrations, a name coined by Dr. Harrison-Ross, have been held in New York City, Houston, and New Orleans and have created a coveted space for fellowship and collective storytelling about what people traversed and were able to overcome.

CREATING PLATFORMS AND EXPOSURE FOR DISASTER-RELATED DISCUSSION FOCUSED ON COMMUNITIES OF COLOR

Creating platforms and exposure for disaster-related discussion focused on communities of color is another role that AHMHA has embraced. AHMHA has organized conferences to focus on the impact of human-caused disasters such as the Flint water crisis, supporting community leaders and advocates in their efforts to fight for social justice and ameliorate the damage caused by lead poisoning in their Michigan community. Lead is a toxic metal, and lead poisoning can have devastating health consequences for children, including impacts on brain development and behavior (CDC 2022). AHMHA organized a conference at Howard University in Washington, D.C., bringing together scholars in different fields from across the nation to tackle the issues of lead contamination of water, particularly in urban communities with crumbling infrastructure. AHMHA's goal has been to assist in the identification and utilization of opportunities to educate and stimulate change to protect the mental health and well-being of some of Flint's residents. Many members of this community are still going through the nightmare of lead-tainted water 8 years after the beginning of the water crisis.

The Flint crisis is just one example of the risks across the nation of too little clean water, especially in vulnerable communities where water crises add insult to injury. In 2020, cities across Texas and Jackson, Mississippi, experienced significant hardship when a power grid failure compromised access to clean water. The stress generated by not having this basic need met was an impetus for AHMHA to join with representatives of Southern areas affected by water disasters to share strategies and lessons learned from the community-based organizations that had been active in responding to the Flint crisis.

AHMHA's first conference in June 2019 in Baltimore focused on culturally appropriate disaster response, featuring experts in emergency management, social work, psychiatry, engineering, farming, logistics management, and other fields. All of these disciplines have a role to play in preventing and responding to a wide range of disasters and hazards, whether they are natural in origin or human caused. Every person in this professional "village" can also contribute to restoring mental health and well-being in disaster-affected communities.

PREPARING BLACK CONTRACTORS TO CATCH THE BALL

AHMHA also helps position Black vendors to "catch the ball" by providing crisis counseling, disaster case management, and other resources to the Black community and other communities of color. These populations are at risk of being overlooked by the usual sources of support such as FEMA, the American Red Cross, national and state voluntary organizations active in disasters, and state emergency management. AHMHA has undertaken this positioning role in order to equip churches, contractors, and other groups to be prepared to receive funding and to raise awareness among disaster agencies about the need to serve the Black community and other communities of color that may be left out of the first waves of support.

DEALING WITH DISPROPORTIONATE EFFECTS OF COVID-19

COVID-19 has been a devastating scourge in the Black community in the United States, with disproportionate rates of death, the inability to work from home, and overrepresentation among essential workers experiencing high exposure to the coronavirus, accompanied by increased levels of unemployment and financial hardship. The totality of these harms has been superimposed on the accumulated stressors associated with four centuries of racism and racial discrimination as well as disasters such as Hurricane Florence, Hurricane Harvey, historic flooding, and other disasters from which Black families have still not recovered after years of reverberating effects. The confluence of these disasters has had a devastating impact on Black and other racially marginalized communities (Mack et al. 2021).

There has been considerable hesitancy among communities of color regarding testing and vaccination given the lack of trust in the medical establishment. The long history of racism in the United States against Black people, particularly in the medical establishment, with egregious acts against Black patients, undergirds this distrust. This is a critical issue because Black and Indigenous communities are experiencing COVID-19 deaths at a higher rate than other Americans, and adverse social determinants of health have fueled these disparities (Hill and Artiga 2022). This is truly a paradox in which the people who need help the most are the least likely to receive support. The conundrum is being fueled by deliberate disinformation in what many see as a depopulation strategy and outright genocide in order to consolidate power as the country becomes more racially diverse without a white majority in many states, as evidenced by the 2020 U.S. Census (Jensen et al. 2021).

AHMHA partners have worked hard to keep up with their response to multiple successive disasters of all types while engaging in efforts to help Black communities grapple with the COVID-19 pandemic. Organizing COVID-19 testing sites in Black communities, educating people about the importance of wearing masks, distributing masks and hand sanitizer to communities without them, advocating for unhoused individuals to have means for washing their hands on the street and access to hotel rooms for their safety, distributing free COVID-19 home testing kits, making appointments for seniors to receive COVID-19 vaccinations, driving members of communities without their own personal vehicles to vaccine appointments, and developing public service announcements to raise awareness about the importance of vaccination are all examples of how AHMHA's multidisciplinary partners and community volunteers have been active in supporting their communities to combat the COVID-19 disaster. These acts of strategic engagement in communities hit hard by the pandemic underscore the importance of Black communities being their own solutions to disaster.

The AHMHA Education Task Force focused on the deleterious impact of virtual education for children faced with school closures due to the risks associated with COVID-19, providing information important to parents, students, educators, and administrators of school systems. This displacement was devastating given that many public school districts with large percentages of children of color residing in segregated areas were already underresourced. School closures and virtual education placed pressure on families headed by essential workers who could not be at home teleworking during the school day, unleashing a second disaster on top of the pandemic. Children from these households would be left behind academically unless additional supports were brought in to offset these setbacks. Churches and other community organizations stepped into this breach to avert further crises that would not bode well for the futures of children of color. The lack of computers and internet access exposed the digital divide and placed in harm's way the education of children of color in economically fragile households. It is devastating that some children disengaged from their education completely during this period, frequented fast food restaurants in order to have Wi-Fi connectivity, or did not have a place to study at all. These are all manifestations of the disaster that the COVID-19 pandemic exposed, and AHMHA and other organizations need to speak out and advocate for change for the betterment of the social determinants of health among vulnerable populations.

ADDRESSING RACIAL VIOLENCE

Racial violence and the tragic deaths of Michael Brown, Eric Garner, George Floyd, Breonna Taylor, and others have prompted a key AHMHA partner, the Community Healing Network, to create a mechanism for healing from the human-caused disasters of racism and white supremacy. This organization was motivated to develop its mission by the American Psychiatric Association's position statement on racism (American Psychiatric Association 2018), which discussed the impact of racism and racial discrimination on mental health, including the point that "racism and racial discrimination adversely affect mental health." The Community Healing Network, in collaboration with another AHMHA partner, the Association of Black Psychologists, has developed community-based in-person and virtual support groups to process and heal from historical and contemporary collective trauma in Black communities. Examples of such racial trauma include the unnecessary killing of unarmed Black people and innumerable examples of inhumane treatment that Black people have experienced, from 1619 to COVID-19. These support groups, called Emotional Emancipation Circles, were implemented starting in 2006 in Tuskegee, Alabama. Tuskegee, like many other places across the nation, was the site of a horrific event leading to collective trauma among Black people. This location was the site of the infamous Tuskegee experiment in which Black men who had contracted syphilis were observed over time without benefit of the prevailing standard treatment, penicillin, which was widely available at that time.

Each of the episodes of violence mentioned in the previous paragraph resulted in the homicide of one individual, but these deaths have had reverberations across the nation that are associated with collective racial trauma. In the aftermath of these occurrences, Black people realize that these murders could have involved them or their family members. Ferguson, Missouri; Baltimore, Maryland; and New York City all have in common widely publicized killings of unarmed Black people. The mass murder of 10 Black people in a Buffalo, New York, supermarket by an 18-year-old white supremacist shooter prompted the AHMHA to partner with the Community Healing Network and other organizations to respond to this attack on the Black community. The groups organized rapid response virtual healing circles modeled after the emotional emancipation circles to give members of the Black community in Buffalo an opportunity to process their trauma and grief in response to this heinous act of terrorism.

The succession of racially motivated episodes has created a growing demand for emotional emancipation circles, which provide safe spaces and culturally comfortable forums for processing the psychological sequelae of structural racism against Black people. These circles also provide another benefit: They carry the potential for forging a path forward for healing, principled leadership, and action to make things better in Black communities. The emotional emancipation circles have ushered in a movement for people to work through, in an organized and culturally grounded way, the assaults on the Black community and to overcome the internalized racism in Black communities. These emotional emancipation groups are occurring in the United States, Europe, Africa, and South America, giving people of the African diaspora the space to process, overcome, and collectively heal from more than 400 years of oppression and internalized racism in the aftermath of enslavement—the ultimate disaster.

The collaboration between the Community Healing Network and AHMHA has made possible the deployment of emotional emancipation circles training to increase the capacity for facilitators to offer these forums in their own communities. The killing of George Floyd during the first few months of the COVID-19 pandemic led to an increase in emotional emancipation circles being provided virtually. These remote circles facilitated healing among hurting Black people across the nation who yearned to come together in fellowship because physical distancing was required because of the pandemic. AHMHA collaborated with the BPA to establish emotional emancipation circles for BPA members, most of whom were psychiatrists dealing with their own racial trauma while steeling themselves to help others process trauma and pain. This offering for Black mental health professionals underscored, once again, the importance of caring for the caregiver. The use of technology in the form of videoconferencing for the purpose of bringing Black people together to heal collectively from widespread societal harms driven by systemic racism is emblematic of the vision of Dr. Phyllis Harrison-Ross. Early on in the evolution of AHMHA, she saw the value of using "telepresence" to bring people together to foster mental health.

Takeaways

Black psychiatrists working in concert with people from a wide variety of other disciplines, through an organization such as AHMHA, can promote mental health and community well-being postdisaster in the Black community and other communities of color. This is not about pathology or psychiatry in a professionally orthodox sense. Rather, this is true culturally aligned community mental health. AHMHA's disaster-focused efforts have extended over a 16-year period and counting. AHMHA will continue to connect the Black community and other communities of color with creature comforts, which lets them know that their needs have not been overlooked. These communities are seen, heard, and valued, and, as a result, a "for us, by us" approach is necessary, even if to augment what federal, state, nongovernmental organization, and local authorities provide. Interdisciplinary, collaborative approaches ensure that disaster response is comprehensive in addressing unmet community needs. It is essential to engage local community leaders in collaborative and inclusive efforts to develop strategies to meet community needs in a culturally appropriate way, as in the mantra "Nothing about us without us."

References

American Psychiatric Association: Position statement on resolution against racism and racial discrimination and their adverse impacts on mental health, July 2018. Available at: www.psychiatry.org/File%20Library/About-APA/Organization-Documents-Policies/Policies/Position-2018-Resolution-Against-Racism-and-Racial-Discrimination.pdf. Accessed October 10, 2021.

American Red Cross: Culturally sensitive DMH services, in Disaster Mental Health Handbook. Washington DC, Disaster Services, American Red Cross, October 2012, pp 154–157. Available at: www.cuny.edu/wp-content/uploads/sites/4/page-assets/about/administration/offices/ovsa/disaster-relief/hurricanes-harvey-irma/Disaster-Mental-Health-Handbook.pdf. Accessed October 10, 2021.

Arenson A: The Dred Scott case said Blacks had no rights "the white man was bound to respect." But in the West things turned out differently. Washington, DC, History News Network, George Washington University, March 3, 2015. Available at: https://historynewsnetwork.org/article/158681. Accessed, May 5, 2022.

Brymer M, Jacobs A, Layne C, et al: Psychological First Aid: Field Operations Guide, 2nd Edition. Los Angeles, CA, National Child Traumatic Stress Network and National Center for PTSD, July 2006. Available at: www.nctsn.org/resources/psychological-first-aid-pfa-field-operations-guide-2nd-edition. Accessed March 5, 2023.

Carroll C: Mundane extreme environmental stress and African American families: a case for recognizing different realities. J Comp Fam Stud 29(2):271–284, 1998

CDC: Health effects of lead exposure. Atlanta, GA, Centers for Disease Control and Prevention, March 9, 2022. Available at: www.cdc.gov/nceh/lead/prevention/health-effects.htm. Accessed May 4, 2022.

Compton MT, Shim RS: The Social Determinants of Mental Health. Focus 13:419–425, 2015

Flavelle C: Why does disaster aid often favor white people? New York Times, June 7, 2021. Available at: www.nytimes.com/2021/06/07/climate/FEMA-race-climate.html. Accessed October 10, 2021.

Fullilove MT: Root Shock: How Tearing Up City Neighborhoods Hurts America and What We Can Do About It, 2nd Edition. New York, New Village Press, 2016

Geronimus AT, Hicken M, Keene D, Bound J: "Weathering" and age patterns of allostatic load scores among blacks and whites in the United States. Am J Public Health 96(5):826–833, 2006 16380565

Harrison-Ross P: I Am a Fact, Not a Fiction. Solomon Carter Fuller Award lecture, American Psychiatric Association Annual Meeting, New York, May 3, 2004

Hill L, Artiga S: COVID-19 cases and deaths by race/ethnicity: current data and changes over time. San Francisco, CA, Kaiser Family Foundation, August 22, 2022. Available at: www.kff.org/coronavirus-covid-19/issue-brief/covid-19-cases-and-deaths-by-race-ethnicity-current-data-and-changes-over-time. Accessed March 5, 2023.

Hobfoll SE, Watson P, Bell CC, et al: Five essential elements of immediate and mid-term mass trauma intervention: empirical evidence. Psychiatry 70(4):283–315, discussion 316–369, 2007 18181708

Jensen E, Jones N, Rabe M, et al: 2020 U.S. population more racially and ethnically diverse than measured in 2010: the chance that two people chosen at random are of different race and ethnicity has increased since 2010. Suitland, MD, U.S. Census Bureau, August 12, 2021. Available at: www.census.gov/library/stories/2021/08/2020-united-states-population-more-racially-ethnically-diverse-than-2010.html. Accessed June 30, 2022.

Jones CP: Edward Mazique Symposium, National Medical Association Annual Conference (online), August 2021a

Jones CP: Racism denial is "a black hole" that hurts our ability to get a handle on COVID. Ali Velshi Show, MSNBC, March 7, 2021b. Available at: https://www.msnbc.com/ali-velshi/watch/dr-camara-jones-racism-denial-is-a-black-hole-that-hurts-our-ability-to-get-a-handle-on-covid-102232133732. Accessed May 4, 2022.

Mack DH, Hughes C, Douglas M, Gaglioti A: Disaster preparedness and equitable care during pandemics. J Natl Med Assoc 113(2):220–222, 2021 33268104

Millar H: What is environmental racism? Medical News Today, November 14, 2021. Available at: www.medicalnewstoday.com/articles/environmental-racism. Accessed May 4, 2022.

Pierce C: Extreme environments: the ghetto and the South Pole. Washington, DC, Educational Resources Intervention Center, 1981. Available at: https://eric.ed.gov/?id=ED242428. Accessed October 10, 2021.

Raypole C: A savior no one needs: unpacking and overcoming the white savior complex. Healthline, July 13, 2021. Available at: www.healthline.com/health/white-saviorism. Accessed October 10, 2021.

U.S. Department of Health and Human Services: For community and faith leaders: creating community connections for mental health. MentalHealth.gov, April 6, 2022. Available at: www.mentalhealth.gov/talk/faith-community-leaders. Accessed May 4, 2022

PART II

Responding to the Realities of Racism

6

Application of an Emotional Competence Framework to Racism

Loma K. Flowers, M.D.

In this chapter I describe the development and application of a practical approach to building personal frameworks for the development of comprehensive social and emotional skills (Jones and Flowers 2019). These skills are known collectively as emotional competence (EC), which enhances an individual's ability to respond constructively to everyday life events (Goleman 1995). Moreover, this framework approach to EC enables individuals to adapt successfully to unexpected challenges. African Americans, for example, face the double burdens of social and economic disadvantages; the COVID-19 pandemic and health care disparities; and organized reactivation of white supremacy and unpredictably fatal racist encounters with law enforcement and civilians, as well as the all too common mass shootings and tragic suicides that affect everyone.

The routine application of this EC approach to emotionally important events is essentially *preventive* psychiatry, building skills systematically before devastating crises occur. To demonstrate the application of relevant aspects of this approach, I present an event with racism in action and analyze it from this EC perspective. This discussion illustrates how the approach can be used to provide a constructive perspective to understand the dynamics of any event, large or small; process the impact; and tailor individualized, effective responses. Finally, I discuss broader implications.

Curriculum Development

Historically, clinical observations and experience are well known for their contributions to medicine and psychiatry (Freud 1951) as well as providing context for improving quality of care. In that tradition, my experience as a psychiatrist treating diverse patients in public, private, and federal health care systems using pragmatic, goal-oriented, collaborative psychotherapy with individuals, couples, and groups is invaluable (Flowers 1972, 1993; Flowers and Zweben 1996). I have applied that experience to the development of various programs involving mental health education including the EC framework (Flowers 1976, 2015; Flowers and Zweben 1996, 1998).

In 1994, Lanette Brown, a creative educator and old Cleveland friend, recruited me to teach, as she phrased it, "everything my students need to know, psychiatrically, to be successful" in an innovative program, 3-1-3. The low-income, high-potential but low-performing high school freshmen in the program aimed to complete high school and college in 7 years, becoming first-generation college graduates. I had no idea what they needed. However, the invitation was very explicit: "Come talk to them. You can talk about dreams [my current project]; you'll figure it out" (Flowers 1988). Collaborative process I could do. Tailored content would follow.

I am a psychiatrist trained primarily in psychopathology, and my 1960s Case Western Reserve training in biology research under Norman Rushforth, Ph.D., and the medical school Family Clinic Program teaching normal baseline body functioning under stress (pregnancy) served as models. Being a Black mother raising Black boys (Grier and Cobbs 1968), teaching and mentoring (Fernandez et al. 2019; Grier and Cobbs 1968; Mahoney et al. 2008) were other reference points. Although success is a universal concept, in practice it is highly individual. So I began monthly success-focused classroom conversations about troublesome incidents in the students' lives, small to large, in and out of school.

Asking questions and carefully listening to answers and comments, I sorted out the students' thinking and feelings that led to actions, both constructive and destructive. This guided me to relevant dynamics, common themes, and individuality. By integrating the students' baseline knowledge and practices, I identified universal concepts and principles and designed protocols for teaching and learning individual skills (Flowers 2005). Presenting this curriculum in a similar process to other groups nationally and in the United Kingdom enabled additions, adaptations, and refinements for wider applicability (Fernandez et al. 2019; Flowers et al. 2014; Thomas-Squance et al. 2011).

Much later, I learned that this process resembles an Afrocentric approach, the group conversation method (DuBois and Li 1971). In Western culture, reason is valued over emotions and spirit; the African view sees these three as a unit (King and Mitchell 1995). With a gifted community liaison, Howard Willis, who knew every family connection and circumstance, we built cohesion by keeping the class together for all subjects; held Saturday classes and provided tutoring; and offered parallel student, parent, and teacher workshops about emotions. The 3-1-3 program went on to win a statewide award in 1998 (Flowers and Brown 2000).

The excitement in learning this approach to success is in the delivery system. It is as if emotions fill the spaces between thoughts to complete the experiences. The emotional connections that develop in collaboration-focused workshops create cohesion and relationships. Those relationships are integral to the program development, which is why I have included the names of key leaders. In this open context of parallel learning and teaching, participants can relate both their own progress and the progress of others to their individual self-development interests. In comparison, any written description of the whole system reads like a methods section. Nonetheless, in contrast to regrets, disappointment, blame, and excuses, EC mastery brings the excitement of achievements. Like every practice, expertise develops from replication, on demand, of various aspects within this integrated system outlined in the curriculum: "Practice on small stuff, rehearse for big stuff" (Jones and Flowers 2019).

Curriculum Terminology

The curriculum was originally titled Emotional Education, but educators preferred the name Emotional Empowerment, which highlights the outcome of emotional education. Modeling EC in action, we adopted their suggestion. After Goleman (1995) popularized the work of Gardner (1999) and Solway et al. (2002) on various types of intelligence as emotional quotient (EQ), Ruth Thomas-Squance and I founded a nonprofit organization, Equilibrium Dynamics, in California in 2005 to teach this approach. We shortened the name of the organization to EQDynamics (EQD) and also used it for the curriculum approach. In 2018, psychiatrist Jabari Jones in New York succeeded Dr. Thomas-Squance as executive director.

In publications, we use EC to describe our work. In addition, we use the words *feelings* and *emotions* interchangeably as people do in everyday life, and we treat all emotions equally, including the basic few that researchers use. This approach defines EC as a moderate to high level of understanding of concepts and principles related to intrapersonal (emotional, internal) and interpersonal (social, external) dynamics, as well as the mastery and application of relevant skills for *constructive* everyday action. The most fundamental of these EC skills involves the *integration* of thinking, feeling, and good judgment *before* action, which is particularly relevant to navigating contemporary challenges of being Black in America.

Curriculum Outline

For ease of teaching and learning, the EQD curriculum is divided into five giant steps (self-awareness, self-development, relationships, self-responsibility, and reflections and feelings), each with substeps covering important aspects of EC development. In managing the normal events and interactions of everyday life, one can select from multiple concepts, principles, and skills in the steps and substeps as needed, often out of order, as you will see. Racism increases both stakes and emotions, requiring considerable mastery of EC skills to manage the complexities of troubling events smoothly and successfully.

Individuals can gradually increase their level of EC by progressing from step 1 to step 5 and back to step 1 again like ascending a spiral staircase. Nonetheless, there are inevitable overlaps—and occasional rapid surges in mastery, or regressions between steps and substeps. Because individuals have a lifelong process of growth and development, unintended or intentional, this approach was designed to keep pace and can be initiated, paused, or resumed at any stage of life.

Step 1 is *self-awareness*, the cornerstone of EC. It includes the following substeps: individual diversity (e.g., physical, habits, talents, styles); verbal and nonverbal communication; Feeling Management, a 10-step protocol that extends beyond containing feelings to constructive responses; and dreams and nightmares using Delaney's dream interview method (DIM) (Flowers 1993, 1995, 2015; Flowers and Zweben 1996, 1998).

Step 2, *self-development*, addresses the continual need for adaptations and change. This step includes the following substeps: identity, change, phases of grief, the alternatives-benefits-costs (A-B-Cs) of decisions, dependency-interdependence-independence, and balance in life.

Step 3, *relationships*, covers three major aspects. The basics include emotional connection, three components (self, other, and what happens between the two), and sequential process. Facets of relationships include type and level of intimacy, which is a key dynamic in the #MeToo movement; boundaries; and vulnerability. Skills include communication; goals; multitasking; and other-awareness, which includes culture competence (Flowers 1972).

Step 4, *self-responsibility*, involves autonomy; self-reliance; plans and structure, such as time management or this curriculum; accurate, kind self-assessment without blame or excuses; limit setting; community responsibility and leadership; routine good judgment and minimizing bad judgment, both of which are crucial to effective action; and values and judgments around such elements as integrity, privacy, power, politics, money, sexuality, religion, ethics and morality, health, and lifestyle.

Step 5, *reflections and feelings*, includes journaling facts and feelings and integrating additional skills, such as mindfulness, yoga, and meditation.

Overall, this approach to EC provides a broad platform of universally applicable concepts and principles to support the development of a personalized combination of skills into a systematic, effective, constructive approach to life's challenges. Although the content can be taught, each individual has the responsibility to develop a personalized adaptation with a cohesive integration of the concepts, principles, and skills into a systematic, easily accessible, personally valuable repertoire. That is the last mile challenge.

Emotionally Competent Responses

The curriculum also describes three interdependent levels of response to events: instant, considered, and developmental.

The *instant response* is an immediate reflex reaction to an event (e.g., an unexpected difficult conversation). The effectiveness of instant responses is dependent largely on previous experience and level of mastery of EC skills.

The *considered response* to an emotional event allows individuals to precisely target success with constructive, well-thought-out actions. It is the workhorse of EC, a skill development tool identical to the Feeling Management 10-step protocol. Regular practice with this sequential process leads to more competent instant responses.

The *developmental response* is a directed growth step designed to meet specific challenges such as learning to collaborate instead of compete. It may be used to fill a skill gap, such as limit setting or asking *explicitly* for what you need, or to process complex emotions, such as Grier and Cobbs's (1968) concept in their book *Black Rage*, which can interfere with achieving constructive results. Developmental responses incorporate many considered responses and other emotional and social skills.

EC concepts and principles, rather than rules, allow for both universality and individuality and intentionally link content and process to provide a framework for developing lifelong personal and professional EC in different contexts. In addition to the personalized development of basic EC skills, this framework holds a continuing expectation of upgrades to handle changing demands, a hallmark of resilience.

In addition to the usual lumps and bumps of life, African Americans in the United States are generally destined for encounters with multiple varieties of individual and/or systemic racism at any time. Such encounters are inherently fraught with emotions for everyone involved, particularly the most vulnerable. Many encounters also challenge identity in new ways, testing both external and internal skills. Managing this well requires all three EC responses.

The following snippet of a now-infamous encounter with racism illustrates some relevant EC considerations.

An Illustrative Encounter With Racism

The proliferation of video recordings with instant and irrevocable global distribution by social media in the almost 30 years between the videos of the 1991 Rodney King beating and the May 25, 2020 George Floyd murder by police provides us with multiple incidents to examine.

> In an encounter in the Ramble section of New York's Central Park, also on May 25, 2020, a birder, an African American man, asked a new dog owner, a white woman, to leash her dog as the rules required. She did not. The birder began video recording the woman and her dog.
>
> The dog owner countered with a command tone of voice, not a request, that he stop recording and advanced toward him holding her still unleashed dog by the collar.
>
> The birder continued to record video without responding verbally to the dog owner's demand. He physically backed up repeatedly, saying, "Please don't come close to me."
>
> The dog owner's response was to continue to advance on the birder, threatening to call the police, and pointing her finger directly at him.
>
> The birder responded, "*Please* call the cops. *Please* call the cops."
>
> The dog owner took out her phone and called the police. The birder captured her on video saying, "There is an African American man. I am in Central Park. He is recording me and threatening me and threatening my life and my dog."

Emotional Competence Considerations for the Moment and the Aftermath

In the moment, EC requires you to hear what is audible and see what is clearly visible, including actions and impacts. The primary visible problem in the example above is the interaction between these two people. Identifying the problem focuses our analysis in this case on the basic three components of a relationship: two individuals and their interactions.

In my experience, unreasonable responses such as the dog owner's refusal to leash her dog indicate that *emotional logic* is operating: she did not *want* to leash her dog; therefore she shouldn't have to. When the birder also firmly refused to concede, the dog owner's instant response was escalation. The absurdity of her fabricated report of a lethal threat indicates a racist dynamic, recognizable to millions who saw the video. Less blatant evidence of racism is a continuing challenge of being Black in America because even mentioning instances is often met with "Oh, I'm sure there's another [more acceptable, less threatening] explanation." That response is one of many reflex denials of racism that reinforce the status quo. A move toward greater self- and other-awareness would be "Really? I wouldn't have considered that."

It is well known that brief encounters between strangers vary widely, from combat and road rage or mask rage (notorious on airplanes) to emergency rescues, heartwarming kindnesses, and hookups. The video shows no hint of any mutual emotional connection, the essential ingredient of any viable relationship. The birder might have been open given his measured responses. The dog owner definitely was not.

Encounters leading to mutual positive emotional connections between strangers can ease negotiations and even mark the beginning of sustainable relationships in which those connections become reciprocal sustaining forces that fuel both individuals (e.g., doctor-patient relationships, best friends). During the early social isolation periods of the COVID-19 pandemic, people's self-awareness of the importance of close physical contacts increased considerably. However, in this case, two strangers were caught in a conflict of needs, exacerbated by her behavior and the absence of an emotional connection.

On reflection, I realized that the dog owner possibly felt a *threat to her life of white privilege* (DiAngelo 2018), that is, her legacy of the right to have her needs met on demand *without question* and to flaunt rules with impunity. People publicly commented on social media below the videos I watched that the dog owner's deliberately misleading report that threatened the birder's life indicated she had precedents to expect police officers to enforce her lawless position against a Black man.

EC recognizes that feelings are the driving force of life, but, like electric engines, they are often out of sight and not audible. Nonetheless, we can infer from the video that this interaction was driven by powerful feelings. On the dog owner's side, I see strident entitlement to an exemption from the rules. This dynamic is now so recognizable that current urban slang refers to any middle-class white woman with this dynamic as a "Karen." On the birder's side, I see a twenty-first-century African American expectation that everyone must follow the rule of law, skillfully supported with courteous self-defense against her bullying.

Understanding the power of feelings and the dynamics they produce underscores the need to keep track of these feelings. This requires emotional literacy, the ability to recognize, describe, and/or name dozens of feelings, and self-awareness (step 1 of EC) to acknowledge and *include* them in all choices of action and inaction. The corollary is that containment, suppression, disassociation, denial, and repression of feelings are temporary crisis or expediency measures only. For emotional health, hidden feelings need to be gently explored and processed as soon as practical to reduce periodic explosions, meltdowns, anxiety and depression, substance use disorders, and/or somatic leaks (e.g., stress-related illnesses).

For EC, these feelings are first organized by thinking about what happened. Then, possible responses are filtered through good judgment, a specialized thinking for risk assessment. The incident with the birder and dog owner showcases good judgment by the birder and bad judgment by the dog owner. Both good judgment and bad judgment are part of self-responsibility in the EC curriculum. When teaching an EQD workshop series at San Francisco's county jail charter high school, we covered good judgment points like a pilot's checklist as part of step 4, self-responsibility. There was little engagement from this lively group. As a result, we requested the inmates' help to design a bad judgment protocol derived from actions they had taken that led to bad outcomes. That worked. This list of destructive or risky actions based on poor or no risk assessment is now a permanent part of teaching judgment. The dog owner made a number of bad judgments, including walking her new dog off leash where prohibited without considering all the possible negative consequences, then acting impulsively on strong feelings without reflection, which could have led to legal consequences had the birder been less gracious.

One self-awareness concept related to what happens between people is that nonverbal communication can be deliberate or inadvertent.

Both participants in the dog owner–birder encounter seemed intentional toward each other. The white dog owner's nonverbal and verbal communications to the Black birder sought to intimidate him. Her yanking her dog around was a secondary issue, which seemed to me—as a witness after the fact—to be a thoughtless response to her agitation. That behavior also inadvertently suggests both a self-absorbed character and an unempathetic relationship with her dog, contradicting the usual reasons for letting a dog off leash.

The birder made a verbal request before the start of the video, then nonverbally asserted his position by using the video recording to document the interaction with the dog owner to provide an unedited account to the police and the internet. He avoided any physical threat with process: politeness and distance. He backed up but did not back down. His instant response was so poised and the video so steady (despite his voice possibly indicating anxiety when setting his distance limits) that I suspect he had considerable experience with assertiveness, his own and that of others. The nonviolent protesters in the 1960s evinced a similar calm process, but for documentation activists had to rely on news reporters and organizations for choices of what was filmed, recorded, and aired.

Self-awareness also includes insight into one's own dynamics and mindfulness of behavior, past and present. The 10-step Feeling Management protocol begins with a time-out because emotional events often require a pause (e.g., a few deep breaths) both to avoid destructive impulsive reactions and to process the impact of an event. The dog owner might have benefited from this step. Processing feelings also enables us to recognize internal changes and the skills needed to achieve positive outcomes.

The second step of Feeling Management is to analyze what happened. I relied on a video clip and news snippets to describe the encounter in chronological order. This helps distinguish cause and effect, which is essential for understanding the dynamics and each person's role and the decision points in their behavior.

This event also raises the self-development concept of identity. Internally, identity is a uniquely personal matter, a combination of temperament, style, personality, character, values, family, and culture. Developmentally, identity is formed at the confluence of many forces, including values, and commonly changes with context. Each African American's identity develops and exists in a powerful force field created by at least two distinct clusters of forces. One cluster is individual and institutional racism, which includes prejudice, presumptions, politics, policies, precedents, and even prescriptions—large and small—for

Black identity. Externally, these racist forces have ever-shifting configurations that affect each African American differently depending on multiple variables such as externally visible factors (e.g., skin color, speech, gender identity). The internal impact of racist forces can reshape an identity (Cobbs 2005).

The other cluster of forces arises within the Black community and can be positive or negative (and mixed). The impact is visible as a pull toward warmly connected, mutually supportive, familiar groups with constructive goals, such as churches and social groups. These powerful forces can extend to strangers, from passing nods to warm support of achievements and success that I still treasure. How Lonnie Bunch III created the Smithsonian National Museum of African American History and Culture in Washington, D.C., is a spectacular example of this dynamic (Bunch 2019).

In contrast, the familiar destructive forces of gangs and groups undercutting individual success exert an explicit gravitational pull on members. In seeking to explore broader alternatives, they risk exclusion, leaving them isolated but free to pursue their goals—a catch-22. For instance, both parolees and first-generation college students can experience alienation and stress when returning home. Such experience is a formidable deterrent from essential self-development, particularly without emotional and social competence skills to ease those transitions.

Clarifying the distinctions between these influences as one formulates a current identity enables one to more precisely tailor responses to racist challenges such as being pulled over for "driving while Black." Racism makes simply living one's life hazardous; my young son was once slammed against a wall by a police officer while running flat out for a bus. Because of the overwhelming combination of institutional and individual racism aimed at Black people, sophisticated EC is required for individuals to emerge alive, unharmed, and emotionally balanced. The birder's identity and instant response was up to this challenge and provides a valuable model.

Similarly, individuals who are unwittingly or unwillingly caught up in perpetuating racist policies of institutions and their communities require strong identities and EC mastery to safely navigate the complexities of sidestepping destructive conflicts and supporting or instituting positive change. Inevitably, making changes triggers corresponding changes in identity, which is easier when one's starting identity is carefully adjusted with EC skills.

Step 4 of the curriculum, self-responsibility, includes values and judgments, highlighting values that repeatedly cause trouble over centuries, such as integrity, money, sex, and politics. Individuals learning EC are encouraged to identify and think through their personal values realistically as early in life as possible because values are easier to change before they become embedded in character and a way of life.

Two other values, confidentiality or privacy and power, play significant roles in the encounter between the birder and the dog owner. Everyone who watched the public disputes about confidentiality in the televised Congressional January 6 [2021] investigation saw these values operating. In our illustration, the birder recording his encounter with the dog owner triggered her demand for privacy. The immediate escalation revolved around power values. Who has the most? The rule of law or might (physical, social, economic, religious, or political) makes right? The Black birder asserted and held his rule-of-law power position without deviation, simultaneously maintaining respect, ethics, and integrity despite provocation and the covert threat of lethal force in calling "the cops" for support. Under such conditions, one needs self-confidence in a solid identity and purpose to avoid the temptation to match destructive might-makes-right, "I win, you lose" actions with further escalations.

It is noteworthy that the white dog owner subordinated any values she might have had around integrity, ethics, empathy, humility, respect, and compassion in her attempt to force her will on the Black birder. In that context, her protest of the video implied a wish for secrecy in her power grab, well beyond ordinary privacy. EC skills facilitate not only developing but also negotiating all these values in a conflict. Fortunately for the birder, the police officers discharged their professional responsibility appropriately and charged the dog owner.

The second relationship in this encounter evoked concern and outrage from dog lovers seeing the dog owner's mistreatment of her dog. An appropriate developmental response for her might be to expand her relationship skills, especially other-awareness skills, to respect not only her dog's welfare as the shelter required, but also the rights of her fellow members of the New York community.

Relationships skills, step 3, include other-awareness, which is routinely practiced by people watchers and user-friendly systems. Similarly, mental health professionals use other-awareness daily for quality care and safety. This skill enables anticipation and adjustments to maximize constructive impacts in interactions, and attention to the impact of this curriculum on workshop participants remains an essential part of its continuing relevance (Flowers et al. 2014).

Significant self-development responses evoke grief because change invariably involves loss. If the white dog owner were to both grieve the loss of her white privilege after this incident and broaden her EC repertoire by incorporating relevant upgrades in her emotional and social skills, she could maximize her ability to succeed on level playing fields. That would be one giant self-development step. Her values and identity would determine which skill set she uses in situations where white privilege persists.

Lindemann (1944) identified five phases of grief: 1) shock, 2) yearning, 3) protest/anger, 4) despair, and 5) detachment. For EC, I add 6) anniversary reactions, which occur frequently, 1 year (or more) later, as if out of the blue. These six phases occur at their own pace in overlapping waves, like a tide coming in and receding. The duration of grief often frightens people into deliberately halting it, especially between waves two and three or three and four, to avoid facing despair. In my experience, unfinished grief can lead to a chronic state of rage or yearning for the romanticized past or a fantasized future. The January 6, 2021 attackers of the U.S. Capitol may have been recruited through this emotional vulnerability. In contrast, once despair is processed, the mind is free to relinquish the loss and work creatively toward constructive alternatives.

The encounter in the park highlights the EC relationship principle that motivation and impact are frequently misaligned. The video provides no information about the feelings that drove the birder's actions, but his verbal request and nonverbal insistence on taking the video demonstrate his intent to get the dog appropriately leashed. Instead of answering "Oh, sure" and complying with the request, which would have had a mild impact on her, the dog owner wildly escalated her responses, indicating a disproportionate impact. I assume that unrelenting assertiveness from a Black man evoked her racism. In contrast, his later action, when he declined to cooperate with police on misdemeanor charges filed against the dog owner, suggest forgiveness. His considered response had positive social, legal, financial, and emotional impacts on the dog owner, who had already lost her job because her behavior was publicized.

The dog owner's motivation is also unknown, although I read in an online news report that she said she did not understand her own motivation. Unconscious or unconsidered motivation is very common and is best explored with minor events. However, people often are not motivated until serious trouble occurs. The video was a consequence of her impact on the birder. Both the dog owner and the birder were motivated, for different reasons, to involve the police, and they experienced differential impacts. To avoid presumptions and misconceptions, it is important to understand any motivation-impact picture as best you can prior to any EC response.

For example, confusion around the dynamics of actions and consequences and motivations and impacts is central in COVID-19 mask and vaccination mandates, counter mandates, compliance, indifference, and resistance responses. Moreover, advocating personal choice as a motivational defense of actions that carry unintended but potentially lethal, universal impacts implies poor decision-making skills—the alternatives-benefits-costs of decisions in step 2—and/or limited application of other-awareness skills and community responsibility values.

Resolution of such motivation-impact conflicts requires addressing both motivation and impact on *all* sides. Justifiably or not, we Americans still pride ourselves in pulling together and rising to challenges to succeed as a nation. Unfortunately, like the individual dog walker, Americans demonstrate precedents for choosing unbalanced, short-term, self-interested actions (e.g., climate change denials, persistent corporate pollution, rampant lobbying) over longer-term national win-win outcomes.

In the aftermath of emotionally intense events, the EQD curriculum offers two other skills that facilitate processing impacts of the event: dream interpretation and journaling. First, the Delaney method of dream interpretation, DIM, can increase self-awareness (Flowers 1988, 1993, 1995; Flowers and Zweben 1996, 1998) and provide a framework for constructive action, which is particularly helpful to anyone unfamiliar with routinely incorporating feelings. In addition, interpreting nightmares from events intense enough to produce them often provides lessons useful for feeling management and developmental responses. Although both recall and the interpretative process take practice to master, the steps are easily understood (Flowers 1993, 1995, 2015; Flowers and Zweben 1996).

In the context of racism, many African Americans are constantly vigilant while awake, a "head on a swivel" level of other-awareness, to safely navigate dangers. Safe mentors and friends provide social strategies and support but fewer emotional skills. Not surprisingly, many feelings remain walled off or closeted, contributing to symptoms of emotional distress, acting out, and mental illness. Clinically, anxiety often signals unresolved internal conflicts and unprocessed feelings elucidated in dreams (Flowers 1993, 2015). Somatization exacerbates various physical illnesses (Flowers 1995). DIM with specific presleep suggestions can not only provide emotional and social insights but also result in improvements in physical conditions (Flowers 1988, 1995), and it also has been used in substance use recovery (Flowers and Zweben 1996, 1998).

Because the dreamer is the source of *all* information used in the interpretation, the validity of DIM is often convincing. When done with a group or partner and/or a therapist trained in DIM, support is available for any flood of painful, vulnerable feelings that can follow insight. Those feelings need to be contained while they are named, sorted, and processed with the EC Feeling Management protocol to support a constructive developmental response.

Second, journaling facts and feelings in two columns provides internal perspective on daily events. Research has demonstrated that this process alone, done for at least 20 minutes two to three times a week, can improve both physical and mental health (Ullrich and Lutgendorf 2002). The facts column should contain only descriptions of events, facts, and actions, including speech, verbatim if possible. The feeling entries for EC should include opinions, beliefs, inferences, and speculation because they function similarly to emotions. Journaling improves many EC skills, such as attention to and recall of facts; distinguishing feelings and opinions from facts; fluency in discussing feelings with others; reflection; and analytic skills for considered, instant, and developmental responses. Externalizing inner musings with journaling can assist in restoring resilience and emotional balance, constant challenges that are exacerbated by the impact and divisive political responses to multiple terrifying twenty-first century realities.

Implications for Emotional Competence Action

Mental health in the twenty-first century faces tremendous challenges on many fronts. The international impact of the short video taken by the birder in Central Park is a wake-up call for *all* Americans to be as vigilant about racism as African Americans are. Given the psychological and other burdens of racism, inattention can no longer be treated as a neutral act. We are all in this boat together, and eradicating racism is a shared professional responsibility: the asymptomatic racist carrier could be you or me.

Because EC is essentially about survival and thriving, I propose that EC training is no longer optional. With EC on *both* sides, the event in Central Park could have been a trivial encounter long forgotten by both participants—and the dog—despite the dog owner's racism. At present, most individuals choose actions or inactions that define their roles in conflicts involving racism without pragmatic training in considered responses, a key skill for constructive outcomes that go beyond excessive political correctness and apologies.

In view of the demonstrated importance of EC in interactions, I recommend routine focused collaborations to resolve conflicts at all levels throughout the field of psychiatry. Each party has a responsibility for both self- and other-awareness and other basic EC skills to facilitate discussions in which all parties express what they need, courteously, in order to negotiate win-wins. This uphill challenge is particularly relevant to those in positions of power and responsibility, an indelibly linked pair in EC because although you can delegate authority, you cannot delegate responsibility.

In conclusion, there are five possible interventions in which aspects of the EQD approach to EC could be constructively applied and evaluated to maximize positive outcomes.

- Psychiatry and other mental health professions have recognized a preventive leadership responsibility to expand their teaching of emotional health skills to patients, families, and the public. Providing *interactive* emotional and social health skills classes or workshops similar to those for diabetes and hypertension could extend baseline public understanding of and skill levels in EC. This is EQD's mission. Such classes would address ongoing concerns, complementing the American Psychiatric Association Foundation's 2021 launch of the *Mentally Healthy Nation* podcast.
- Taking health care disparities as a prototype challenge, community engagement projects often use versions of the group conversation model. Additional shared EC training could enhance the skills of group leaders and members in considering facts and feelings, from minor to major, in developing, evaluating, researching, and adapting user-friendly programs explicitly targeting disparities in their communities.
- As burnout and COVID-19 stress illustrate, our traditional unrealistic institutionalized expectations for researchers and practitioners still need improvement, beginning with trainees. Professional training programs have an opportunity and the community responsibility to improve their training in basic EC skills to support emotional health in all professionals. A collaborative focused group discussion process to engage trainees and faculty in choosing their long- and short-term best results, and planning and execution with evaluation of results, would support accountability and begin institutionalizing EC change.
- The "minority tax" on successful African American professionals and other professionals of color in majority white organizations refers to using their insights and other-awareness in ways that exploit and simultaneously sidestep upgrading those and other skills throughout the organization. In these circumstances, regretful exit interviews with burned-out minority professionals seem disingenu-

ous. Alternative approaches could include "minority bonuses" agreed on in a collaborative group conversational process with EC-trained participants. At the same time, the group could decide how to upgrade their own self- and other-awareness skills to deal with African American job applicants and colleagues in a culturally competent way that promotes hiring and retention. Documenting, examining, and publishing successful and unsuccessful experiences could expedite the developmental responses in other institutions.

- White people have long enjoyed privileges with respect to legal, political, and social rules, especially automatic waivers of accountability, whether previously unrecognized or flaunted as "free, white, and 21." Changes resulting from progress in equality will require developmental responses for many white Americans who experience existential threats at the loss of these privileges. Easily accessible emotional competence education classes (e.g., on anxiety in a changing world) as a basic part of health care, like exercise classes for bodies, could support white Americans in feeling management or broader application of self-responsibility in a changing context.

Individual changes in expectations can both support and drive institutional change toward a more diverse, equitable, and inclusive America with its contradictory traditions of savagery and valor, slavery and freedom, greed and generosity.

References

Bunch LG III: A Fool's Errand: Creating the National Museum of African American History and Culture in the Age of Bush, Obama, and Trump. Washington, DC, Smithsonian Books, 2019

Cobbs P: My American Life: From Rage to Entitlement. New York, Atria Books, 2005

DiAngelo R: White Fragility: Why It Is So Hard for White People to Talk About Racism. Boston, MA, Beacon Press, 2018

DuBois R, Li M: Reducing Social Tension and Conflict: The Group Conversation Method. New York, Association Press, 1971

Fernandez A, Chen V, Quan J, et al: Evaluation of a medical student research and career development program to increase diversity in academic medicine. Acad Med 94(8):1220–1228, 2019 30998582

Flowers LKB: Psychotherapy: black and white. J Natl Med Assoc 64(1):19–22, 1972 5061417

Flowers LK: The development of a program for treating obesity. Hosp Community Psychiatry 27(5):342–345, 1976 950221

Flowers LK: The morning after: a pragmatist's approach to dreams. Psychiatr J Univ Ott 13(2):66–71, 1988 3043513

Flowers LK: The dream interview method of dream interpretation in private psychotherapy practice, in New Directions in Dream Interpretation. Edited by Delaney GMV. Albany, NY, SUNY Press, 1993

Flowers LK: The use of presleep instructions and dreams in psychosomatic disorders. Psychother Psychosom 64(3–4):173–177, 1995 8657849

Flowers LK: The missing curriculum: experience with emotional competence education and training for premedical and medical students. J Natl Med Assoc 97(9):1280–1287, 2005 16296219

Flowers LK: Teaching dream interviewing for clinical practice, in Dream Research: Contributions to Clinical Practice. Edited by Kramer M, Glucksman M. New York, Routledge, 2015, pp 14–26

Flowers LK, Brown L: Keys to success in pre-college programs. Opportunity Outlook December:17–20, 2000

Flowers LK, Zweben JE: The dream interview method in addiction recovery: a treatment guide. J Subst Abuse Treat 13(2):99–105, 1996 8880667

Flowers LK, Zweben JE: The changing role of "using" dreams in addiction recovery. J Subst Abuse Treat 15(3):193–200, 1998 9633031

Flowers LK, Thomas-Squance GR, Brainin-Rodriguez JE, Yancey AK: Interprofessional social and emotional intelligence skills training: study findings and key lessons. J Interprof Care 28(2):1–3, 2014 24164409

Freud S: Psychopathology of Everyday Life (1904). Translated by Brill AA. New York, Mentor Books, 1951

Gardner H: Intelligence Reframed: Multiple Intelligences for the 21st Century. New York, Basic Books, 1999

Goleman D: Emotional Intelligence. New York, Bantam Books, 1995

Grier WH, Cobbs PM: Black Rage. New York, Basic Books, 1968

Jones J, Flowers L: The Power of Emotional Competence: A Universal Framework for Life (self-pub), 2019

King JE, Mitchell CA: Black Mothers to Sons. New York, Peter Lang, 1995

Lindemann E: Symptomatology and management of acute grief. Am J Psychiatry 151(6 suppl):155–160, 1944 8192191

Mahoney MR, Wilson E, Odom KL, et al: Minority faculty voices on diversity in academic medicine: perspectives from one school. Acad Med 83(8):781–786, 2008 18667896

Solway P, Meyer JD, Caruso D: The positive psychology of emotional intelligence, in Handbook of Positive Psychology. Edited by Snyder CR, Lopez ASJ. London, Oxford University Press, 2002, pp 159–171

Thomas-Squance GR, Goldstone R, Martinez A, Flowers LK: Mentoring of students from under-represented groups using emotionally competent processes and content. Med Educ 45(11):1153–1154, 2011

Ullrich PM, Lutgendorf SK: Journaling about stressful events: effects of cognitive processing and emotional expression. Ann Behav Med 24(3):244–250, 2002 12173682

*Contributors and Black
Psychiatry Leaders*

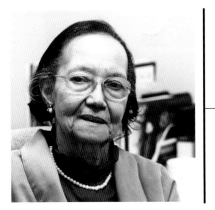

Mildred Mitchell-Bateman, M.D.

Courtesy of Michelle Mitchell-Bateman.

Carl Bell, M.D.

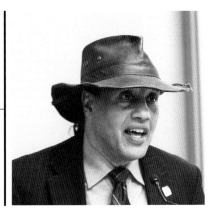

Courtesy of David Hathcox.

June Jackson Christmas, M.D.

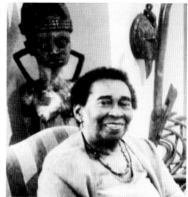

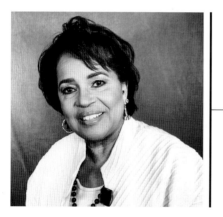

Michelle Clark, M.D., DLFAPA

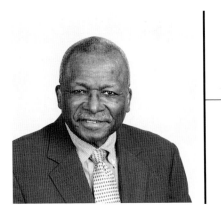

H. Westley Clark,
M.D., J.D., M.P.H.

Pamela Y. Collins,
M.D., M.P.H.

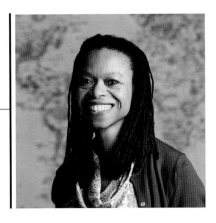

James P. Comer, M.D.,
M.P.H.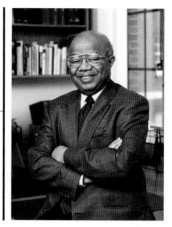

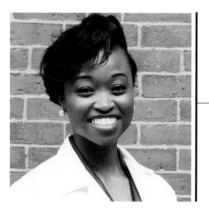 *Devin Cromartie, M.D.,*
M.P.H.

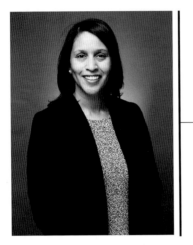

Michelle P. Durham,
M.D., M.P.H., DLFAPA,
DFAACAP

Loma K. Flowers, M.D.

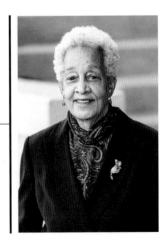

Keith Hermanstyne,
M.D., M.P.H.,
M.S.H.P.M.

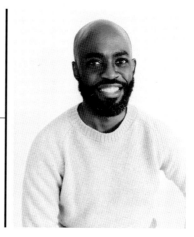

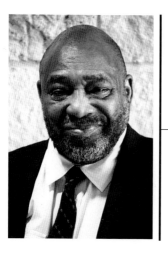

William Lawson, M.D.,
Ph.D., DLFAPA

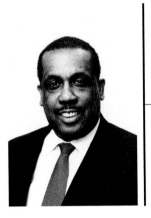

Hassell H. McClellan, Ph.D.

Stephen A. McLeod-Bryant, M.D.

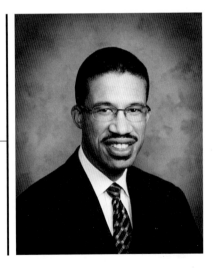

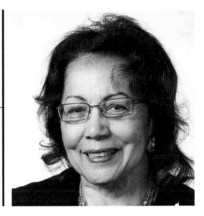

Donna M. Norris, M.D.

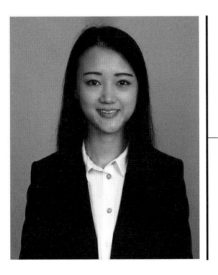

Nicola Park, M.D.

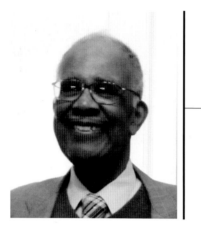

Chester Pierce, M.D.

Courtesy of Dr. Orlando Lightfoot.

Charles Pinderhughes,
M.D.

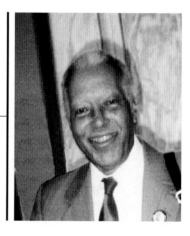

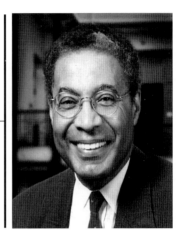

Alvin Poussaint, M.D.

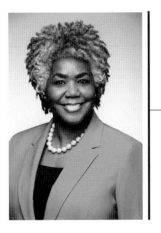

Annelle B. Primm, M.D., M.P.H.

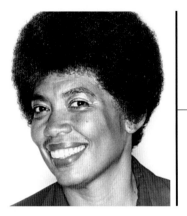

Phyllis Harrison-Ross, M.D.

© New York Medical College.
Used with permission.

*David Satcher, M.D.,
Ph.D.*

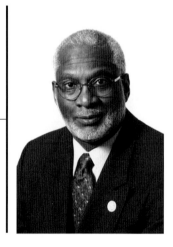

Ruth S. Shim, M.D., M.P.H. —

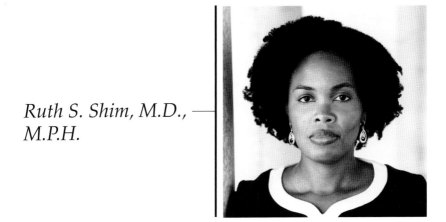

— *Jeanne Spurlock, M.D.*

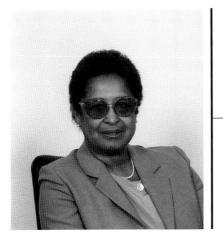

Courtesy of David Hathcox.

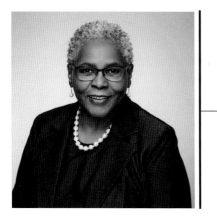

Altha J. Stewart, M.D.

Johnny Williamson, M.D.

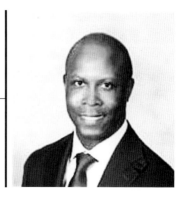

Centering Blackness in Mental Health Equity

Michelle P. Durham, M.D., M.P.H., DFAPA, DFAACAP
Devin Cromartie, M.D., M.P.H.

*What most whites perceive as an orderly American social system, most
Black [people] experience as unresponsive, unremitting, dehumanized,
well-rationalized, quiet, courteous, institutionalized violence not unlike colonialism.*
Dr. Charles Pinderhughes (1969, p. 109)

For decades, research has shown inequities in how, when, and whether
Black people access mental health care (Ayalon and Alvidrez 2007). Dr.
David Satcher's *Mental Health: Culture, Race, and Ethnicity*, a supplement to his 1999 *Mental Health: A Report of the Surgeon General* clearly
presented the barriers to care for Black people, starting with stigma, followed by access and misdiagnosis, regardless of socioeconomic status
(Satcher 2001). In 2021, 47.2 million people in the United States identified their race as Black, either alone or as part of a multiracial or ethnic
background. That was up from 36.2 million in 2000 (Lopez and Mosli-

mani 2023). The 2020 U.S. Census showed that the population of non-Hispanic whites who identify with a single race shrank by 3%—or about 5.1 million people—from 2010 to 2020 (Krogstad et al. 2021). The history of racial inequities and changing demographics of our society should push each of us to center the experience of Black people in our workplace, clinics, communities, and research.

In this chapter, we define what it means to center Blackness to address mental health inequities, providing a brief overview of how racial and economic inequities have affected mental health equity. We then describe ways to center the Black experience, culture, attitudes, and beliefs through culturally responsive care. Finally, we provide examples of how academic training programs and researchers can shift to centering Blackness in their pursuit of mental health equity, especially through partnership with the community.

Why Is Centering Blackness Necessary to Address Mental Health Inequities?

Racism is a system of structuring opportunity and assigning value on the basis of the construct of race (Jones 2002). Racism has worked historically (and presently) through interpersonal interactions (i.e., prejudice) and institutionally through differential access to resources and opportunities (i.e., discrimination), and it can manifest internally in members of the stigmatized race when they accept negative beliefs about their worth (Jones 2000). Therefore, anti-Black racism specifically "voids Blackness of value," marginalizes Black people and Black issues, and disregards the anti-Black institutions and policies that reinforce adverse outcomes for Black people (Movement for Black Lives 2020).

Mental health systems are particularly vulnerable to perpetuating racist views of patients because access to care, screening, diagnosis, treatment, and crisis response are all at the clinician's discretion (Merino et al. 2018). Health care inequities exist in part because of the flawed individuals who determine need, treatment, and solutions on the basis of the race of individuals who interact with the system.

Structural racism refers to the "totality of ways in which societies foster [racial] discrimination, via mutually reinforcing [inequitable] systems…(e.g., in housing, education, employment, earnings, benefits, credit, media, healthcare, criminal justice) that in turn reinforce discriminatory beliefs, values, and distribution of resources," reflected in history, culture, and interconnected institutions (Krieger 2014, p. 650). Racism becomes a self-propelling system when mutually reinforcing institutions propagate a culture that further energizes racism on institutional, interpersonal, and internal levels; this process is called structural racism (Bailey et al. 2017). When we do not acknowledge structural racism as a factor in health inequity and give implicit bias, microaggressions, and other terms more meaning and research value, this hinders our ability to find lasting solutions to end racial inequity (Boyd et al. 2020).

The field of mental health has to evaluate the role that social and environmental factors play in bringing about poor mental health and causing and worsening mental illness (Compton and Shim 2015). Anti-Black racism affects all sectors of life, from employment, housing, and access to healthy foods to community engagement and supports. Decades of research have shown how anti-Black racism affects the ability of Black people to obtain economic and health equity. For example, federal agencies report that Black Americans are almost four times more likely than white Americans to be suspended between kindergarten and twelfth grade, five times more likely to be denied a loan, and seven times more likely to be incarcerated as adults (Love and Hayes-Greene 2018). The zip code an individual is born into shapes educational attainment, economic opportunity, and health throughout their life. The racial wealth gap has a clear impact on health and health outcomes.

Black people are not a monolith. *Blackness* refers to race—a social construct to describe a group of people on the basis of shared characteristics (an array of brown skin tones, in this case). Ethnicity is more aligned with the variables that shape cultural identities, such as language, geographical descendance, worldviews, values, and traditions. The Black diaspora in the United States contains a great diversity of ethnicities with different cultures, including American Descendants of Slavery, Afro-Latinx, and Afro-Caribbean. The diaspora also includes African immigrants from numerous African countries. It is important to note that these cultures have continued to evolve through the mixing of immigrant and "American" cultures across time and descendant generations.

When we center Blackness, we recognize, validate, and prioritize the multiple identities Black people hold. When we recognize the humanity in each individual, we can create programming and services that speak to and acknowledge the intersectional identities of Black people while recognizing the structures and policies that have prevented economic and health equity. The many inequities we see in mental health result from devaluing Blackness, so centering Blackness places the value back on Black bodies to reverse the inequities that occur because of anti-Black racism.

How Do We Center Blackness?

Many well-intentioned providers understand why centering Blackness is essential to addressing mental health inequities. However, many are unsure (and even hopeless) when confronted with the prospect of addressing the inequities built into centuries-old racist structures. In the following sections, we define terms and outline recommendations and best practices that psychiatrists can consider in research, training, and education. Finally, we discuss engaging with Black communities, which is vital to integrate with the other practices we discuss.

Definitions

The cultural manifestations of racism make cultural competence and humility necessary for solving racial mental health disparities. The Substance Abuse and Mental Health Services Administration (2014) defines *cultural competence* as the attainment of cultural awareness, cultural knowledge, and culture-related skill sets for the discipline of practice (e.g., mental health care). Notably, cultural competence requires an understanding of the distinctions between the many cultures within the Black diaspora. It also involves knowledge of the cultural effects of racism, which affect the Black diaspora as a whole.

The term *cultural humility* has gained favor more recently in place of cultural competency. The use of the term *humility* acknowledges the responsibility of the culturally competent provider to defer to the patient's description of their culture and to partner with the patient to frame their culture in treatment. The concept of cultural humility can improve interactions with different cultures at the provider level, clinical level, and organizational level.

However, a focus solely on culture would not adequately address the issues of mental health inequities, which are rooted in structural racism. The ability to discern how structural racism relates to the social determinants of health that have clinical manifestations on patient attitudes, symptoms, and diseases is called *structural competence* (Metzl and Hansen 2014). Metzl and Hansen summarized five steps for providers to gain structural competence as follows:

1. Recognize the extraclinical structures (i.e., social determinants) that shape clinical interactions and outcomes.

2. Explore the (nonmedical) social science literature that has researched and explained how the identified structures from the first step manifest as clinical observations and outcomes.
3. Use the knowledge from the second step to translate cultural presentations into structural terms (e.g., a Black patient may be skeptical of a psychiatric diagnosis because of the history of misdiagnosis of Black patients in the mental health care system).
4. Consider structural interventions for clinical issues.
5. Practice *structural humility*. In a structural framework, the practice of humility requires acknowledgment of the medical model's limitations in addressing structural issues. We may need to think outside the medical framework to address these disparities.

Competence and humility within the cultural and structural frameworks are foundational prerequisites for addressing the inequities that affect Black mental health outcomes. However, *culturally and structurally responsive care* integrates these foundations into action by accounting for the interpersonal, sociocultural, and socioeconomic realities in which Black people live (Kaholokula et al. 2018; Resnicow et al. 1999). This responsiveness can occur on two dimensions: surface and deep. A surface-level response meets the target population where they are in terms of their culture and experience. These responses include reflecting the community and their structural needs in audiovisual materials, using targeted advertising channels, and recruiting ethnically matched staff. These responses may seem superficial, but they are vital to provoking reception and acceptance from the target community. Deep-level response requires incorporating the cultural, social, historical, environmental, and psychological forces that influence the target community's behavior into care structures. Deep-level responses stand out in the community's eyes and determine the true impact of an intervention.

It is imperative to use partnerships with Black communities to operationalize humility while providing culturally and structurally responsive care. Representatives from the community are the experts on their communities, and expert consultation is key to ensuring the success of any intervention. These representatives are best suited to determine the surface-level engagements their communities embrace or to identify the deep-level forces that would resonate if evoked during an outreach to and interactions with the target community. An example of this is having youth, community, and patient advisory boards as part of any system to ensure the development of equitable policies for target communities.

Research

If evidence matters, we must care how it gets made. Right or wrong, research can drive decisions. If we do not address the power dynamic in the creation of research, at best, we are driving decision making from partial truths. At worst, we are generating inaccurate information that ultimately does more harm than good in our communities.

Chicago Beyond (2018, p. 6)

It is often stated that Black people mistrust the health care system without rightfully validating that they have endured centuries of mistreatment and inequitable access to that system. When Black people are excluded from research, whether as participants in a study or active members in creating the research questions, this creates a system that does not understand and then inadequately diagnoses and treats Black people (Moore et al. 2020).

The Chicago Beyond Health Equity Series proposes a structure to get beyond making statements of decreasing inequities in health (Chicago Beyond 2018). It illustrates how researchers, community members, and funders can have an equal say in how the study operates, what to measure, study tools, and questions related to how the study will improve or bring value to individuals participating in the research. Figure 7–1 outlines each inequity created by a power imbalance and poses questions that can create an opportunity to change the power dynamic.

Training and Education

It is well known that the leaky educational pipeline inhibits many Black people and other marginalized groups from making it through the system to pursue higher education such as college, much less medical education. Systemic and anti-Black racism are core to the various ways that Black people have difficulty achieving higher education. Only 2% of psychiatrists and 3% of psychologists in the United States identify as Black (American Psychological Association 2017; Lin et al. 2018). Furthermore, recruitment to the mental health field requires antistigma and recruitment efforts to occur from elementary through graduate school. Medical students are confronted with barriers when applying to residency programs, which often depend on United States Medical Licensing Examination step scores and clerkship evaluations that historically have been biased (Low et al. 2019).

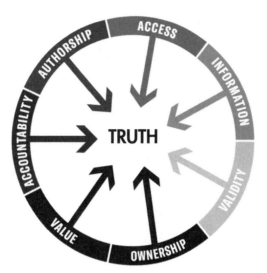

Access	Could we be missing out on community wisdom because the community is not at the table when decisions are made?
Information	Can we effectively partner to get to the full truth if information about research options, methods, inputs, costs, benefits, and risks are not shared?
Validity	Are we valuing community organizations and community members as valid experts?
Ownership	Are we valuing research processes that take from, rather than build up, community ownership?
Value	What value is generated, for whom, and at what cost?
Accountability	Are we holding funders and researchers accountable if research designs create harm or do not work?
Authorship	Whose voice is shaping the narrative, and is the community fully represented?

Figure 7–1. Seven inequities standing in the way of impact, each held in place by power dynamic.
Source. Chicago Beyond 2018.

To address these barriers, psychiatry residency programs need to make a concerted effort to recruit, retain, and support Black students because the experience can be isolating when racism, microaggressions, and bias permeate medicine. *Code switching* has long been a strategy for Black people to successfully navigate interracial interactions and has implications for well-being, economic advancement, and even physical survival (McCluney et al. 2019). Code switching involves adjusting one's style of speech, appearance, behavior, and expression in ways that allow others to feel comfortable in exchange for fair treatment and other opportunities within the system. Training programs and medical institutions can play a pivotal role in cultivating spaces that value inclusion and differences by creating environments where code switching is not necessary for residents' success.

An example of recruitment efforts that help applicants from diverse backgrounds is the Boston Medical Center (BMC) psychiatry residency program, which takes a holistic approach to evaluating medical students who apply to the program. This approach takes a stance that standardized scores do not equate to a competent, compassionate physician. The program focuses instead on applicants' demonstrated passion and commitment to working with marginalized communities. BMC's patient population is 70% Black and Latinx; therefore, it is important for the program to recruit applicants who reflect the patient population served. BMC thus changed the criteria for interview selection, which led to an increase in the number of residents in the program who are typically underrepresented in medicine (URiM). The Association of American Medical Colleges (2021) reports that nationally, 13.8% of residents are URiM, but since 2017, the average percentage of URiM individuals in the BMC psychiatry residency program is 50%, compared with 19% at other BMC residency programs. The change in application review, in addition to efforts at the department level to hire faculty who reflect the applicants the program wanted to bring in, helped to recruit new residents and ensure that they had mentors and saw a reflection of themselves in the department.

Last, training and education in psychiatry must include a curriculum that incorporates discussion of the racial and mental health inequities that affect Black and other marginalized communities. Mental health professionals must know how to respond to the needs of Black people in a culturally responsive manner. Culturally responsive care can be provided when mental health professionals understand how systemic and structural racism impact Black people.

Engaging With Black Communities

Building academic and community partnerships is extremely important if we plan to center Black people in programming and research. We have to reimagine ways to provide care and break down programs that have been built around white supremacy ideals. True partnership with the community entails academic centers remembering who is not at the table when questions are posed or decisions are made.

What are the best ways to operationalize engagement with Black communities? Deciding how deep the engagement process can go involves a continuum from informing to empowering, which is outlined in Figure 7–2.

The first level of the community engagement process involves *informing* and *consultation* with the community (the *stakeholders* in Figure 7–2). In these processes, touch points are made with community members to provide information and obtain feedback about the topic and related plan. The second level of community engagement is *involvement*, where the informing and consultation processes happen consistently and longitudinally. Finally, the deepest levels of community engagement happen with *collaboration*, where a partnership with the community occurs at each level of assessment and decision-making, and *empowerment*, where the community can make final decisions. Considering the benefits of cultural and structural humility, the deeper levels of engagement are preferred when attempting to truly *center* Blackness.

Can the community engagement approach be used successfully to center Blackness in a health care system or clinic setting? Typically, the quality improvement framework is used in health care to improve care delivery (Knox and Brach 2013). One example of successful community engagement in quality improvement to address depression disparities in minority and underresourced communities is the Community Partners in Care (CPIC) project in Los Angeles (Arevian et al. 2019; Wells et al. 2013), a group-level randomized comparative effectiveness trial. Participating programs were randomly assigned to one of two groups: a resources for services (RS) or a community engagement and planning (CEP) intervention. The RS intervention provided programs with a depression collaborative care toolkit and individualized program technical assistance in using the toolkit. The CEP intervention provided support to build multisector coalitions that adapted, improved, and implemented the depression collaborative care toolkits. The CEP intervention used a community-based participatory research (CBPR) framework, which uses structures to ensure equitable community participation in a research endeavor (Wallerstein and Duran 2010). They did this through use of multisector coalitions made up of academic and community members that adapted, improved, and implemented the depression collaborative care toolkits. After 6 months, CEP programs were more effective than RS programs at improving mental health–related quality of life, increasing physical activity, reducing homelessness risk factors, reducing the rate of behavioral health hospitalizations and medication

	INFORM	CONSULT	INVOLVE	COLLABORATE	EMPOWER
GOAL	Provide stakeholders with balanced and objective information to assist them in understanding the problem, alternatives, and solutions.	Obtain stakeholder feedback on analysis, alternatives, and/or decisions.	Work directly with stakeholders throughout the process to ensure that their concerns and aspirations are consistently understood.	Partner with stakeholders in each aspect of the decision from development to solution.	Shared leadership of community-led projects, with final decision-making at the community level.
STYLE	"Here's what's happening."	"Here are some options; what do you think?"	"Here's a problem; what ideas do you have?"	"Let's work together to solve this problem."	"You care about this issue and are leading an initiative; how can we support you?"

Figure 7-2. **Community engagement continuum.**

Source. Adapted from IAP2 2018. and Tamarack Institute 2017.

visits, and increasing the rate of primary care depression visits. After 4 years (3 years after intervention support ended), CEP was more effective than RS at increasing depression remission.

Considering structural humility, we should attempt to decenter the health care system in our quest to improve mental health outcomes for Black populations. For example, the CPIC study found that CEP programs had a greater increase than RS programs in the use of faith-based and park programs for depression after 6 months. How can we reach outside clinic walls in this way and engage Black communities where they are to address mental health disparities?

For centuries, scholars have acknowledged Black church institutions (known as the Black Church) as a source of resilience for Black communities. They are spaces where Black communities meet for spiritual strength and secular community building and resource sharing. For these reasons, the Black Church is a prime space for promoting mental health in Black communities, especially because Black Americans are less likely to use traditional clinic-based mental health services (Hankerson and Weissman 2012).

For example, the Bridges to Care and Recovery (BCR) program in St. Louis, Missouri, is a partnership between the Behavioral Health Network of Greater St. Louis and the Black Church community that has a goal of improving mental health in the African American community there (Scribner et al. 2020). The BCR program uses wellness champions who participate in longitudinal training to recognize mental illness and substance use disorders and refer people to affordable mental health services. Black church leaders were part of the stakeholder group that conceptualized the idea for the BCR program. Infrastructure and staff are in place to facilitate ongoing relationship building, training of the wellness champions, and advocacy for the communities the program serves.

In another example, the Black Church Project uses a CBPR framework with the Black Church community in New Haven to complete a needs assessment and conceptualize a substance use disorder intervention within Black churches. The intervention, under the direction of academic principal investigator Dr. Ayana Jordan of Yale University, uses Black church leaders trained as health advisers to lead groups in which participants complete computer-based cognitive-behavioral therapy for substance use disorder that is integrated with spiritual exercises. A pilot study of the intervention showed that participants were adherent to the intervention and showed reduction in substance use over time verified through urine samples (Jordan et al. 2021).

In addition to the success of the above interventions, one of us (D.C.) is the principal investigator of a Black Church and mental health project based in the historically Black neighborhood of Roxbury in Boston, Massachusetts. The project explores how the Black Church can mobilize to address the mental health needs of their community in the context of the COVID-19 crisis and racial stress exposures. The project operationalizes the CBPR model by partnering with a community advisory board of Black church leaders and congregants. Together, the academic team and advisory board conduct a needs assessment and address community mental health needs by developing an intervention. This project focuses on studying the process of academic partnerships between Black and religious communities and the development and sustainability of culturally and structurally responsive interventions. There is a paucity of literature on implementing the CBPR model in Black religious communities in a sustainable manner. In addition, most of the literature on the process of CBPR centers on building a partnership for already existing medical interventions through involvement and collaboration with communities. This project is novel because it will study the empowerment of the community as the primary decision-makers toward mental health equity in their communities, from designing a needs assessment to prioritizing the issues they want to address. We will facilitate the empowerment of the community not only through power sharing but also through training and education, collaboration with other stakeholders when necessary, and provision of resources. The lessons learned in the study can catalyze replication of more academic-community partnerships with Black churches or other institutions in the Black community.

Summary

When we center Black people in the pursuit of health equity, we ensure they are at the center of decisions being made about their lives and their community. Research, training, education, and community-based partnerships require that we center Black voices to move away from systems that have harmed Black people to systems that are culturally and structurally responsive and relevant to their lives.

References

American Psychological Association: Data tool: demographics of the U.S. psychology workforce. Washington, DC, American Psychological Association, 2017. Available at www.apa.org/workforce/data-tools/demographics. Accessed March 5, 2022.

Arevian AC, Jones F, Tang L, et al; Community Partners in Care Writing Group: Depression remission from community coalitions versus individual program support for services: findings from Community Partners in Care, Los Angeles, California, 2010–2016. Am J Public Health 109(S3):S205–S213, 2019 31242001

Association of American Medical Colleges: Table B5: Number of active MD residents, by race/ethnicity (alone or in combination) and GME specialty, in 2021 Report on Residents. Washington, DC, Association of American Medical Colleges, 2021. Available at: www.aamc.org/data-reports/students-residents/interactive-data/report-residents/2021/table-b5-md-residents-race-ethnicity-and-specialty. Accessed March 25, 2022.

Ayalon L, Alvidrez J: The experience of Black consumers in the mental health system—identifying barriers to and facilitators of mental health treatment using the consumers' perspective. Issues Ment Health Nurs 28(12):1323–1340, 2007 18058337

Bailey ZD, Krieger N, Agénor M, et al: Structural racism and health inequities in the USA: evidence and interventions. Lancet 389(10077):1453–1463, 2017 28402827

Boyd RW, Lindo EG, Weeks LD, McLemore MR: On racism: a new standard for publishing on racial health inequities. Health Affairs blog, 2020. Available at: www.healthaffairs.org/do/10.1377/forefront.20200630.939347/full. Accessed March 5, 2022.

Chicago Beyond: Why Am I Always Being Researched? Chicago Beyond Equity Series, Vol 1. Chicago, IL, Chicago Beyond, 2018

Compton MT, Shim RS: The social determinants of mental health. Focus 13:419–425, 2015

Hankerson SH, Weissman MM: Church-based health programs for mental disorders among African Americans: a review. Psychiatr Serv 63(3):243–249, 2012 22388529

IAP2: IAP2 Spectrum of Public Participation. Toowong, QLD, Australia, IAP2 Australasia, 2018

Jones CP: Levels of racism: a theoretic framework and a gardener's tale. Am J Public Health 90(8):1212–1215, 2000 10936998

Jones CP: Confronting institutionalized racism. Phylon 50:7–22, 2002

Jordan A, Babuscio T, Nich C, Carroll KM: A feasibility study providing substance use treatment in the Black church. J Subst Abuse Treat 124:108218, 2021 33771290

Kaholokula JK, Ing CT, Look MA, et al: Culturally responsive approaches to health promotion for Native Hawaiians and Pacific Islanders. Ann Hum Biol 45(3):249–263, 2018 29843522

Knox L, Brach C: The practice facilitation handbook: training modules for new facilitators and their trainers (Handbook No AHRQ Publ No 13-0046-EF). Rockville, MD, Agency for Healthcare Research and Quality, 2013

Krieger N: Discrimination and health inequities. Int J Health Serv 44(4):643–710, 2014 25626224

Krogstad JM, Dunn A, Passel JS: Most Americans say the declining share of white people in the U.S. is neither good nor bad for society. Washington, DC, Pew Research Center, 2021. Available at: www.pewresearch.org/fact-tank/2021/08/23/most-americans-say-the-declining-share-of-white-people-in-the-u-s-is-neither-good-nor-bad-for-society. Accessed March 5, 2022.

Lin L, Stamm K, Christidis P: How diverse is the psychology workforce? Monitor on Psychology 49(2):19, 2018

Lopez MH, Moslimani M: Key Facts about the nation's 47.2 million Black Americans. Washington, DC, Pew Research Center, February 10, 2023. Available at: www.pewresearch.org/fact-tank/2023/02/10/key-facts-about-black-americans. Accessed March 13, 2023.

Love BP, Hayes-Greene D: The groundwater approach: building a practical understanding of structural racism. Greensboro, NC, Racial Equity Institute, 2018

Low D, Pollack SW, Liao ZC, et al: Racial/ethnic disparities in clinical grading in medical school. Teach Learn Med 31(5):487–496, 2019 31032666

McCluney CL, Robotham K, Lee S, et al: The costs of code-switching. Harvard Business Review, 2019

Merino Y, Adams L, Hall WJ: Implicit bias and mental health professionals: priorities and directions for research. Psychiatr Serv 69(6):723–725, 2018 29493411

Metzl JM, Hansen H: Structural competency: theorizing a new medical engagement with stigma and inequality. Soc Sci Med 103:126–133, 2014 24507917

Moore Q, Tennant PS, Fortuna LR: Improving research quality to achieve mental health equity. Psychiatr Clin North Am 43(3):569–582, 2020 32773082

Movement for Black Lives: Glossary. Cleveland, OH, Movement for Black Lives, 2020. Available at: http://web.archive.org/web/20200109004008/https:/policy.m4bl.org/glossary. Accessed March 5, 2022.

Pinderhughes CA: Understanding Black power: processes and proposals. Am J Psychiatry 125(11):1552–1557, 1969 5776864

Resnicow K, Baranowski T, Ahluwalia JS, Braithwaite RL: Cultural sensitivity in public health: defined and demystified. Ethn Dis 9(1):10–21, 1999 10355471

Satcher D: Mental Health: Culture, Race, and Ethnicity: A Supplement to Mental Health: A Report of the Surgeon General. Rockville, MD, Substance Abuse and Mental Health Services Administration, 2001

Scribner SS, Poirier RF, Orson W, et al: Bridges to care and recovery: addressing behavioral health and mental health needs through the faith community. J Relig Health 59(4):1946–1957, 2020 32020383

Substance Abuse and Mental Health Services Administration: Improving Cultural Competence (HHS Publ No (SMA) 14-4849), Treatment Improvement Protocol (TIP) Ser No 59. Rockville, MD, U.S. Department of Health and Human Services, 2014

Tamarack Institute: Index of Community Engagement Techniques. North Waterloo, ON, Canada, Tamarack Institute, 2017

Wallerstein N, Duran B: Community-based participatory research contributions to intervention research: the intersection of science and practice to improve health equity. Am J Public Health 100(suppl 1):S40–S46, 2010 20147663

Wells KB, Jones L, Chung B, et al: Community-partnered cluster-randomized comparative effectiveness trial of community engagement and planning or resources for services to address depression disparities. J Gen Intern Med 28(10):1268–1278, 2013 23649787

8

The Media Is the Message

FILM AND TV INFLUENCES ON BLACK MENTAL HEALTH

Keith Hermanstyne, M.D., M.P.H., M.S.H.P.M.

Visual media are powerful tools in which people can see themselves and their experiences reflected through others. For members of underrepresented groups, such as Black Americans, viewing a character's experience or seeing people of color portraying key roles that previously were filled predominantly by white actors on the screen not only can give a person insight into their lives and how others may cope with similar opportunities or stressors but also can affect how others think about them (Bobolitz and Yam 2017; Lawson 2018). For much of the twentieth century, American film and television were limited in their representation, focusing primarily on white characters as the lead story line drivers, with people of color relegated to secondary roles. Even incidental events, such as the controversy surrounding Will Smith and Chris Rock after the famed comedian made a joke about actress Jada Pinkett Smith, show that press coverage around Black Americans can often center on "hot takes," age-old stereotypes, privilege, and systemic racism within America.

Widely disseminating evocative or salient images of Black people in film and television can positively improve the lives of not only Black

Americans but individuals in society as a whole. One notable pioneer of using media messaging with a specifically targeted Black American lens is Dr. Alvin Poussaint, whose work often focused on media presentations of Black Americans, examined the ways in which Black people were depicted in popular media, and analyzed the impact these depictions had on all who viewed them.

Dr. Poussaint's interest in improving what Black viewers saw on the screen contributed to his extensive consultation work in television, including for *The Cosby Show* and *A Different World*, along with his leadership of the Media Center of the Judge Baker Children's Center. He noted the importance of media coverage during the arc of his career, beginning with the mid-twentieth-century American civil rights movement, emphasizing how documenting protests in support of racial equality was instrumental to the success of key legislation (e.g., the 1965 Voting Rights Act) and affected the political ebbs and flows of several Black politicians, from Shirley Chisholm's historic run for president in 1972 all the way to Barack Obama's meteoric rise from televised guest speaker at the Democratic National Convention in 2004 to two-term president in 2016 (A. Poussaint, personal communication, March 14, 2022).

Although progress has been made in terms of more diverse characters and writers crafting movies and television shows, positive depictions of mental illness or substance use disorders in entertainment media remain limited. Previous research has noted that whereas representations of behavioral health disorders may be frequent in American television programming, people with mental illness are often portrayed as more violent than characters who are not mentally ill, with levels of violence that are not supported by real-life data (Stuart 2006). Often, television characters with mental illness have limited social connections and have no professional identity or life outside their condition (Stuart 2006). Movies have also had a role in stigmatizing psychiatric treatment. These television and film images can shape how a person views someone with a behavioral health condition or their views on psychiatric treatment in detrimental ways. In addition, media coverage of certain events, such as instances of anti-Black violence or systemic racial injustice, can also have a significant impact on Black mental health.

Research has demonstrated the damage a lack of representation can cause for Black Americans. For example, a report noted that for Black men, there is a pattern of overall media underrepresentation in which negative depictions outweigh positive examples, which can contribute to antagonism and result in others being more likely to associate Black men with violence and criminal activity (The Opportunity Agenda 2021). Media images can also have direct impacts on Black men, contributing to lower self-esteem and diminished views of themselves (The Opportunity Agenda 2021). Similarly, a longitudinal survey of Black and white elementary school children showed an association between television exposure and reduced self-esteem for all except white boys, which the researchers hypothesized could be influenced at least partially by gender and racial stereotypes (Martins and Harrison 2012).

In this chapter, I briefly review the history of the impacts of film and television on Black Americans, then examine the state of the television and film industry since the end of the twentieth century to provide context on what is shaping current entertainment media representations of Black people. In subsequent sections, I examine recent examples of Black characters in television and film in which mental health or substance use disorders were a key aspect of their characterizations and also briefly discuss the role of media coverage and its impact on Black mental health as it relates to highly publicized traumatic events involving Black people.

Brief History of Black Americans and the Film and Television Industry

Minstrelsy, which involved white performers wearing blackface and costuming, became a popular form of American entertainment in the first half of the nineteenth century and provided a caricatured view of Black Americans (National Museum of African American History and Culture 2021). Some Black performers also engaged in minstrelsy because this form of entertainment was the sole route available for Black entertainers during this period, and some Black minstrel performers such as Bert Williams and George Walker infused political commentary within their routines (Clark 2021).

The Black stereotypes from minstrelsy in theatrical, musical, and dance productions heavily influenced later American media, such as radio, advertising, film, and television (Nelson 2008). These types of performances disseminated various stereotypes of Blacks as being dedicated to servitude, prone to malfeasance, or teeming with ignorance (National Museum of African American History and Culture 2021). For example, one of the first sitcoms that focused predominantly on Black characters, *Amos 'n' Andy*, had roots in radio minstrelsy and became a television show in 1951 (Burr 2001). Similarly, the television series *Beulah*, which debuted in 1950, centered on a Black maid to a white family and furthered the common "Mammy" stereotype of Black women (Burr 2001). Although stereotypes were not the only depictions of Black people in the

1950s, the depictions of Black characters such as the ones found in *Amos 'n' Andy* and *Beulah* had a long-lasting impact (Burr 2001).

The 1960s brought programming that broadened the types of Black characters seen on television with shows such as *Julia* and *I Spy*, and the 1970s brought a wealth of Black-focused shows, including *The Jeffersons*, *Good Times*, *Diff'rent Strokes*, and *Sanford and Son* (although some of the key character portrayals trafficked in stereotypical depictions of Black Americans) (Burr 2001). *The Cosby Show* was a massive success in the 1980s and was notable for its positive depictions of an upper-middle-class Black American family. However, *The Cosby Show* also received criticism from people who thought it did not sufficiently delve into the complicated realities of modern Black American life (Giorgis 2021). In contrast, *A Different World*, which was a spin-off from *The Cosby Show*, tackled challenging issues, including racism (with one of its later episodes exploring the aftermath of the Los Angeles riots resulting from the acquittal of police officers involved in the Rodney King beating), and the writing room hired several Black writers who went on to create significant Black sitcoms, including Yvette Lee Bowser (*Living Single*) and Cheryl Gard (*The Fresh Prince of Bel-Air*) (Giorgis 2021). In the 1990s, several new networks, including Fox, UPN, and the WB, aired notable Black-led shows such as *Martin*, *In Living Color*, *Moesha*, and *Sister, Sister* (Giorgis 2021), but the decade nearly concluded with an NAACP-led boycott of one of the four major networks due to the lack of Black and minority characters in the new fall prime-time television lineup (Burr 2001).

The history of American film also followed a similar pathway of limited and often damaging representations of Black people and a lack of Black creators during its earlier phases. The influential film *Birth of a Nation* by D.W. Griffith used blackface to depict Black Americans as immoral and savage, and its popularity was so successful in disseminating these stereotypes that the film became a recruiting tool for the Ku Klux Klan (Clark 2021).

Although there were pioneering Black filmmakers such as Oscar Micheaux, who launched his own film studio in 1919, American film was primarily made by and geared toward white viewers (Whitten 2021). The 1939 film *Gone With the Wind* is but one example of this narrow perspective given that Black actors in the film depict slaves during the Civil War era. Yet the film was historic for the 1940 Oscar award for Hattie McDaniel, the first Black actor to win this honor (Abramovitch 2015). The context of her win also reflected the racism and discrimination inherent during that time in the American film industry and the United States as a whole: The hotel hosting the awards had a "no-Blacks" policy that almost prevented McDaniel's entrance into the building. The film's producer, David O. Selznick, intervened, and McDaniel was seated at a separate table, isolated from the rest of the *Gone With the Wind* cast (Abramovitch 2015).

The Oscar win did not open new opportunities for Hattie McDaniel, whose predominant film roles represented the Mammy stereotype. The 2011 release of *The Help* echoed the mixed blessing of what types of performances receive wide recognition in the American film industry and the gearing of film stories toward white viewers despite being decades removed from *Gone With the Wind*. *The Help*, which focused on the struggles of Black maids in 1960s Mississippi, garnered 2012 Best Supporting Actress Oscar nominations for Viola Davis and Octavia Spencer (who went on to win the award), but the movie's exploration of the civil rights movement primarily via a white protagonist was controversial. Davis later noted her regret in participating in the film, stating that it was "created in the filter and the cesspool of systemic racism" and that film narratives often are "invested in the idea of what it means to be Black, but…it's catering to the white audience" (Saraiya 2020).

One notable period of Black-centered film was the Blaxploitation era, a cultural film movement in the 1970s that focused predominantly on urban Black characters who sought justice on their own terms outside the law (Oxford African American Studies Center 2021). As a genre, these films received a mixed reception, as demonstrated by the term *Blaxploitation* itself, with the person who coined the term, Junius Griffin of a local NAACP chapter, believing these films took advantage of Black Americans' desire to see Black stories and characters in film by focusing on derogatory depictions (Oxford African American Studies Center 2021). However, others saw films that centered on strong male and female Black characters who were the lead drivers of their narratives and fighting oppressive systems in realistic urban settings, a combination of factors that were not often depicted in cinema at the time (Oxford African American Studies Center 2021). Subsequent decades saw the pioneering work of Black directors, including Spike Lee, John Singleton, and Julie Dash. In recent years, such filmmakers as Tyler Perry, Ava DuVernay, Barry Jenkins, and Steve McQueen have found both critical and commercial success (Whitten 2021).

Film and Television Industry in the Twenty-First Century

When Dr. Poussaint contributed to *The Cosby Show* and *A Different World*, the American television industry catered predominantly to white viewers. There have been shifts in terms of entertainment media representation and creators since that time, but recent analysis shows that although the

United States is increasingly more diverse than in previous decades, with projections that people of color will become the majority population in upcoming years (Hunt and Ramón 2020), the television industry remains overwhelmingly white. The 2020 UCLA Hollywood Diversity Report showed that in spite of America's increasing diversity, people of color remain underrepresented as narrative leads in broadcast, digital, and cable television programming, with close to proportional representation for cable television when compared with the percentage of people of color in the American population (Hunt and Ramón 2020).

Unsurprisingly, when examining who is creating this television programming, people of color are also underrepresented as program creators, network heads, credited writers, and directors. The film industry showed comparatively greater progress when considering proportional minority representation in regard to film actors, but there was a similar lack of minority representation in film writers and directors (Hunt and Ramón 2021). Although the Hollywood Diversity Reports for both television and film show overall progress in terms of minority representation compared with past years, the dearth of people of color shaping narratives, creating film and television programming, and being cast as lead characters affects the types of stories that are viewed by the general public, which has implications for how stories about minority behavioral health are depicted.

In addition to a lack of diversity both behind and in front of the camera in the film and television industry, there is also a deficit of behavioral health depictions in film and television programming. A recent study examining popular films and television series estimated that less than 2% of film characters and approximately 7% of television series characters were portrayed with these conditions (Smith et al. 2019). In addition, most of the portrayals centered on addiction, and the majority of characters were white and male, with very limited LGBTQ+ representation. A significant percentage of these characters were treated in a derisive or mocking manner, and a notable percentage of these film and television characters were depicted as violent perpetrators. Overall, the report demonstrated the lack of behavioral visibility in popular entertainment and noted that current depictions are limited, unrepresentative of the general population, and frequently stigmatizing.

Notable Entertainment Media Depictions of Black Mental Health

Representation in television and film can be a useful tool in educating people about behavioral health conditions and related treatment. However, people with mental illness or addiction challenges are often depicted in films or television as characters whose whole lives are defined by their behavioral health conditions. This narrow presentation can lead to stereotyping and provides limited insight into how chronic behavioral health conditions can be manageable with treatment and support. In recent years, television and film have had notable depictions of key characters experiencing behavioral health struggles. An exhaustive list of Black film and television characters with behavioral health conditions as a primary component of their depiction is beyond the scope of this chapter, but in this section I highlight some notable characterizations since the start of the current century.

In *This Is Us*, one of the main characters, Randall Pearson, struggles with an anxiety disorder in the show's initial season (culminating in a significant panic attack at his workplace), and subsequent episodes show him receiving treatment, including individual therapy. Besides the significance of Randall being one of the show's primary characters, this depiction is also rare in that this is only one facet of his characterization; he is also a successful business executive who is married with three children and eventually enters politics. In season 4, he discusses his mental health journey with another Black male character, Darnell, who shares how therapy helped him in the past. As noted in a research article by Stamps (2021), this type of vulnerable interaction between two Black male characters in a scripted television show is significant. The potential viewer impact from seeing Randall's journey is also significant; as the actor portraying Randall, Sterling K. Brown, noted, "…the power of media is, once you see somebody else do it, then it sort of makes it a little bit easier for you to envision yourself taking that step on a personal level" (Jackson 2020). The scope of this portrayal of a Black man receiving treatment for anxiety, including the exploration of his formation of Black identity and working with a racially discordant therapist, has led others to cite its utility as a teaching tool for behavioral health trainees (Wooten et al. 2021).

In the popular television show *Empire*, a main character, Andre Lyon, grapples with bipolar disorder while experiencing business success as a music industry executive. White (2015) noted that Andre "is a rare TV or movie character with a chronic mental illness who is shown managing his illness by taking his medication and managing his symptoms (with the support of his wife) while functioning at a very high level." This contrasts with other common portrayals of people who are unable to reach their full potential because of their behavioral health condition or who refuse treatment because they are in denial (White 2015). The depiction of bipolar disorder in *Empire* is also unique in the intersection of race and class prevalent in its demonstration of treatment and recovery (Smith-Frigerio 2017). At the same time, there has been criticism about the accuracy of this portrayal of bipolar disorder, with Harris (2015) noting that the rapidity of Andre's mood swings may not be consistent with how a person generally experiences this condition.

In the television series *A Million Little Things*, a lead Black male character experiences another significant behavioral health condition, depression. In fact, the first episode of the series begins with this character, Rome Howard, attempting suicide via a drug overdose before stopping his attempt after learning of a friend's unexpected suicide. Later in the series, viewers see Rome become increasingly open about his emotions with those closest to him while receiving both therapy and antidepressant treatment. The show also depicts how Rome's efforts to improve his mental health are not universally well received, including a challenging conversation with the character's father when he unexpectedly discovers his son's antidepressant medication (Stamps 2021).

Another show that presents a significant depiction of suicidal ideation (and, eventually, a completed suicide) with one of its Black characters is *Being Mary Jane*, in which the titular character's friend Lisa ends her life. Lisa's suicide becomes the centerpiece of an episode that explores various characters' views on depression, psychiatric medication, and mental illness in general (Bastién 2016).

Other notable television Black characters shown with behavioral health conditions include Annalise Keating on *How to Get Away With Murder*, who spends several seasons showing the complicated aspects of a severe alcohol use disorder, and Miranda Bailey on *Grey's Anatomy*, who struggles with obsessive-compulsive disorder in later seasons. *Insecure* reveals a secondary character's bipolar disorder and shows a primary character receiving individual therapy from a Black woman therapist, with the latter story possibly contributing to increased interest in therapy among Black Americans (Smith 2020). Season 4 of *In Treatment* centers on a Black woman therapist, Dr. Brooke Taylor, who is shown treating several patients (including two patients of color) while also receiving her own recovery support (Harris 2021). As Dr. Alfiee Breland-Noble, a clinical psychologist, noted in a recent *New York Times* article, having a show like *In Treatment* that centers on a highly effective Black therapist may encourage people of color to seek out behavioral health care, which is in line with the show's desire to reduce the stigma associated with receiving behavioral health care in communities of color (Soloski 2021). At times, however, television portrayals of Black characters involving mental illness or addiction have been criticized for further stigmatizing these conditions or affecting primarily supporting characters (Bastién 2017).

During the same period of the twenty-first century, one notable example of a film with a Black lead character that explores behavioral health issues is *The Soloist*, which was released in 2009. This film is based on the friendship between a *Los Angeles Times* journalist, Steve Lopez, and a Black musician, Nathaniel Ayers, who is grappling with paranoid schizophrenia. The film shows the onset of Nathaniel's illness during his music studies at Juilliard and displays how his racial identity intersects with his perceptual disturbances (Maia 2021). In a critical analysis, Maia (2021) noted that the film does not portray Nathaniel as a violent individual, which counters other depictions that tend to present people with psychosis as dangerous individuals to be feared. In addition, the film crafts a portrait that is clinically accurate in terms of Nathaniel's expressed symptoms and his schizophrenia subtype, creating a well-rounded and human depiction of his struggle (Clyman 2009; Maia 2021).

The popular 2017 horror film *Get Out* also has a psychological underpinning. The depiction of the *sunken place*, a trancelike state in which the film's Black characters become trapped, provides insight into the psyche of the protagonist, Chris, and is triggered via hypnosis and using the traumatic death of his mother. Writers have examined how the sunken place references W.E.B. Du Bois's concept of *double consciousness*, which represents the internalized conflict that Black Americans experience as they view themselves in the way that the dominant culture sees them (Darden 2017; Wilkinson 2017). By structuring the film in such a way that Chris and other characters become victims of white objectification, *Get Out* highlights the psychic challenges that Black Americans navigate in a white-centered world.

Power of Film and Television Representation

Depictions of behavioral health conditions in film and television programs are not the only ways that entertainment media can have impacts on Black mental health. The power of representation, of a person seeing characters who resemble their own lived experiences, can have its own significant impact.

A recent study by the National Research Group highlighted the importance of media representation. Almost two-thirds of Black Americans sampled stated that there was insufficient representation of themselves on screen (Turchiano 2020). A high percentage (91%) of all survey respondents noted that media can have impacts on society, and 87% of Black Americans surveyed stated that media depictions of Black Americans can influence the lives of Black Americans (Turchiano 2020). A similar survey found that 71% of Black women felt that media diversity had a huge influence in making them "feel more confident and proud," but many of them felt that stereotypes of Black women contribute to being judged as stronger than others and being "held to a higher standard" (Tapp 2021).

The release of the film *Black Panther* in 2018 was a transformational moment in film history. The film is based on the Marvel comic book hero who is the leader of the fictional African kingdom Wakanda. The character debuted during the civil rights era and was revolutionary in its depiction of a wealthy and technologically sophisticated Black-populated world. As Jamil Smith noted, the release of the film "serv[ed] a black audience that has long gone underrepresented," with a Black director (Ryan Coogler) and a mostly Black cast (Smith 2018). The power of Black Americans seeing well-rounded characterizations of themselves has impacts not only on them directly but also on how people who are not Black view them.

Within the past two decades, there also has been an increase in television programming centered on Black lead characters. Shonda Rhimes has been a key producer in this effort, with the massive success of *Grey's Anatomy*, followed by such shows as *Scandal* and *How to Get Away With Murder* that were led by Black women. When *Scandal* launched in 2012, Kerry Washington's starring role as Olivia Pope was one of the few instances since the 1970s of a Black woman leading a television program (Aurthur 2021). With her history of casting Black people in key roles as high-powered professionals, Rhimes has been hailed as a revolutionary force in television; as she recently stated in an interview, "We changed the faces that you see on television" (Aurthur 2021). With her recent transition to the streaming platform Netflix, Rhimes has continued her track record of diverse casting choices through her production company Shondaland, as evidenced by the 2020 hit series *Bridgerton*.

Following Rhimes's move to Netflix, Kenya Barris, creator of the television show *Black-ish*, also made a production deal with this streaming platform, and Ava DuVernay has created several programs for Netflix, including a series on the Central Park Five (*When They See Us*), a film on structural racism and the American carceral system (*13th*), and a series on the life of Colin Kaepernick (*Colin in Black and White*). One factor that may be driving this exodus of Black production talent to streaming platforms, including Amazon Prime and Hulu, is that compared with traditional broadcast formats, the streaming business model may not be as dependent on ratings success (Giorgis 2021).

Media Coverage of Anti-Black Violence and Its Impact on Black Mental Health

Within the past decade, there has been increased media coverage on police killings of unarmed Black people in the United States. The names have arrived in a torrent: Eric Garner, Tamir Rice, Alton Sterling, Walter Scott, Philando Castile, Breonna Taylor, and others, with the murder of George Floyd in 2020 contributing to a national reckoning regarding race and police misconduct. The video recording of George Floyd's death was widely disseminated, and a Census Bureau survey noted that significant symptoms of anxiety and depression increased in Black Americans 1 week after the video's release (Fowers and Wan 2020). According to a Gallup survey, Black Americans experienced a significant increase in anger and depression, and U.S. Census data showed a greater increase in depression and anxiety symptoms among Black Americans as compared with white Americans following Floyd's murder (Eichstaedt et al. 2021).

The loss of life has had an immeasurable impact on people directly connected to those who died, and there is increasing evidence that police killings and their media exposure can have more widespread effects on Black Americans as well. A research study examined the effect of police killings of unarmed Black Americans on the mental health of a sample of Black Americans surveyed in the same state where a specific killing occurred, with exposure defined to include various forms of media, including television, print, radio, and social media (Bor et al. 2018). Using a comparison sample of Black Americans who were temporally distanced from the police killings, Bor et al. (2018) noted that police killings were associated with an increase in poor mental health days, suggesting that these violent events can have a negative impact on a population level. Another research article noted that exposure to two or more publicized incidents of Black racial violence was associated with poorer mental health days for Black Americans (Curtis et al. 2021).

Similarly, researchers have also shown the detrimental impact on adolescent Black Americans of viewing traumatic events online. Tynes et al. (2019) examined data from a survey of Black and Latinx adolescents that assessed their online viewing of events that affected their specific racial/ethnic groups, including arrests, assaults, and shootings, and discovered that viewing such events was associated with increases in depressive and PTSD symptoms. Overall, this emerging branch of literature demonstrates that the publicizing of events that are related to anti-Black violence can have widespread impact even on those Black Americans who are not directly affected by these traumatic events. Future research will be crucial for examining whether this negative impact on emotional well-being can lead to longer-term behavioral consequences and whether the American health care system can sufficiently screen, prevent, and treat any mental health sequelae.

Conclusion

Entertainment media can have both positive and negative impacts on a viewer's perception of behavioral health conditions and their associated treatment. Despite advances in recent years, significant challenges in representation of Black people and other people of color still remain within the film and television industry. Although recent years have seen significant television and film portrayals in which Black characters manage mental illness or a substance use disorder, at times these portrayals have received criticism of how they depict mental health. In addition, recent entertainment programs have also centered on Black therapists or Black people seeking therapy. Increasing visibility of Black characters in film and television programming can have a positive impact on Black mental health, but emerging research has shown that media coverage of anti-Black violence can have a detrimental impact on a Black population level.

References

Abramovitch S: Oscar's first Black winner accepted her honor in a segregated "no Blacks" hotel in L.A. Hollywood Reporter, February 19, 2015. Available at: www.hollywoodreporter.com/movies/movie-news/oscars-first-black-winner-accepted-774335. Accessed February 5, 2022.

Aurthur K: Shonda Rhimes on creating hit TV at Netflix, "Inventing Anna" and whether Regé-Jean Page will ever return to "Bridgerton." Variety, November 4, 2021. Available at: https://variety.com/2021/tv/news/shonda-rhimes-netflix-bridgerton-inventing-anna-shondaland-1235102790. Accessed December 1, 2021.

Bastién AJ: Why don't women of color get to be mentally ill on TV? Splinter, September 8, 2016. Available at: https://splinternews.com/why-dont-women-of-color-get-to-be-mentally ill-on-tv-1793861756. Accessed October 18, 2021.

Bastién AJ: Claiming the future of Black TV. The Atlantic, January 29, 2017. Available at: www.theatlantic.com/entertainment/archive/2017/01/claiming-the-future-of-black-tv/514562. Accessed October 19, 2021.

Bobolitz S, Yam K: Why on-screen representation actually matters. HuffPost, February 24, 2017. Available at: www.huffpost.com/entry/why-on-screen-representation-matters_n_58aeae96e4b01406012fe49d. Accessed on December 1, 2021.

Bor J, Venkataramani AS, Williams DR, Tsai AC: Police killings and their spillover effects on the mental health of Black Americans: a population-based, quasi-experimental study. Lancet 392(10144):302–310, 2018 29937193

Burr S: Television and societal effects: an analysis of media images of African-Americans in historical context. Journal of Gender, Race, and Justice 4:159–182, 2001

Clark A: How the history of blackface is rooted in racism. New York, History, April 20, 2021. Available at: www.history.com/news/blackface-history-racism-origins. Accessed December 1, 2021.

Clyman J: The Soloist: part II. Psychology Today, May 14, 2009. Available at: www.psychologytoday.com/us/blog/reel-therapy/200905/the-soloist-part-ii. Accessed October 19, 2021.

Curtis DS, Washburn T, Lee H, et al: Highly public anti-Black violence is associated with poor mental health days for Black Americans. Proc Natl Acad Sci USA 118(17):e2019624118, 2021 33875593

Darden J: "Get Out" gets in our heads about African Americans and mental health. HuffPost, March 14, 2017. Available at: www.huffpost.com/entry/get-out-gets-in-our-heads-about-african-americans_b_58c7489de4b022817b291685. Accessed December 1, 2021.

Eichstaedt JC, Sherman GT, Giorgi S, et al: The emotional and mental health impact of the murder of George Floyd on the US population. Proc Natl Acad Sci USA 118(39):e2109139118, 2021 34544875

Fowers A, Wan W: Depression and anxiety spiked among Black Americans after George Floyd's death. Washington Post, June 12, 2020. Available at: www.washingtonpost.com/health/2020/06/12/mental-health-george-floyd-census. Accessed December 1, 2021.

Giorgis H: Not enough has changed since "Sanford and Son": the unwritten rules of Black TV. The Atlantic, September 13, 2021. Available at: www.theatlantic.com/magazine/archive/2021/10/the-unwritten-rules-of-black-tv/619816. Accessed December 1, 2021.

Harris A: How accurate is Empire's treatment of bipolar disorder? Slate, March 10, 2015. Available at: https://slate.com/culture/2015/03/how-empire-handles-andres-bipolar-disorder-is-the-show-realistic-or-overly-dramatic-video.html. Accessed October 18, 2021.

Harris A: "Black lady therapists" are still a TV trope. But now they have more depth. NPR, October 8, 2021. Available at: www.npr.org/2021/10/08/1041882856/black-lady-therapists-ted-lasso-white-lotus-in-treatment. Accessed October 19, 2021.

Hunt D, Ramón A: Hollywood diversity report 2020 part 2: television. Los Angeles, CA, UCLA College of Social Sciences, 2020. Available at: https://socialsciences.ucla.edu/wp-content/uploads/2020/10/UCLA-Hollywood-Diversity-Report-2020-Television-10-22-2020.pdf. Accessed October 18, 2021.

Hunt D, Ramón A: Hollywood diversity report 2021 part 1: film. Los Angeles, CA, UCLA College of Social Sciences, 2021. Available at: https://socialsciences.ucla.edu/wp-content/uploads/2021/04/UCLA-Hollywood-Diversity-Report-2021-Film-4-22-2021.pdf. Accessed October 18, 2021.

Jackson A: Sterling K. Brown on fighting the stigma around mental health through Randall's journey on "This Is Us." Variety, March 24, 2020. Available at: https://variety.com/2020/tv/news/sterling-k-brown-this-is-us-mental-health-stigma-1203544221. Accessed October 20, 2021.

Lawson K: Why seeing yourself represented on screen is so important. Vice, February 20, 2018. Available at: www.vice.com/en/article/zmwq3x/why-diversity-on-screen-is-important-black-panther. Accessed December 1, 2021.

Maia A: Breaking the stigma. New York, New York University, February 20, 2021. Available at: https://confluence.gallatin.nyu.edu/context/interdisciplinary-seminar/breaking-the-stigma. Accessed October 19, 2021.

Martins N, Harrison K: Racial and gender differences in the relationship between children's television use and self-esteem: a longitudinal panel study. Communic Res 39:338–357, 2012

National Museum of African American History and Culture: Blackface: the birth of an American stereotype. 2021. Available at: https://nmaahc.si.edu/blog-post/blackface-birth-american-stereotype. Accessed December 1, 2021.

Nelson A: African American stereotypes in prime-time television: an overview, 1948–2007, in African Americans and Popular Culture. Edited by Boyd T. Westport, Praeger, 2008, pp 185–216

The Opportunity Agenda: Media portrayals and Black male outcomes. New York, The Opportunity Agenda, 2021. Available at: https://opportunityagenda.org/messaging_reports/media-representations-black-men-boys/media-portrayals-black-men. Accessed December 1, 2021.

Oxford African American Studies Center: Photo essay: Blaxploitation cinema. Oxford African American Studies Center, 2021. Available at: https://oxfordaasc.com/page/photo-essay-blaxploitation-cinema. Accessed December 1, 2021.

Saraiya S: Viola Davis: "My entire life has been a protest." Vanity Fair, July 14, 2020. Available at: www.vanityfair.com/hollywood/2020/07/cover-story-viola-davis. Accessed February 5, 2022.

Smith J: The revolutionary power of Black Panther. Time, February 19, 2018. Available at: https://time.com/black-panther. Accessed December 1, 2021.

Smith RA: For some Black Americans, therapy is gradually losing its stigma. Wall Street Journal, July 13, 2020. Available at: www.wsj.com/articles/for-some-black-americans-therapy-is-gradually-losing-its-stigma-11594657327. Accessed October 19, 2021.

Smith SL, Choueiti M, Choi A, et al: Mental health conditions in film and TV: portrayals that dehumanize and trivialize characters. Los Angeles, CA, USC Annenberg, May 2019. Available at: https://assets.uscannenberg.org/docs/aii-study-mental-health-media_052019.pdf. Accessed October 18, 2021.

Smith-Frigerio S: Intersectionality of race, class and gender: the complex representation of bipolar disorder on Fox Network's Empire. Howard J Commun 29:1–16, 2017

Soloski A: "In Treatment" is back. How does that make you feel? May 19, 2021. Available at: www.nytimes.com/2021/05/19/arts/television/in-treatment-uzo-aduba.html. Accessed October 19, 2021.

Stamps D: B(l)ack by popular demand: an analysis of positive Black male characters in television and audiences' community cultural wealth. J Commun Inq 45:97–118, 2021

Stuart H: Media portrayal of mental illness and its treatments: what effect does it have on people with mental illness? CNS Drugs 20(2):99–106, 2006 16478286

Tapp T: Black women want to see "more complex portrayals" of themselves on-screen, says new survey from OWN and NRG. Deadline, November 10, 2021. Available at: https://deadline.com/2021/11/black-women-own-nrg-study-complex-portrayals-1234871479. Accessed December 1, 2021.

Turchiano D: Two in three Black Americans don't feel properly represented in media (study). Variety, September 17, 2020. Available at: https://variety.com/2020/tv/news/representation-matters-study-nrg-black-americans-media-1234772025. Accessed December 1, 2021.

Tynes BM, Willis HA, Stewart AM, Hamilton MW: Race-related traumatic events online and mental health among adolescents of color. J Adolesc Health 65(3):371–377, 2019 31196779

White R: Empire: a new model for bipolar disorder on TV. Psychology Today, February 23, 2015. Available at: www.psychologytoday.com/us/blog/culture-in-mind/201502/empire-new-model-bipolar-disorder-tv. Accessed October 18, 2021.

Whitten S: 20 Black filmmakers who have changed Hollywood in the last century. CNBC, February 19, 2021. Available at: www.cnbc.com/2021/02/19/20-black-movie-directors-that-changed-hollywood-in-the-last-century.html. Accessed December 1, 2021.

Wilkinson A: "Get Out" is a horror film about benevolent racism. It's spine-chilling. Vox, February 25, 2017. Available at: www.vox.com/culture/2017/2/24/14698632/get-out-review-jordan-peele. Accessed December 1, 2021.

Wooten L, Jordan A, Simon KM, Gold J: This Is Us: a case examination on Black men in therapy. Acad Psychiatry 45(6):763–767, 2021 34494205

PART III

A Call to Research

The Work and Legacy of Dr. Carl Bell

Part 1: Building a Better Village

Johnny Williamson, M.D.

My mentoring relationship with Carl C. Bell, M.D., dates to April 1998 at the 151st Annual Meeting of the American Psychiatric Association (APA). As a resident in training, I participated in an APA-sponsored mentorship program. Naive of organized psychiatry and its national infrastructure, I was unsure of what to expect. In my discussions with other mentees from around the country, it became immediately clear to me that Dr. Bell's reputation preceded him. He was clearly revered by many individuals he had mentored at some point in the past. I could as-

Editors' note: The late Dr. Carl Bell was the American Psychiatric Association Solomon Carter Fuller awardee and lecturer in 2011. His lecture was titled "Public Health Efforts: Successful and Failed." For this chapter, we have enlisted two psychiatrists who knew him personally, benefited from his mentorship, and were inspired by him in their own career development.

certain that Dr. Bell had a charismatic personality and commanded the room when he spoke. I learned that he was highly informed, exceedingly well accomplished, and intolerant of the trivial.

Dr. Bell's demeanor was calm. His style was laid-back; he wore jeans, a printed T-shirt, and a hat. His comments were concise, and he chose simple wording to explain complex ideas. He urged us to be analytical in our thinking and deliberate in our career decisions, while also urging us to think about public health and preventive measures in our clinical practice. He directly addressed challenges that lie ahead of us as early career psychiatrists. He covered mental health stigma and challenges related to studying, living, and working in the profession as an African American. He explained how mentorship would help us develop confidence and character while pushing us out of our comfort zones. He urged us to bring our entire selves to our jobs and daily lives. Finally, he encouraged us to "do something" more than merely treat patients. He dared us to have an impact that would be of greater benefit to our respective communities above our efforts to heal our patients.

Carl Compton Bell was born in Chicago, Illinois, to Pearl Debnam and William Yancey Bell Jr. He earned a medical degree from Meharry Medical College and completed training in psychiatry at the Illinois State Psychiatric Institute, located within the University of Illinois Hospital system. Dr. Bell loved his family, his people, and his profession. He opposed conventional beliefs that many challenges African Americans face originated simply from their failure to succeed. Driven to understand the poor outcomes in mental health care among African Americans, he became a staunch advocate for systemic changes to eliminate health disparities.

Dr. Bell was among the most prominent psychiatrists in the country, and he poured his heart and soul into his South Side community. There, he built an African American–run service organization that served a community of the people of the same culture. The Community Mental Health Council, established in 1987, evolved into one of the country's largest community mental health clinics. This clinic was a center of treatment, training, and research where African American students and professionals could learn and work in an environment in which their cultural identities and professional accomplishments were celebrated openly. A bastion of treatment and education, the Community Mental Health Council connected community with university, bringing evidence-based treatment to a community otherwise forgotten.

Prolific in his achievements, Bell authored more than 500 publications. He was the coauthor of *Suicide and Homicide Among Adolescents* (Holinger et al. 1994). He authored *The Sanity of Survival: Reflections on Community Mental Health and Wellness* (Bell 2004) and *Fetal Alcohol Expo-*

sure in the African-American Community (Bell 2018). Bell dedicated his life to worthy causes, and the highest distinctions have been bestowed on him. His APA awards include the Solomon Carter Fuller Award, the Distinguished Service Award for exceptional meritorious service, the Adolf Meyer Award for lifetime achievement in psychiatric research, the Agnes Purcell McGavin Award for Prevention in child and adolescent psychiatry, and a Special Presidential Commendation in recognition of outstanding advocacy for mental illness prevention and person-centered mental health wellness and recovery. In honor of his extraordinary achievements in advancing human rights, he was awarded the American Association for Social Psychiatry's Abraham L. Halpern Humanitarian Award.

Bell's prolific scholarship granted him inclusion in several key national organizations with mental health oversight. He was a member of the National Academy of Sciences Board on Children, Youth, and Families and of the National Advisory Mental Health Council of the National Institutes of Health (NIH). The council collectively advises the Secretary of Health and Human Services, NIH, and the National Institute of Mental Health on all policies and activities relating to the conduct and support of mental health research, research training, and other programs. Furthermore, Dr. Bell worked as a consultant for several correctional departments; colleges; and local, state, and federal government organizations, including the U.S. Department of Justice, the National Institute of Mental Health, and the Office of the Surgeon General. He gaven talks internationally and was interviewed by a variety of news organizations.

Bell believed in the African maxim "It takes a village." This principle was emblematic of his commitment to mentorship throughout his career. His strategy for strengthening the mental health of African Americans was to increase the involvement and influence of the future generation of African American psychiatrists.

A Leader I Could Trust

Leadership is a process of social influence, which maximizes the efforts of others, towards the achievement of a goal.

Kruse (2015)

Leadership is derived from social influence on others; however, it is dependent not on authority but rather on the personality of the individual (Kruse 2015). My mentoring relationship with Dr. Bell taught me that the path to developing the ability to lead is a process of internal maturation. It includes the transformation of self into an effective communicator and a critical thinker and the ability to identify clear goals and a path to attaining them. In his various research projects, forensic cases, and joint publications, Dr. Bell consistently prompted clarity of goal. Over time, when I would become uncertain on how to proceed, I could often discover the answer simply by reflecting on my overarching goal. In the initial phases of mentorship, I would ask a question and Dr. Bell would answer. Eventually, he responded to questions with prompts to motivate a reconsideration of the goal. In the end, he would answer my questions by saying, "Why are you asking me?" This maturation weaned me from my dependence on his approval, allowing me to achieve a sense of independent competence.

Bell emphasized that effective leadership is required to build a safer community. Central to any mentorship relationship is the question "What kind of leader will you be?" This is more than an academic question because a person's leadership style may determine how effective they will be and how great an influence their leadership can have. Leadership generates measurable change in individuals, groups, and even communities. In addition to clarity of goal, Bell's leadership demonstrated change through action. "The ultimate test of practical leadership is the realization of intended, real change that meets people's enduring needs" (Burns 1978, p. 461). Leadership is so much more than the willingness to stand in front and have someone follow you. Being an effective leader requires having a followership. A followership consists of people who have the capacity or willingness to follow a leader. As a leader, Dr. Bell often made things look easy. One strategy he used when helping followers develop clarity about the meaning of their actions was to ask them to describe a real-life occurrence in which their work had directly affected another person. It was this ability to translate large-scale, complicated concepts into examples of daily living that bridged the gap for many of us who enjoyed following his stewardship.

In a guidance on leadership, Dr. Bell related the interdependent function between leadership and followership. He once described a discussion he had about followership with a patient. Essentially, the person made the statement that "I could be a follower, if I could find a leader I could trust." Dr. Bell strongly believed that "understanding the concept of followership better is likely to improve training and organizational performance" (Crossman and Crossman 2011, p. 481).

Dr. Bell's leadership is exemplary and deserving of study. He understood that for leaders to lead, they need have not only exceptional talent but also the ability to attract people who can contribute. The leadership role typically has glamour and attracts attention. However, followership is key to reciprocal mentorship relationships. Given that we are more often followers than leaders, followership plays a more frequent and impactful role in our work and lives.

Followership, defined by active participation in the pursuit of common goals, is best achieved when there is an understanding of how the leader makes decisions and an awareness of critical challenges that the leader faces. Dr. Bell encouraged proactivity, critical thinking, independence, and cultural competence in his mentees. He sought to inspire colleagues to work toward the mental health benefit of the larger African American community. He made himself personally available for others, nationally and internationally, on a continual basis. Effective followers are more than passive participants. Being receptive to followership encouraged me to think for myself and become a self-starter. I learned to maintain dynamic commitment and actively fill roles. Dr. Bell supported the followership role of his mentees by encouraging productivity, assertiveness, and aspiration in those who pursued the path that he was charting.

In my review of Bell's leadership style, I recognize that, consistent with his personality, his style was eclectic. In describing the prominent aspects of his leadership style, I have borrowed from several theories of leadership. Acknowledging the contradictions and limitations of these theories, you can find elements of each of them in Dr. Bell's leadership. In a research paper on African American leadership, Watson and Rosser (2017) offered details of various theories of leadership, including the great man theory, which posits that hereditary background explains inherited leadership. Essentially, you were born into greatness and, thus, leadership by bloodline. This theory suggests leaders are born, not made. This is a largely debunked theory, and Dr. Bell himself humbly stated, "It doesn't really matter where you came from, doesn't really matter that you're able to trace some great accomplishments or achievements by your forebears" (Bell 2008). To be clear, Dr. Bell felt that everyone has something of value. Nevertheless, the fact remains that Bell obtained an M.D.; his father, William Y. Bell Jr., earned a Ph.D. in sociology; and his grandfather, William Y. Bell Sr., received a Ph.D. from Yale Divinity School. Dr. Bell often shared pictures of his father with President John F. Kennedy, his grandfather with President Harry S Truman, and himself with President Bill Clinton. In each of these photographs, the Bells were serving in an advisory role to their respective president.

Situational Leadership

The principle in situational leadership is that there is no one best style of leadership. Effective leadership is relevant to the task. Leaders who are most successful adapt their leadership style to the needs of the individual or group they are attempting to lead (Crossman and Crossman 2011). In many of the accomplishments credited to Dr. Bell, his leadership style emerged or was adjusted on the basis of the needs of the particular circumstance. For example, he is known for leading efforts to address the misdiagnosis of psychosis in African Americans and the underdiagnosis of fetal alcohol spectrum disorder in young African Americans with learning and behavioral problems, both of which were causes that confronted failings of the mental health system as it relates to populations of color. Additionally, Dr. Bell contributed to broadening the current understanding of the impacts of implicit and other racial biases and health disparities. These perspectives were not always readily accepted. However, they have become more broadly accepted thanks to his advocacy.

Having the chance to observe Dr. Bell lead on these difficult issues allowed me to appreciate how universal his impact was. To be clear, Dr. Bell had a unique and resilient personality. At times, his persona seemed to serve as a catalyst to his message. Conversely, it was not unheard of for him to take a direct, unflinching approach to difficult topics, even when some people felt his message was controversial. In our discussion of this approach, he described how he was once told he was irreverent. He agreed with this assessment and wholly accepted this aspect of his personality. He always remained true to himself. Yet, he could simultaneously adjust his focus, strategy, perspective, and anything necessary to meet the needs of the individuals he was attempting to lead and to attend to the communities he was intent on serving. He could lead a highly assenting crowd enthusiastically in support of his impatient denouncement of unfair and biased impacts on the mental health of African Americans. Equally, he could lead a dissenting group to develop a more empathic, broadened perspective on these issues. Independent of the characteristics of his followership, he supported all perspectives with objective evidence, supportive literature, and critical thought.

Transformational Leadership

The concept of transformational leadership has been described as being integral to developing change in both individuals and social systems. Northouse (2003) defined transformational leadership as the process whereby an individual engages with others and creates a connection that raises the level of motivation and morality in both the leader and the follower. Northouse contended that this type of leader is attentive to the needs and motives of followers and tries to help followers reach their fullest potential. As a leader, Bell's authenticity and willingness to connect with others for mutual benefit stand out. He sought to inspire others to be pioneering in their efforts to develop greater knowledge and insight. The product of such efforts was to be purposed for generating positive change within the followers' communities.

Getting Rid of the Rats

Getting rid of the rats was a metaphor used by Dr. Bell to illustrate his vision of benefiting the community through public health advocacy. Dr. Bell often gave the example that when a patient has a rat bite, a doctor should treat it. However, if the doctor finds several individuals with rat bites in a community, the doctor should help get rid of the rats. Although this metaphor had multiple purposes, Dr. Bell used it to bring focus to public health prevention within our health systems. He also used the metaphor to reflect his desire for psychiatrists of color to become involved in the health of their communities beyond the direct care of their patients. He modeled research, organizational leadership, and public health awareness and invited all to join him.

Dr. Bell did not buy into the idealized images of him held by many of his followers. Despite being vocal in his advocacy for numerous mental health concerns, he was humble at heart. He was often quoted saying, "I don't know what I am doing," a reference to the idea that he was simply following his inner guiding spirit and working to improve the health and lives of others. He was grounded in his beliefs and commitments.

Mentorship: We Are All Bent Nails

Dr. Bell could see the capacity for meaningful contribution in everyone, often in individuals who could not see it in themselves. He often stressed that the competencies of leadership can be learned. He was able to foster and develop such contributions in people of highly diverse interests and qualities, at the same time maintaining consideration for the perspective of the mentee. He understood that determination and curiosity are often stifled by caution and a sense of lack of merit in many early career mental health professionals. He helped these professionals understand their experience, only to challenge them to capitalize on their years of work and sacrifice. He admonished us all to "do something."

Bell often used the term *"bent nail" research* to describe his style of pragmatic, community-based studies that led him to many discoveries. In using the term *bent nail*, he was referring to the usefulness and power that reside in things, people, and processes that consist of imperfect elements (see the section "'Bent Nail' Research" in Part 2 of this chapter). Although his bent nail research may not have always met the standards of a double-blind, placebo-controlled trial, Dr. Bell was able to identify patterns that led to novel considerations that have stood the test of time. He brought this principle into his mentorship. Countless times he empowered his mentees to engage their ideas actively, risking being wrong in the service of finding what is right. His mentorship sought to illuminate strength within each of us, in essence to use our bent nails to build a better village for all.

Unfortunately, not everyone has the benefit of a strong mentoring relationship. Formal mentorship opportunities are lacking in education of African American medical students. This is partly due to the scarcity of physicians of color (Redd et al. 2015). The numbers of Black, Hispanic, Latinx, Native American, Alaska Native, Native Hawaiian, and Pacific Islander physicians remain far below their percentages in the general U.S. population. African Americans make up only 5% of doctors and about 8% of students accepted into medical school (Association of American Medical Colleges 2022). The path to a medical education for an individual of color is wrought with challenges from the start. Poverty, adverse life events, lack of exposure to medical role models, inequities, and racism are but a few of the barriers that must be overcome. Many persons of color find their way through secondary education only to face isolation and racial microaggressions in the workplace. This makes attainment difficult, and consequently, there are simply too few African Americans in medicine (Whaley 2021). Improvements in ethnic and racial diversity and other inequities within the systems of education are warranted and would increase access to medical education.

Dr. Bell's painstaking awareness of these disparities led him to be infinitely generous with his time. Through personal experience, he understood the rigors of medical training and medical practice. He saw firsthand the multitude of obstacles facing African Americans. Most notably, he knew that the negative impacts of these hardships were well healed through a relationship with someone who has knowledge, experience, fortitude, and concern for each individual as a human being of worth.

Advocacy for Black Mental Health

Beyond leadership through mentoring, Bell was a consistent voice within the psychiatric community, representing the mental health needs of African Americans within the organized power structures of psychiatry. Through advocacy and personal observation, he was able to raise national awareness of the health needs of African Americans. Dr. Bell introduced and/or championed several key concerns in mental health, largely on the basis of literature review and his own investigative actions.

Bell engendered a more universally accepted understanding of the impact of violence on children. The mental health community had previously understood traumatic stress–related conditions. However, this understanding was primarily independent of the consideration of the differential impact of chronic and repeated exposure to violence in children. Dr. Bell understood that children with cumulative exposure and adaptation to violence were much more susceptible to various emotional and behavioral consequences. This newly defined clarity gave birth to understandings and interventions that target the causes and impacts of cumulative violence. Ultimately, Dr. Bell introduced the concept of cultivating resiliency as a protective factor in combating the impacts on children of exposure to violence. Consequently, in 2004, he was the first winner of the APA Foundation's Minority Service Award for his efforts to prevent violence.

Bell was a vocal leader in correcting the misconception that Blacks demonstrate higher occurrences of schizophrenia-related disorders than bipolar disorder and mood disorders when compared with whites. African Americans had frequently been misdiagnosed as primarily psychotic when they were manifesting a primary mood disorder. Misdiagnosis can lead to mistreatment and poorer outcomes. Dr. Bell vehemently urged clinicians to become familiar with the cultural distinctions, racial identity, and biological characteristics that affect treatment response and adherence among Blacks. He encouraged the implementation of standardized diagnostic tools for screening and assessment of mental illness in Black communities to combat that disparity. He also identified the increased association between isolated sleep paralysis and panic disorder in Blacks.

Raising Awareness for Prevention

African Americans benefit from health care advances at a diminished rate. This fact haunted Dr. Bell throughout his career. He raised the collective awareness of the need for primary prevention strategies to address violence in the Black community. His lifelong commitment to violence prevention and his role as one of the nation's foremost specialists on the impact of violence on children in disadvantaged areas did not go unrecognized. In 2018, he was awarded the Bernard P. Harrison

Award of Merit by the National Commission on Correctional Health Care, the field's highest honor.

Dr. Bell led a collaborative team in addressing high rates of child removal in African American families exposed to the Illinois Department of Children and Family Services. Dr. Bell and the Community Mental Health Council collaborated with the department and other agencies to provide intervention that improved the social fabric of the community. This significantly reduced the number of children placed in protective care overall, most dramatically among the Black population (Redd et al. 2015).

Bell led a team that demonstrated that individual, family, and community protective factors could help youth avoid risky behaviors that can lead to HIV-positive status in South Africa. HIV risk behaviors were reduced by strengthening family relationship processes as well as targeting peer influences through enhancing social problem-solving and peer negotiation skills for youth (Bell et al. 2008).

Dr. Bell pioneered the awareness of unrecognized high prevalence of fetal alcohol spectrum disorder in African American children as a causative factor in childhood difficulties with speech, language, social skills, and behavioral issues. This was something of a primary prevention discovery because many of these developmental difficulties have permanent impacts and were not being associated with in utero alcohol exposure. This awakening has provided opportunities to develop effective strategies to prevent the disorders altogether.

Legacy and Wisdom

Dr. Bell's alma mater awarded him the 2018 President's Circle of Scholars Award with a presentation of his "50 Years of Lessons Learned Thanks to Meharry Medical College" (Meharry Medical College 2018). In June 2019, the Carl C. Bell Community Wellness Scholarship and Award was established to recognize a resident of the North Lawndale, Chicago, community committed to addressing the multifaceted impacts of trauma on underserved people in the community via the Trauma Response and Intervention Movement. In July 2019, Dr. Bell was presented with the National Medical Association's Scroll of Merit (the association's highest honor). Just days later, on August 2, 2019, Carl Compton Bell, M.D., died at his home.

The accolades for Dr. Bell have continued after his passing, and he has been awarded many honors for his remarkable service in the fight for mental health across the United States. The Inaugural Carl Bell Memorial Lecture was held in September 2020, with former U.S. Surgeon

General David Satcher, M.D., Ph.D., as the first lecturer. In 2021, the Carl C. Bell Memorial Award was developed in his honor to continue to champion mental health disparities, work to prevent community violence, and inspire youth to future greatness. Dr. Bell was well known for having an unparalleled work ethic, which led to a highly productive career with a high volume of publications, including books, chapters, and articles. He always welcomed the opportunity to discuss the state of mental health in the nation and would often recommend many of his works for further study. He never shied away from the spotlight or the opportunity to enlighten people who were unconvinced and unconcerned, yet to know Dr. Bell was to know that he humbly accepted public recognition and felt strongly that his accomplishments did not elevate him to any status above another individual. Through it all, he maintained a balance between gregariousness, irreverence, and humility.

Dr. Bell, never a dull personality, sometimes spoke in paradoxes. When people praised his work or bestowed accolades on him, he would deflect the compliment with the statement "Nobody cares." In my understanding of him, this antiphrasis was his way of acknowledging the significance of his work while remaining grounded in the humility of his spirit. It also served as a reminder and motivation for others because we often are most committed to action when we feel that nobody cares.

Bell left us with many pearls of wisdom. Of all of these pearls, the following quotation may be the most resounding:

> I've recently realized that a major problem with psychiatry is that it's too focused on what we were trained to do. It sometimes feels like psychiatry is stuck in a box that only recognizes diagnosis and treatment. Unfortunately, being in this box precludes psychiatrists from involving themselves with prevention and from focusing on strengths and characteristics of resilience and resistance. These are just as much a part of the human condition as is the psychopathology we were trained to identify and treat. Fortunately, some of us are blessed enough to be on the fringe, which allows us to occasionally leave the box and get a different perspective. This brings new paradigms and models that benefit the human condition. (Bell 2004, p. 466)

Conclusion

Carl Compton Bell, M.D., led a distinguished career. The sheer quantity of his achievements, the lives changed, communities impacted, and accolades bestowed are nearly incomprehensible. His example of effective leadership presents an opportunity for self-reflection on the scope of impact of the physician as leader. Most emblematic of Bell's intentions was his desire to inspire mental health practitioners to lead a vision-inspired existence. It is the intent of this chapter to elevate his legacy in order to bring contemplative focus to how people can live their lives in relation to their goals and aspirations. The challenges of medical training, practice, and leadership faced by communities of color are various and are complicated by race. African Americans also suffer some of the worst health disparities. Bell found these truths intolerable, and he was not alone in that. Ever mindful of the dearth of African American physicians, he used mentorship to provide opportunities to foster the development of African American physician leaders. He hoped that his mentorship would pay forward humanitarian advocacy. He believed there is space for everyone to participate, be it as a leader or a follower. Bell's leadership guaranteed that there was an advocate for the health needs of the African American community throughout his life.

Effective leadership can be learned, but it demands many things. First among them is willingness. The ability to perform in circumstances that are nonideal is required. Keeping well informed and applying a critical thought process are consistent aids to successful change. Remaining undeterred by perceived limitations and taking advantage of opportunities to benefit others will generate leadership opportunities. The necessary complement to leadership is followership. Leadership paired with competent, committed followership and combined with committed action holds the potential for great change.

African American culture has historically suffered great loss of intergenerational knowledge, history, and resources. Further losses of this nature can be prevented with strategic and intentional efforts. The contributions and accomplishments of distinguished African American physicians are worthy of formal documentation and stand to benefit all Americans. The lessons their stories tell must be shared and remembered. Mentorship is vital to the retention and continual expansion of knowledge of health care concerns of the African American community. Mentorship also supports the success of African American physicians who are charged with the responsibility for providing quality care to African Americans. The formal and informal networks of connectivity created by mentorship extend the potential for influence and increase opportunities for wide impact.

There is an aphorism in medical training that goes, "See one. Do one. Teach one." The idea is to learn first by watching. Of course, this principle requires that someone who has come before you is willing to lead you on your educational journey. Once you have been taught, your responsibility is to then do. In this case, it would be to care for the lives of your patients. The circle is then completed with teaching. That is, you then become the physician leader with the responsibility to reach back and pull forward those who come after you. Bell's modern vision of rebuilding the village is a worthy one. His lived experience of leadership presents an opportunity for growth and reflection. Dr. Carl Bell, as acclaimed as he was, would likely have traded every single honor for the opportunity to mentor another person toward a vision-centered life. His accomplishments did not hold tremendous value within themselves so much as they were examples of what is possible. A final point of clarity comes from a Zen Buddhist principle that Dr. Bell routinely paraphrased: "Don't follow the master. Follow the path the master took."

References

Association of American Medical Colleges: ERAS statistic preliminary data—residency October 5, 2022. Washington, DC, Association of American Medical Colleges, 2022. Available at: www.aamc.org/media/6231/download. Accessed May 3, 2022.

Bell CC: The Sanity of Survival: Reflections on Community Mental Health and Wellness. Chicago, IL, Third World Press, 2004

Bell CC: Dr. Carl Bell. Chicago, IL, HistoryMakers, November 3, 2008. Available at: www.thehistorymakers.org/biography/dr-carl-bell-41. Accessed May 3, 2022.

Bell CC: Fetal Alcohol Exposure in the African-American Community. Chicago, IL, Third World Press, 2018

Bell CC, Bhana A, Petersen I, et al: Building protective factors to offset sexually risky behaviors among Black youths: a randomized control trial. J Natl Med Assoc 100(8):936–944, 2008 18717144

Burns JMG: Leadership. New York, Harper and Row, 1978

Crossman B, Crossman J: Conceptualizing followership—a review of the literature. Leadership 7(4):481–497, 2011

Holinger PC, Offer D, Barter JT, Bell CC: Suicide and Homicide Among Adolescents. New York, Guilford, 1994.

Kruse K: What is leadership? Forbes, September 2, 2015. Available at: www.forbes.com/sites/kevinkruse/2013/04/09/what-is-leadership/?sh=4fc2f6ac5b90. Accessed October 11, 2021.

Meharry Medical College: Carl C. Bell, M.D. '71 named 2018 President's Circle of Scholars Award winner. Nashville, TN, Meharry Medical College, April 12, 2018. Available at: https://home.mmc.edu/carl-c-bell-m-d-71-named-2018-presidents-circle-of-scholars-award-winner. Accessed October 11, 2021.

Northouse PG: Leadership Theory and Practice. Thousand Oaks, CA, Sage, 2003, pp 169–199

Redd J, Suggs H, Gibbons R, et al: A plan to strengthen systems and reduce the number of African-American children in child welfare. Milton Keynes, UK, CORE, March 14, 2015. Available at: https://core.ac.uk/display/101764891. Accessed May 3, 2022.

Watson AC, Rosser M: The emergence of African American leaders in American society. Mission Viejo, CA, Association of Leadership Educators, February 14, 2017

Whaley M: Importance of mentorship for Black medical students. Cleveland, OH, Center for Reducing Health Disparities, April 28, 2021. Available at: https://reducedisparity.org/2021/04/28/importance-of-mentorship-for-black-medical-students. Accessed October 11, 2021.

The Work and Legacy of Dr. Carl Bell

Part 2: Public Health Efforts

Ruth S. Shim, M.D., M.P.H.

Carl C. Bell, M.D., was at the forefront of merging public health and mental health in research. In fact, throughout his distinguished career, he led and shifted narratives and directions of research study because he would often pursue an important topic of research in improving outcomes for populations many years before other experts in the field identified these issues. In Part 2 of this chapter, I describe three such examples of Dr. Bell's prescience, although there are many more to draw from.

In the early 1980s, Bell raised the alarm and concern about community violence and its impact on people of color. Then, Dr. Bell sounded the alarm about the devastating impact of early childhood trauma on outcomes for young people, long before the renowned Adverse Childhood Experiences (ACE) Study (Felitti et al. 1998). And finally, at the time of his death, Dr. Bell was advancing an important narrative about the detrimental effects of fetal alcohol exposure in the Black community. It is unclear how Dr. Bell was able to so consistently prophesize on the direction that public health and mental health research needed to go, but his vision was often years, if not decades, ahead of its time. Dr. Bell certainly had an uncanny ability to observe the needs of Black communities and effectively research and design effective interventions to improve outcomes. Consideration of his distinguished career may serve as an example of how to boldly seek solutions to complex and wicked problems.

Bent Nail Research

Perhaps Dr. Bell's ability to understand the specific research questions in mental health that were most pressing for Black communities was because of his creation of and reliance on the concept of "bent nail" research. He often spoke about this concept in detail, including in a chapter in the groundbreaking book *Black Mental Health: Patients, Pro-*

viders, and Systems (Bell 2019). As the story goes, a young Carl Bell was given a book filled with activities to try at home. As he attempted to build a piece of furniture, a bookcase, as described in the book, he ran into some challenges because he did not have all the necessary equipment. Ever the industrious child, he managed to find all the supplies—wood and nails—that he needed by rummaging through the alleys and streets of Chicago, but these supplies were not in pristine condition. He had to hammer the used, bent nails straight before he could use them. When he completed the construction of his bookcase, it was functional but leaned a little to the right—it was, as Dr. Bell described, a "bent nail bookcase."

In his adulthood, and throughout his career, Dr. Bell thought often of the bent nail bookcase and its applications to research in the Black community. He has described his career as one in which he did not always have the most sophisticated infrastructure or funding mechanisms to conduct state-of-the-art research, yet his research findings and observations have been remarkably functional. Often unspoken in Dr. Bell's observations was the toll of structural racism on brilliant Black scientists like Dr. Bell. Recent data have shown a greater than 2 to 1 funding disparity between Black scientists and white scientists who are principal investigators applying for funding from the NIH (Stevens et al. 2021). Nevertheless, Dr. Bell developed a highly effective workaround, in which his bent nail research allowed for significant findings and helped guide the field toward the most important outcomes and interventions to improve the mental health of Black people and other people of color.

Violence Prevention in Black Communities

In the mid-1980s, Dr. Bell began to research the detrimental effects of neighborhood violence on Black communities. In an article published in the *Community Mental Health Journal* in 1987, titled "Preventive Strategies for Dealing With Violence Among Blacks," Dr. Bell laid out the issue in stark terms, describing the high rates of homicide among Black people and effectively linking some of these terrible outcomes to head injuries (Bell 1986, 1987). Indeed, this issue has recently become the forefront of the investigation of the association between aggressive behavior and chronic traumatic encephalopathy, as examined in former boxers and football players (Martin and McMillan 2020).

Over time, Dr. Bell honed his arguments about the detrimental impacts of community violence on outcomes and focused more on the toxic effects of violence in young people. Using bent nail research techniques, Dr. Bell examined the impact of community violence on children in South Side Chicago (Bell and Jenkins 1993), among adolescents (Jenkins and Bell 1994) and school-age children (Shafii and Shafii 2008), in children in correctional facilities (Bell and Jenkins 1995), and among other special populations of young people (Bell and Jenkins 1991).

Ultimately, this extensive research led to comprehensive prevention, intervention, and postvention strategies to end community violence and its detrimental impact on Black youth and families. The article "Lessons Learned from 50 Years of Violence Prevention Activities in the African American Community," published in the *Journal of the National Medical Association* in 2017, was the culmination of these efforts, delivering the most comprehensive summary of interventional science and surveying and assessing current violence prevention initiatives. Dr. Bell summarized the article by stating, unequivocally, that "to withhold violence prevention programs that have been shown to be effective from communities that need them is unethical" (Bell 2017, 233).

Early Childhood Trauma

Before the ACE Study, Dr. Bell (in collaboration with Dr. Esther Jenkins) was attuned to the dangers of toxic stress in developing children (Bell and Jenkins 1991). Surveys administered to Black school-age children in South Chicago identified students who had witnessed violence, with 26% of children reporting that they had witnessed someone getting shot and 29% of children reporting that they had seen someone stabbed (Bell and Jenkins 1991). These early childhood traumas were then linked directly to a number of poor outcomes, including PTSD (Pynoos and Nader 1988), poor cognitive performance (Pears and Fisher 2005), and lower self-esteem (Hyman et al. 1988). Additionally, Bell and Jenkins (1991) highlighted problems of repeated, chronic exposure to trauma, before the concept of complex PTSD was identified or defined (Herman 1992).

Dr. Bell described the role of community-based participatory research in addressing early childhood trauma. He described this practice as "rebuilding the village" and described how these interventions could minimize the effects of trauma, provided that these research methods were implemented with a culturally competent framework (Bell et al. 2009). With colleagues, he also successfully connected the trauma of racism to early childhood trauma in children, one of the first clinician-researchers to make this important connection (Vaughans and Spielberg 2014). Specifically, he directly linked the work of Dr. Charles Pinderhughes and Dr. Jeanne Spurlock on the detrimental developmental effects of racism to various social determinants of mental health, highlighting Black children's vulnerability to childhood trauma when raised by Black parents who are discriminated against in the racist society of the United States (Douglas et al. 2014). He also discussed differences in the types of early childhood trauma that Black children experience (secondary to racism, which leads to family and community violence), contrasting this with traditional criteria for PTSD (Douglas et al. 2014). Even as he observed these findings and noted the inequities in research perspectives, he also emphasized the importance of protective factors in the mental health and wellness of Black children.

Dr. Bell excelled in providing actionable recommendations to improve outcomes. Regarding the harmful effects of childhood trauma, he encouraged mental health practitioners to perform a childhood trauma history as part of their initial psychiatric evaluation (Bell 2013), a practice that has been widely adopted as a standard of current appropriate clinical practice (Thakur et al. 2020).

Fetal Alcohol Syndrome

The monograph *Fetal Alcohol Exposure in the African-American Community*, written by Dr. Bell and published in 2018 (Bell 2018), is a gift for any psychiatrist or mental health practitioner who wants to understand the impactful and extensive career of Dr. Carl Bell. For me, the small book is a precious gift that I received directly from Dr. Bell during the American College of Psychiatrists meeting in February 2019, one of the last times I had the pleasure to interact with him. As with many of our conversations toward the end of his life, we discussed our differing opinions about the prevalence of alcohol use among pregnant Black people. He respectfully (and often) disagreed with me with the knowledge of someone who is certain they are right. And he was. The genius of this work is not only is it a beautiful retrospective of a deeply impactful career, but it also highlights the same prescience that Dr. Bell always had when approaching all problems impacting African American communities:

> I have finally figured some of what is going on with this problem of Fetal Alcohol Exposure and how widespread it is, and what African-American people can do about it. I should add, my main concern is African-American people living within the United States of America where in one community the rate of Fetal Alcohol Exposure is 388/1,000 people. (Bell 2018, p. 7)

In this brief, easy-to-read book, Dr. Bell described the origins of his career, from his education at Meharry Medical College to his work with the Community Mental Health Council and with the 16th surgeon general of the United States, Dr. David Satcher, and his growing knowledge of the pervasive nature of the problem of fetal alcohol exposure in his clinical and research experiences. And, as always, he presented actionable solutions to address this public health crisis, including advocacy and increased awareness, increasing choline in prenatal vitamins (as an effective universal prevention strategy to reduce the detrimental effects of fetal alcohol exposure), and, importantly, hope.

Again, the book, like all other things Dr. Bell did, was prescient. In the final chapter, he noted, "The reason I hope you 'get it' is because I am getting old. This may be my last crusade for African-Americans. I am tired" (Bell 2018, p. 137). The work, as well as the crusade to address fetal alcohol exposure in Black communities, is a powerful mantle that has already been picked up. In 2018, a study published in *JAMA* asserted that the prevalence of fetal alcohol spectrum disorders was far higher in the population than previously thought, with prevalence rates similar to those of autism spectrum disorders (May et al. 2018).

The Legacy of Dr. Carl Bell

Perhaps the greatest legacy of Carl Bell was the vision to merge public health with mental health and, in doing so, defining and clarifying the field of community psychiatry as one in which public health efforts are applied to populations to improve mental health at the community level. At his core, Dr. Bell was a preventionist, and he often spoke of considering the primary, secondary, and tertiary preventive interventions in populations. This prevention focus is a fundamental principle of public health. Out of this merging of public health and mental health, he developed the seven field principles of the theory of triadic influence as a strategy for effective behavioral change in communities (Table 9–1) (Bell et al. 2002).

Conclusion

Carl Bell had a vision for a society in which all people, especially those from oppressed and marginalized communities, are able to experience greater mental wellness. He pursued this vision by merging the fields of public health and mental health, developing and honing the concept of community-based participatory research, inventing the concept of bent-nail research, and always championing the mental health needs of

Table 9-1. Seven field principles of the theory of triadic influence

Principle	Description
Rebuild the village	Research has shown that when children and adults are surrounded by social fabric such as a tight-knit community, nearly everyone in the community benefits from collaboration
Provide access to all forms of modern and ancient technology	Computerized or modern medical technologies can spark preventive interventions
Facilitate connectedness	Resilience depends on connections to a variety of people who serve as best-interest models (or mentors)
Develop social skills	Having social skills helps youth and adults gather support to overcome challenges in life
Encourage self-esteem	Engaging children in activities that create a sense of power, produce a sense of connectedness, develop of sense of models, and generate a sense of uniqueness leads to increased self-esteem
Reestablish the adult protective shield	Parents can shield children from trauma by giving them a sense of routine, safety, and the calming influence of reassurance
Minimize the effects of trauma	Trauma does not cause anxiety, distress, and traumatic stress, but helplessness in the face of trauma does, which turns traumatic helplessness into learned helpfulness

the most vulnerable and marginalized communities in the United States. Long before there was any formal discussion of the social determinants of mental health, Carl Bell was describing these social determinants and analyzing their impact on the mental health of communities. In his lifetime, great progress was made toward tackling the most challenging problems in psychiatry—he cleared a path, and it is up to future generations to venture down this path toward progress in improving mental health outcomes.

References

Bell CC: Coma and the etiology of violence, part 1. J Natl Med Assoc 78(12):1167–1176, 1986 3100816

Bell CC: Preventive strategies for dealing with violence among Blacks. Community Ment Health J 23(3):217–228, 1987 3677590

Bell CC: Trauma associated with living in violent neighborhoods. Psychiatr Times 30:16, 2013

Bell CC: Lessons learned from 50 years of violence prevention activities in the African American community. J Natl Med Assoc 109(4):224–237, 2017 29173929

Bell CC: Fetal Alcohol Exposure in the African-American Community. Chicago, IL, Third World Press, 2018

Bell CC: The importance of bent nail research for African American population, in Black Mental Health: Patients, Providers, and Systems. Edited by Griffith EEH, Jones BE, Stewart AJ. Washington DC, American Psychiatric Association Publishing, 2019, pp 257–268

Bell CC, Jenkins EJ: Traumatic stress and children. J Health Care Poor Underserved 2(1):175–185, 1991 1685908

Bell CC, Jenkins EJ: Community violence and children on Chicago's southside. Psychiatry 56(1):46–54, 1993 8488212

Bell CC, Jenkins EJ: Violence prevention and intervention in juvenile detention and correctional facilities. J Correct Health Care 2:17–38, 1995

Bell CC, Flay B, Paikoff R: Strategies for health behavior change, in The Health Behavioral Change Imperative: Theory, Education, and Practice in Diverse Populations, edited by Chunn JC. Boston, Springer, 2002, pp 17–40

Bell CC, Wells SJ, Merritt LM: Integrating cultural competency and empirically based practices in child welfare services: a model based on community psychiatry field principles of health. Child Youth Serv Rev 31:1206–1213, 2009

Douglas KI, Bell CC, Williamson JL: Race and trauma in African American children, in The Psychology of Black Boys and Adolescents. Edited by Vaughans KC, Spielberg W. Santa Barbara, CA, ABC-CLIO, 2014, pp 297–311

Felitti VJ, Anda RF, Nordenberg D, et al: Relationship of childhood abuse and household dysfunction to many of the leading causes of death in adults: the Adverse Childhood Experiences (ACE) Study. Am J Prev Med 14(4):245–258, 1998 9635069

Herman JL: Complex PTSD: a syndrome in survivors of prolonged and repeated trauma. J Trauma Stress 5:377–391, 1992

Hyman LA, Zelikoff W, Clarke J: Psychological and physical abuse in the schools: a paradigm for understanding post-traumatic stress disorder in children and youth. J Trauma Stress 1:243–267, 1988

Jenkins EJ, Bell CC: Violence among inner city high school students and post-traumatic stress disorder, in Anxiety Disorders in African Americans. Edited by Friedman S. New York, Springer, 1994, pp 76–88

Martin A, McMillan A: Concussion killjoys: CTE, violence and the brain's becoming. Biosocieties 17:229–250, 2020

May PA, Chambers CD, Kalberg WO, et al: Prevalence of fetal alcohol spectrum disorders in 4 US communities. JAMA 319(5):474–482, 2018 29411031

Pears K, Fisher PA: Developmental, cognitive, and neuropsychological functioning in preschool-aged foster children: associations with prior maltreatment and placement history. J Dev Behav Pediatr 26(2):112–222, 2005 15827462

Pynoos RS, Nader K: Psychological first aid and treatment approach to children exposed to community violence: research implications. J Trauma Stress 1:445–473, 1988

Shafii M, Shafii SL: School Violence: Assessment, Management, Prevention. Washington, DC, American Psychiatric Publishing, 2008

Stevens KR, Masters KS, Imoukhuede PI, et al: Fund Black scientists. Cell 184(3):561–565, 2021 33503447

Thakur N, Hessler D, Koita K, et al: Pediatrics adverse childhood experiences and related life events screener (PEARLS) and health in a safety-net practice. Child Abuse Negl 108:104685, 2020 32898839

Vaughans KC, Spielberg W: The Psychology of Black Boys and Adolescents. Santa Barbara, CA, ABC-CLIO, 2014

10

Will Advances in Research Address Racial Disparities?

William Lawson, M.D., Ph.D., DLFAPA

Disparities in health outcomes continue to be persistent for African Americans. Mental disorders are no exception. Poorer outcomes are seen compared with white counterparts even when controlling for various socioeconomic factors. Inappropriate diagnostic practices, suboptimal services, and lack of access to treatment account for some of these differences in outcome. Recent advances in diagnosis and treatment have improved diagnostic reliability and accuracy. Advances in behavioral interventions and neuroscience have led to more effective and safer treatments. Various psychological treatments have led to improved outcomes and have made recovery meaningful. Newer pharmacological agents may be more helpful for African Americans because they are better tolerated, produce fewer side effects, and have better efficacy. However, several challenges continue to limit access to these new treatments. They include systemic racism, historical distrust of the medical system, costs, and social policies that address substance use disorders and/or mental illnesses with criminalization or deinstitutionalization without adequate follow-up treatment. Improving access in the context of newer nonpharmacological and pharmacological interventions can improve the outlook for African Americans. New systemic delivery systems, using new treatment modalities, may finally reduce these persistent disparities.

The Diagnostic Dilemma

From the earliest periods in American history, when enslaved Africans were brought to this country, racism had an oversize impact on thinking about mental disorders in African peoples. Such thinking was clearly used to justify subhuman treatment as well as slavery and was broadly extended to all people of color (Schwartz and Blankenship 2014). Mental disorders were particularly vulnerable to political views because even though, at that time, advances were being made for physical disorders, there was no physical test or indicator for mental illness. Causal theories, legislation, and public opinion determined thinking about mental disorders.

On the basis of the zeitgeist of that time, African Americans were thought not to have a sophisticated mental life, if they had any at all. Such thinking, that African Americans were subhuman, easily justified slavery and denial of basic services. African Americans were considered by some to be immune to mental illness because they did not own property, engage in commerce, or participate in civic affairs such as voting or holding public office (Davis 2018). Others believed that certain mental disorders were peculiar to enslaved men and women, including drapetomania, the tendency to run away from slave owners. Samuel Cartwright in 1851 described dysaesthesia aethiopis, which was thought to be a type of mental disorder of biological origin in which afflicted persons exhibited "rascality" and "disrespect for the master's property," for which the cure was severe physical punishment and removal of toes (Metzl 2010), p. 30). The assumptions behind the racial attitudes borne out of slavery, limited mental life, and disorders consistent with the politics of the time continue to determine the diagnosis and treatment of African Americans to the present. Slavery was believed to be justified because of the inferior mental status and childlike behavior of enslaved people. It was thought that without the institution of slavery, or its equivalent, mental disorders would increase. The notorious 1820 census was believed to show that mental disorders were more common among freed slaves than among enslaved people. Up through the twenty-first century, medical professionals commonly believed segregation was justified because the stress of being in an integrated society would lead to mental disorders (Misra et al. 2022).

Long after slavery had ended, African Americans were thought to have limited mental and emotional capacity (Primm and Lawson 2010;

Thomas and Sillen 1972). Depression and other mood disorders were long thought to be rare or nonexistent in African Americans because of either limited mental apparatus or impoverished lives (Adebimpe 1994). If African Americans had mental disorders at all, they were much more likely to be diagnosed with disorders such as psychosis and schizophrenia, while rarely being diagnosed with affective disorders such as depression and bipolar disorder (Adebimpe 1994; Bell and Mehta 1980). In clinical settings, African Americans with clear-cut symptoms of bipolar disorder were diagnosed with schizophrenia (Akinhanmi et al. 2018). Patients with depression, PTSD, and anxiety disorders were either diagnosed with schizophrenia or not diagnosed at all. Because there is no blood test or biological marker for mental disorders, reliable and valid diagnostic systems continue to be a challenge for psychiatry and have increased the likelihood that social beliefs influence diagnostic decisions. Nevertheless, in recent years, diagnostic systems were built on clinical consensus and later modeled after structured instruments. These models were based on advances in behavioral sciences with diagnostic systems developed from empirical observations and biostatistical formulations that have strong reliability and evidence-based validation. Development of successive generations of the various iterations of the *Diagnostic and Statistical Manual of Mental Disorders*, including the most recent version, DSM-5-TR (American Psychiatric Association 2022), have led to progressively more improvements in diagnostic validity and reliability.

Despite advances in diagnostic systems, misdiagnosis of African Americans has continued to persist (Adebimpe 1994; Akinhanmi et al. 2018; Bell and Mehta 1980). The overdiagnosis of schizophrenia is especially disturbing. Schizophrenia has some of the worst outcomes of any mental disorder, and individuals with this disease clearly benefit from early intervention and targeted treatment to prevent increased risk of suicide, violence, joblessness, homeless, or prolonged institutionalization. Misdiagnosis may impede treatment strategies that can directly address illness morbidity and has led to a general recognition that some of the more serious disparities in mental disorders may, in fact, be due to these disparities. African American individuals with bipolar disorder, in comparison to white individuals with bipolar disorder, have been reported to have significantly higher rates of receiving an initial clinical diagnosis other than bipolar disorder (Johnson and Johnson 2014). Misdiagnosis limits the opportunity for treatment with lithium and/or mood-stabilizing anticonvulsants, as well as access to evidence-based psychotherapies for bipolar disorder. In addition to issues related to misdiagnosis, patients who receive correct diagnoses of bipolar disorder are inadequately treated. Thus, morbidity of serious mental illness may be magnified by racial disparities in access to or provision of health care.

As noted previously, African Americans were more likely than the white population to receive a diagnosis of schizophrenia and less likely to be diagnosed with affective disorders in clinical settings. Yet empirical studies have shown that racial differences tend to disappear when structured interviews, which force strict adherence to diagnostic criteria, are used. Large epidemiological studies do not find any diagnostic categories with a higher prevalence among African Americans than other racial or ethnic groups, even when socioeconomic status is controlled (Kessler et al. 1994; Regier et al. 1984). However, clinical reports continue to show overdiagnosis of schizophrenia, usually at the expense of affective disorder (Akinhanmi et al. 2018).

The reasons for the misdiagnosis remain unclear, but reviews suggest information variance (i.e., the quality or type of history and symptoms used), rather than criterion variance (i.e., disagreement about the diagnostic criteria used), among other factors (Haeri et al. 2011; Strakowski et al. 1997). It is not that African Americans have different symptoms or even describe their symptoms differently. It is how providers use the information that they gather. Consistently, clinicians tend to discount affective symptoms (Strakowski et al. 1997). This should not be surprising because there has been a historical precedent to reinforce the idea that African Americans lack feelings or emotions. Ongoing differences in help-seeking behaviors and access to care have meant that African Americans receive treatment later in the course of illness or when the symptoms are more severe, thus increasing the likelihood the illness is more severe and difficult to identify clearly (Primm and Lawson 2010). Also, clinicians disagree about the presentation of symptoms on the basis of race. Many clinicians simply refuse to believe people of color have affective feeling states (Thomas and Sillen 1972).

The Gara multisite study directly addressed the problem of misdiagnosis by carefully evaluating and controlling for various factors that might contribute to misdiagnosis (Gara et al. 2012). As noted, patients with affective disorders often are misdiagnosed as having schizophrenia, perhaps because of differences in symptom presentation, severity of illness, or misinterpretation of symptoms. Moreover, African Americans may present with greater severity of illness due to treatment delay. The focus of the study was to determine if overdiagnosis still occurred after controlling for age, sex, income, site, and education, as well as the presence or absence of serious affective disorder, as determined by experts blinded to race and ethnicity. The data collection included diagnostic data from six sites from four sources: 1) medical records, 2) structured interviews, 3) interview transcripts, and 4) blinded expert consensus. Ethnic cues were deleted from medical records, and these edited records were reviewed to identify the primary psychiatric diagnoses as formulated by treating clinicians, who were psychiatrists. Medical records were blinded to subjects' race and ethnicity to guard against investigator bias. Structured interviews provided the second set of diagnostic data by using the Diagnostic Interview for Genetic Studies (DIGS). A second independent interviewer at each site reviewed the transcripts and unblinded medical records and provided an independent diagnostic assessment and symptom ratings. Editors carefully reviewed each set of medical records and transcripts and removed racial and ethnic cues. Interview text was edited to eliminate references to people, names, and places and linguistic idiosyncrasies, phrasing, or syntax describing personal histories or situations that could cue the diagnostic rater to specific ethnicities. Secondary editors reviewed redacted documents and compared the modified text with the original transcript to ensure both adequate blinding and equivalence of meaning. If there was not agreement, the second editor completed a second level of redaction and then sent the text to a third editor for final approval. The redacted records and transcripts were then distributed to two independent diagnostic experts, who rated symptoms and diagnosis independently and then discussed the case by telephone to achieve a consensus assessment. The experts reviewed diagnostic criteria and the basis for each of their decisions and then discussed disagreements until a consensus could be reached. The fourth source of study data comprised expert consensus diagnoses and ratings.

Despite these careful controls, African American individuals continued to exhibit significantly higher rates of clinical diagnoses of schizophrenia than non-Latinx white subjects, even after controlling for covariates such as serious affective disorder. Improved assessment technology, therefore, did not resolve the diagnostic issue. Overdiagnosis continued to occur despite extensive attempts to control for most factors that contribute to misdiagnosis. These findings also raised the issue that the cultural climate that perpetuates racism has become embedded in the diagnostic process.

It must also be noted that problems occur even when nonaffective disorders are examined. A number of anxiety disorders, including obsessive-compulsive disorder; panic disorder; phobic disorders; and the fear circuitry disorder, PTSD, are often underrecognized or underdiagnosed in African Americans (Alim et al. 2006; Randle et al. 2013). Despite advances in psychometrics, misdiagnosis continues to be an issue.

African Americans with depression and anxiety disorders often receive treatment in primary care settings. Providers in those settings have limited time to address mental health issues, and such issues must compete with the demands of general medical conditions. Opportunities for in-depth diagnosis, assessment, and introduction of new treatments and interventions are far less likely (Primm and Lawson 2010). Our study group and others have noted that patients with major depression, anxiety disorder, bipolar disorder, and PTSD are common in primary care settings (Alim et al. 2006; Graves et al. 2011; Randle et al. 2013). However, these disorders are often unrecognized, and the patients do not typically receive evidence-based care. Additionally, they tend not to be referred to specialized mental health care settings (Alim et al. 2006; Graves et al. 2011). Major depression, bipolar disorder, or frank PTSD are simply not treated (Graves et al. 2011). If African American patients with these disorders are given correct diagnoses, they do not receive optimal treatment or referral to specialized treatment (Gara et al. 2019; Graves et al. 2011; Lawson 1986).

Treatment Outcomes

Racial misdiagnosis often leads to the use of the wrong medications, which in turn can lead to poorer outcomes. As noted in the previous section, African Americans are overdiagnosed with schizophrenia and consequently are more likely to receive antipsychotics when they are not needed and less likely to receive agents such as lithium when they have bipolar disorder (Lawson 1986; Primm and Lawson 2010). They are also less likely to receive antidepressants when they have depressive symptoms (Haeri et al. 2011; Remmert et al. 2022). They are more likely than white patients to receive antipsychotic medication in general. Dosing is more likely to be intermittent, with medication being taken on an as needed basis, more frequent medication interruptions due to poor adherence, or lack of access to regular treatment (Lawson 1986; Randle et al. 2013).

African Americans may require lower doses of a medication yet be prescribed higher doses (Haeri et al. 2011; Lawson 1986). Differences in clinical response and pharmacokinetics have been attributed to ethnic differences in drug metabolism mediated through the cytochrome P450 microsomal enzyme system that is responsible for the metabolism of most psychotropic medication. African Americans may be given excessive medication, especially antipsychotics, for psychosocial reasons that are explored in the section "Treatment Versus Punishment." The pharmacokinetic data therefore do not justify the practice of prescribing excessive dosing.

Ethnic differences have also been reported with lithium (Strickland et al. 1995; Wilson and Grim 1991). The lithium ratio in African Americans has been attributed to the same mechanism that accounts for the increased risk for hypertension in African Americans (Wilson and Grim 1991). The ancestors of today's African Americans had high mortality rates while crossing the Atlantic Ocean when they were originally brought over in slave ships. It has been speculated that many of those deaths were due to hyponatremia. Consequently, the survivors tended to handle sodium differently and were more likely to conserve sodium, which would lead to an increased hypertension risk (Strickland et al. 1995; Wilson and Grim 1991).

Most antipsychotics have been found to show little difference in efficacy. However, the antipsychotic clozapine has consistently been shown to be an exception (Kane et al. 1988). Clozapine is effective in many patients who are unresponsive to treatment with first-generation antipsychotics. It also seems to have minimal extrapyramidal effects and a lower risk for tardive dyskinesia. Unfortunately, clozapine has not been as available to African Americans because of cost, restrictive formularies (Primm and Lawson 2010), and greater risk for agranulocytosis (Mijovic and MacCabe 2020). Regular leukocyte counts are required for clozapine administration, and African Americans are known to have a normal leukocyte count whose range can extend well below listed normal values (i.e., a benign leukopenia). As a result, clozapine is often not prescribed to African Americans because of guidelines that would suggest caution with normal but low white blood cell counts (Dotson et al. 2021). Recent guidelines have attempted to account for these racial differences, but African Americans continue to be less likely to receive clozapine.

Depot or long-acting agents have improved outcomes. This is a benefit for African Americans who are disproportionately in settings with less medication availability. Moreover, atypical antipsychotic agents are now also available in these long-acting forms. Nevertheless, these depot agents are less available for African Americans. Consistent with other treatments, African Americans are less likely to receive the safer atypical agents and less likely to receive the atypical agents that are believed to have better outcomes. African Americans and Hispanics, in particular, are more likely to be on Medicaid. In a study of Medicaid patients, we found that African Americans are less likely to receive atypical agents, including in depot form (Lawson et al. 2015). Medicaid tends to have restrictive formularies, which further limits the availability of new agents even though newer agents may be more cost effective and lead to better clinical outcomes. These findings are significant because only Medicaid patients were used in this study, which controlled for income differences. Income is therefore not the only factor that limits the availability of new treatments. More needs to be done to educate policy makers about assessing total cost of care in determining the cost of including newer agents on formularies.

Treatment Versus Punishment

When compared with whites, African Americans are less likely to have access to mental health care, and Hispanics are more likely to have less care than needed or delayed care (McGuire et al. 2006; Primm and Lawson 2010). African Americans have a significantly lower likelihood of any health care expenditure when compared with whites. African Americans are more likely to have mania, psychosis, and panic disorder, and, along with Hispanics, are less likely to have mental health care coverage compared with whites (McGuire et al. 2006). These findings are especially disturbing because they show that few gains have been made since the surgeon general's report that demonstrated the same results a decade earlier (U.S. Department of Health and Human Services 2001). People of color are far more likely to receive mental health care in the primary care or correctional system, again, related to economic factors (Lawson et al. 1994; Primm and Lawson 2010; U.S. Department of Health and Human Services 2001). Mentally ill African Americans are more likely to be hospitalized and to be involuntarily hospitalized, which works against their willingness to accept treatment. Research shows that prolonged in-hospital stays were counterproductive and that deinstitutionalization would have benefited African Americans (Lawson 1986). However, African Americans, if anything, were more likely to end up in the streets or to be incarcerated (Lawson and Lawson 2013).

A contributing factor is that historically, African Americans were perceived as being more violent than the general population, perhaps in relation to the fear that slaves would attack their oppressive masters (Davis 2018; Thomas and Sillen 1972). Studies show that African Americans are sentenced more harshly than whites. They are 2.17 times more likely to be arrested than white people, 3.5 times more likely to be incarcerated in jail, and nearly 5 times more likely to be incarcerated in prison nationwide, which is likely related to the legacy of perceived dangerousness (Bassett and Graves 2018; Mitchell 2005). We reported that staff on the psychiatric ward consistently perceived African Americans to be more violent (Lawson and Lawson 2013).

The perception of mentally ill African Americans being more violent may have affected the perception of African Americans and schizophrenia. *The Protest Psychosis: How Schizophrenia Became a Black Disease* provides a historical exploration of the means by which schizophrenia became associated with the perceived hostility, rebellion, mistrust, and violence of Black men during the civil rights movement (Metzl 2010). Once considered a nonthreatening disease that targeted primarily white middle-class female populations, schizophrenia, particularly among African American patients, has come to be perceived as especially dangerous. Thus, advances in care can be overcome by the politics of the time.

The AIDS epidemic, which began in the 1980s, also exacerbated existing health disparities among vulnerable populations. This epidemic was associated with racial disparities in outcomes and access to treatment. Recently, the world experienced a pandemic of COVID-19, a novel virus that mutates quickly and spreads easily. African Americans were more likely to be hospitalized and to have higher mortality rates from COVID-19. The AIDS epidemic and the COVID-19 pandemic asymmetrically affected low-income neighborhoods where Black people, Hispanics, and older adults disproportionately face negative health outcomes and experience comorbidities that increase their risk for COVID-19 (Kakolyris et al. 2021). The issues noted earlier, including access to care for mental disorders, have made the impact of the pandemic worse. Moreover, COVID-19 treatment and effective vaccines are less available for African Americans, just as new treatments for mental disorders are not as available. Therefore, larger concerns of access to health care transcend disease state and demonstrate that the historical consequences of racism are very much still present.

Potential Impact of Technology

Innovative technology has improved mental health care, but a barrier to any new technological advance is the willingness of the population to accept it, and African Americans have been slow to accept new health care approaches. African American patients are not as willing to accept psychotropic medication. Moreover, there is an unwillingness to accept nonpharmacological approaches such as electroconvulsive therapy (Lawson 1986; Primm and Lawson 2010). Part of this difficulty in accepting treatment modalities has been the medical mistrust that developed as a result of past research involving African Americans, such as the Tuskegee syphilis study (Alsan et al. 2020). Our group has found that although African Americans may willingly participate in clinical trials, they are more likely to believe that such studies will have unfavorable consequences for them (Nwulia et al. 2011). The good news is that rating scales and other technologies can improve recognition and treatment outcomes (Randle et al. 2013). Unfortunately, it is common that academic and research centers either do not use these advances or disregard the results because of their overall work demands.

The COVID-19 pandemic popularized digital technologies, which are especially useful in psychiatry, where direct patient contact is often unnecessary. Use of medical treatment with digital technologies can ameliorate the effect of the pandemic, including racial disparities (Kakolyris et al. 2021). Technology can address disparities in care, especially when it is used to identify why communities are at a disadvantage and the factors distressing the communities. Understanding epidemiological and socioeconomic conditions that foster the high rates of morbidity and mortality across race/ethnicity and geographical areas could help policy makers manage the impacts of mental disorders. This can provide a way to address ongoing issues in mental health such as the increase in suicide, homicide, and drug overdoses. The challenge is to get these technologies to people of color and improve acceptance of novel approaches and to do so despite the economic factors that promote disparities.

References

Adebimpe VR: Race, racism, and epidemiological surveys. Hosp Community Psychiatry 45(1):27–31, 1994 8125456

Akinhanmi MO, Biernacka JM, Strakowski SM, et al: Racial disparities in bipolar disorder treatment and research: a call to action. Bipolar Disord 20(6):506–514, 2018 29527766

Alim TN, Graves E, Mellman TA, et al: Trauma exposure, posttraumatic stress disorder and depression in an African-American primary care population. J Natl Med Assoc 98(10):1630–1636, 2006 17052054

Alsan M, Wanamaker M, Hardeman RR: The Tuskegee Study of Untreated Syphilis: a case study in peripheral trauma with implications for health professionals. J Gen Intern Med 35(1):322–325, 2020 31646456

American Psychiatric Association: Diagnostic and Statistical Manual of Mental Disorders, 5th Edition, Text Revision. Washington, DC, American Psychiatric Association, 2022

Bassett MT, Graves JD: Uprooting institutionalized racism as public health practice. Am J Public Health 108(4):457–458, 2018 29513591

Bell CC, Mehta H: The misdiagnosis of Black patients with manic depressive illness. J Natl Med Assoc 72(2):141–145, 1980 7365814

Davis K: Blacks are immune from mental illness. Psychiatr News, May 1, 2018. Available at: https://psychnews.psychiatryonline.org/doi/10.1176/appi.pn.2018.5a18. Accessed March 5, 2023.

Dotson S, Shtasel D, Freudenreich O: Race-based medicine, clozapine, and benign (ethnic) neutropenia: a call for nuance. Psychiatr Serv 72(2):232–233, 2021 33517696

Gara MA, Vega WA, Arndt S, et al: Influence of patient race and ethnicity on clinical assessment in patients with affective disorders. Arch Gen Psychiatry 69(6):593–600, 2012 22309972

Gara MA, Minsky S, Silverstein SM, et al: A naturalistic study of racial disparities in diagnoses at an outpatient behavioral health clinic. Psychiatr Serv 70(2):130–134, 2019 30526340

Graves RE, Freedy JR, Aigbogun NU, et al: PTSD treatment of African American adults in primary care: the gap between current practice and evidence-based treatment guidelines. J Natl Med Assoc 103(7):585–593, 2011 21999033

Haeri S, Williams J, Kopeykina I, et al: Disparities in diagnosis of bipolar disorder in individuals of African and European descent: a review. J Psychiatr Pract 17(6):394–403, 2011 22108396

Johnson KR, Johnson SL: Inadequate treatment of Black Americans with bipolar disorder. Psychiatr Serv 65(2):255–258, 2014 24492903

Kakolyris A, DelaCruz JJ, Giannikos CI: COVID-19, race/ethnicity, and age: the role of telemedicine to close the gaps on health disparities. J Econ Race Policy Aug 26:1–11, 2021 35300311

Kane J, Honigfeld G, Singer J, Meltzer H; The Clozaril Collaborative Study Group: Clozapine for the treatment-resistant schizophrenic: a double-blind comparison with chlorpromazine. Arch Gen Psychiatry 45(9):789–796, 1988 3046553

Kessler RC, McGonagle KA, Zhao S, et al: Lifetime and 12-month prevalence of DSM-III-R psychiatric disorders in the United States: results from the National Comorbidity Survey. Arch Gen Psychiatry 51(1):8–19, 1994 8279933

Lawson WB: Racial and ethnic factors in psychiatric research. Hosp Community Psychiatry 37(1):50–54, 1986 2867967

Lawson WB, Lawson AA: Disparities in mental health diagnosis and treatment among African Americans: implications for the correctional system, in Crime, HIV and Health: Intersections of Criminal Justice and Public Health Concerns. Edited by Sanders B, Thomas YF, Deeds BG. Springer, New York, 2013, pp 81–91

Lawson WB, Hepler N, Holladay J, Cuffel B: Race as a factor in inpatient and outpatient admissions and diagnosis. Hosp Community Psychiatry 45(1):72–74, 1994 8125467

Lawson W, Johnston S, Karson C, et al: Racial differences in antipsychotic use: claims database analysis of Medicaid-insured patients with schizophrenia. Ann Clin Psychiatry 27(4):242–252, 2015 26554365

McGuire TG, Alegria M, Cook BL, et al: Implementing the Institute of Medicine definition of disparities: an application to mental health care. Health Serv Res 41(5):1979–2005, 2006 16987312

Metzl J: The Protest Psychosis: How Schizophrenia Became a Black Disease. Boston, MA, Beacon Press, 2010

Mijovic A, MacCabe JH: Clozapine-induced agranulocytosis. Ann Hematol 99(11):2477–2482, 2020 32815018

Misra S, Etkins OS, Yang LH, Williams DR: Structural racism and inequities in incidence, course of illness, and treatment of psychotic disorders among Black Americans. Am J Public Health 112(4):624–632, 2022 35319958

Mitchell O: A meta-analysis of race and sentencing research: explaining the inconsistencies. J Quant Criminol 21:439–466, 2005

Nwulia EA, Hipolito MM, Aamir S, et al; BiGS Consortium: Ethnic disparities in the perception of ethical risks from psychiatric genetic studies. Am J Med Genet B Neuropsychiatr Genet 156B(5):569–580, 2011 21595007

Primm AB, Lawson WB: Disparities among ethnic groups: African Americans, in Disparities in Psychiatric Care: Clinical and Cross-Cultural Perspectives. Edited by Ruiz P, Primm A. Baltimore, MD, Wolters Kluwer, 2010, pp 19–29

Randle AC, Spurlock AL, Kelley S: Depression screening among African American adults in the primary care setting. J Health Care Poor Underserved 24(40):79–93, 2013

Regier DA, Myers JK, Kramer M, et al: The NIMH Epidemiologic Catchment Area program: historical context, major objectives, and study population characteristics. Arch Gen Psychiatry 41(10):934–941, 1984 6089692

Remmert JE, Guzman G, Mavandadi S, Oslin D: Racial disparities in prescription of antidepressants among U.S. veterans referred to behavioral health. Psychiatr Serv 73(9):984–990, 2022 35414191

Schwartz RC, Blankenship DM: Racial disparities in psychotic disorder diagnosis: a review of empirical literature. World J Psychiatry 4(4):133–140, 2014 25540728

Strakowski SM, Hawkins JM, Keck PE Jr, et al: The effects of race and information variance on disagreement between psychiatric emergency service and research diagnoses in first-episode psychosis. J Clin Psychiatry 58(10):457–463, quiz 464–465, 1997 9375599

Strickland TL, Lin KM, Fu P, et al: Comparison of lithium ratio between African-American and Caucasian bipolar patients. Biol Psychiatry 37(5):325–330, 1995 7748984

Thomas A, Sillen S: Racism and Psychiatry. New York, Brunner Mazel, 1972

U.S. Department of Health and Human Services: Mental Health: Culture, Race, and Ethnicity—A Supplement to Mental Health: A Report of the Surgeon General. Rockville, MD, Substance Abuse and Mental Health Services Administration, 2001

Wilson TW, Grim CE: Biohistory of slavery and blood pressure differences in Blacks today: a hypothesis. Hypertension 17(1)(suppl):I122–I128, 1991 1986989

11

Identities at the Intersections of Race, Gender, and Mental Illness

REMEMBERING CHESTER PIERCE

Pamela Y. Collins, M.D., M.P.H.
Nicola Park, M.D.

Professor Chester Pierce delivered the Solomon Carter Fuller lecture in May 1986 in Washington, D.C., at the annual meeting of the American Psychiatric Association. His remarks spoke to the theme of the meeting, "Unity in Diversity," as he framed critical challenges that Black people, and Black professionals specifically, continually confront because of racism. The ongoing stress for Black people, he posited, is to "...make sense of the diversity that being Black, and thereby marginalized, brings with it in all interactions with the general society" (Pierce 1989, 298). This diversity of interactions with society, for Black people in the United States, includes managing outsider experiences or leading in welcoming and supportive situations and in situations in which one's competency is doubted (Pierce 1989). Pierce asserted that the *incessant struggle* for Black people is determining "how and when do we accommodate to racism versus how and when do we resist racism?" (Pierce 1989, p. 296). The *constant problem* is "how and when do we seek assimilation into the total society versus when and how do we insist on separation from the total society?" (Pierce 1989, p. 296). Directing his remarks to Black psychiatrists, he surmised that the *central developmental* task is to manage marginality and fractionation in professional life (Pierce 1989). Pierce believed that one can combat racism and contribute meaningfully to society by distilling and synthesizing the lessons learned through a diversity of professional activities that are often necessary by virtue of being Black, ensuring that those activities have meaning and impact. He emphasized that managing these tasks, which is crucial for navigating the world in a racialized society, consumes time and effort and is itself a source of stress (Pierce 1989). Pierce, an exceptionally accomplished academic, acknowledged the pain and stress of racism that most members of a stigmatized racial group experience, himself included. He expertly drew from personal social and professional experience to generate new concepts that explain these fundamentally human experiences.

In this chapter, we examine Pierce's contributions to our thinking about social stressors associated with racism and sexism and their influence on the mental health of Black people in the United States and globally. We examine the perspectives of Black psychiatrists who participated in Pierce's 2002 convening, The African Diaspora: Psychiatric Issues, and we link the priorities raised by this group to the evolution of the current field of global mental health in subsequent years.

Who Was Chester Pierce?

HISTORICAL CONTEXT IN THE UNITED STATES

In the decades before and after Pierce's birth, the United States was in the throes of a new dynamism with respect to race relations. The Great Migration, the largest movement of humans in the country's history, was well under way as Black people living in the South sought greater freedoms, equity, and economic opportunities in the North. They fled the enduring institutional and cultural racism of the South and the heinous crimes visited on Black communities and discovered that racism thrived in the North as well. The 1920s witnessed the Ocoee massacre, a white mob's murder of about 50 Black people in Ocoee, Florida, after a Black citizen enforced his right to vote. Riots also occurred in the North as the new migrants arrived and racial tensions arose (Momodu 2020). The Chester, Pennsylvania, race riot of 1917 was a symptom of these tensions around the arrival of Black laborers (Mack 2017; Smith 2008). A confrontation among Black residents and a white man that resulted in the death of the white man sparked a 6-day period of violence. Racism pervaded everything, even the responses to crises such as natural disasters. The 1928 Okeechobee hurricane, the first recorded Category 5 storm in the United States, devastated the city of West Palm Beach, Florida (Alexander 2021; Bullard 2008). The deadly storm disproportionately struck Black farmworking and sharecropping communities. An estimated 1,800 to 4,000 people died, 75% of whom were Black. More tragedy followed in the recovery phase as Black survivors entered contaminated water to secure the bodies of friends and family members and were restricted by white landowners in where they could bury their dead.

A BRIEF BIOGRAPHY

Chester Pierce was born in 1927 in Glen Cove, New York, a small town, population 8,000, on Long Island, New York (Griffith 2023). The second of three boys born to Samuel and Hettie Pierce, he was raised in a loving and economically successful family. Consistent with opportunities of the era, his father, an employee at the local country club, specialized in shoe shining. Samuel Pierce was a socially savvy entrepreneur. He studied the wealthy white people in his workplace, marketed his skills as a master restorer of white leather shoes, invested in the stock market, purchased property in Manhattan, and saved for his sons' education. Pierce's childhood and youth were notable for a fertile family environment that enabled him to thrive emotionally and intellectually. Samuel and Hettie Pierce encouraged their sons to envision their futures with "undisguised hope" and explicitly coached them to live wisely "with wily understanding" in a world where opportunities were shaped by racial inequities (Griffith 2023).

Pierce entered Harvard College in 1944 and began his journey to a medical career in 1948 at Harvard Medical School (Griffith 2023). After graduation, he trained in psychiatry at the University of Cincinnati and subsequently joined the faculty there. After formative experiences in Cincinnati, he was drafted in 1954 to serve in the U.S. Navy at the Great Lakes Naval Base. There, his clinical activities provided a rich source of questions that stimulated his intellectual curiosity and launched his research career. By 1968, after several years in a faculty position at the University of Oklahoma, Pierce returned to Harvard as an Alfred North Whitehead fellow in the School of Education and eventually joined the faculty there. He remained at Harvard for the rest of his career. Pierce had an exceptional career, serving as founding president of the Black Psychiatrists of America and in advisory roles for the Peace Corps, the Children's Television Workshop, and the U.S. Arctic Research Commission, to name a few (Organ 2002). Accompanying his professional successes, Pierce was continually aware of his outsider status as a Black man (Pierce 1989).

Chester Pierce's Legacy: Highlights of a Career

The 1986 Solomon Carter Fuller lecture hinted at the breadth of scholarly activities that marked Pierce's life. What he called *fractionation* alludes to a career notable for a diverse set of activities that took him from Ohio to Oklahoma to Antarctica and beyond as a researcher and educator. A common thread linking his studies of extreme environments, high-performing athletes, and enuretic servicemen was performance in stressful circumstances (Pierce 1989). When reflecting on the breadth of his activities, he linked his career trajectory to his race, noting that part of the fractionation he experienced due to involvement in so many distinct projects was related to his attempts to reduce stressful circumstances in daily life. His motivation to "travel great distances in time and space, both literally and figuratively" was a means of discovering how to reduce his stress (Pierce 1989, p. 300) as a professional of color by placing himself in situations that he could enjoy and in which he could manage power dynamics to his satisfaction. In the lecture, he explains the ultimate unifying theme in the diversity of his work: "...wherever I went, whatever I did, and with whomever I worked, my never-ending preoccupation had to be on how to survive as a Black [man]" (Pierce 1989, p. 301). From his experiences as a researcher, educator, administrator, and clinician, he extracted lessons related particularly to the stress associated with incidents of racism, which he equated with extreme stressors of torture and terror (Pierce 1995). In this section, we highlight two strands of his thinking about racism and stress: microaggressions and the similarities among racism, sexism, torture, and terrorism.

MICROAGGRESSIONS

In the latter part of the Solomon Carter Fuller lecture, Pierce discussed concepts of oppression and its operation (Pierce 1995). In 1970, he coined the term *microaggressions* and introduced the concept using the language of psychodynamics (Pierce 1970). *Defensive* mechanisms, he noted, were a central strategy to manage anxiety and were well studied in psychodynamic psychiatry, yet psychiatry did not consider how *offensive* mechanisms operated in society (Pierce 1970). The offenses that arose from feelings of superiority, condescension, and contempt for Black people served as often subtle microaggressive actions (Pierce 1970). Pierce emphasized that to understand public health threats such as racism, social psychiatry and public health were needed to understand the offensive behaviors required to sustain that threat. He wrote, "For racism to be so witheringly effective, strong offensive maneuvers are mandatory" (Pierce 1970, p. 266).

Building on Pierce's conceptualization of microaggressions, researchers later linked microaggressions to the concept of *everyday racism*, that is, routine and chronic incidents of discrimination (Williams et al. 2021). These acts of aggression include overgeneralizations about people of a particular race (e.g., "Black people are good dancers") and any number of behaviors that humiliate or ignore people of a particular race or imply dangerousness (Williams 2020). Despite their sometimes subtle presentation, microaggressions are indeed forms of aggression that are harmful because of their association with stress, anxiety, depression, posttraumatic stress symptoms, low self-esteem, substance use, severe psychological distress, and suicide (Williams 2020). They indicate that an environment is unsafe and, as a chronic stressor, can also lead to hypertension and impaired immunity (Williams 2020).

Pierce described microaggressions as "basic in keeping any Black donating to the quality and perhaps the quantity of life for any White at the expense of the Black's own quality and quantity of life" (Pierce 1989, p. 308). Throughout his writings, he underscored the emotionally challenging and time-consuming effort required to resist racism. The cognitive task, Pierce wrote, of "gauging, titrating, regulating, and expressing appropriate, safe outrage" generated stress for the survivor, who spent a lifetime exposed to microaggressions and the attendant stress of managing racist assaults (Pierce 1989, p. 306).

RACISM, SEXISM, AND DEVALUED IDENTITIES AS SOURCES OF STRESS

Pierce drew parallels between experiences of racism, sexism, torture, terror(ism), and disaster. All involve a relationship between oppressor and oppressed. They evoke similar responses among survivors facing ongoing threat: 1) a requirement to face the stressor with hope and goodwill; 2) a profound need for support—social, emotional, financial, or otherwise—to withstand the stress; and 3) the development of a defensive thinking and continual appraisal of circumstances that keep the oppressed person(s) preoccupied with avoiding danger and less free to think generatively and creatively (Pierce 1995). The sometimes sudden and terrible outcomes of oppression, such as domestic violence, unemployment, or environmental loss (e.g., loss or degradation of land), are disasters because of the magnitude of their impact on individuals and families and the need they create for relief and assistance (Pierce 1995). All, in Pierce's mind, were tied to violence because of their painful, oppressive, dehumanizing, and offensive nature.

Pierce applied both psychodynamic and public health frameworks to understand the interpersonal conflicts that drive the behaviors of oppressor and oppressed and the routes to effective response, respectively. From the psychodynamic perspective, he explained that oppressor and oppressed are locked in conflicts around *entitlement dysfunctions* (Pierce 1978, 1995). Perceived entitlements could include a school system's assumed right to exclude provision of full employment benefits to individuals on the basis of their race and the Black teachers' assumed right to receive equal benefits due them as employees, taxpayers, and citizens. Pierce defined entitlement dysfunctions as "conflicts, real or imagined, microscopic or macroscopic, in which interpersonal confrontation about prestige/status are more salient and expressive than frustrations or obstacles over sex, dependency or aggressions" (Pierce 1978, p. 284, 1995). These entitlements involve each group's (oppressor and oppressed) distinct perceptions of their "rights, duties, privileges or obligations." Typically, entitlement dysfunctions concern which party has the power—"coercive or regulatory hegemony"—in the issue being considered (Pierce 1978, p. 284, 1995). In the context of racism, these conflicts, Pierce explained, usually involve perceived disrespect, "undignified use, misuse or abuse of someone's time, space, freedom of movement or energy" (Pierce 1978, p. 284). Pierce viewed the elimination of these dysfunctions as a challenge for psychiatrists to address as they relate to racism and, more generally, to conflicts in urban life (Pierce 1978).

Pierce underscored the atrociousness of racism and sexism by outlining their proximity to torture and terror. Terrorists and torturers aim to create physical and psychological distress. They seek to control the media and communication channels that influence public perception of their activities in similar ways that racist ideas are propagated. Pierce noted that

> if every textbook, statue, billboard, magazine and newspaper ad, television program, radio newscast and civic ritual reinforces a message, it will be seen as typical, desirable, and probable. There will be little tendency to resist it, and everyone might be persuaded and indoctrinated to its reasonableness and appropriateness. (Pierce 1995, p. 286)

Like racist actors, terrorists and torturers are loyal to a cause, and the loyalty can arise by making ordinary people feel like elites who are superior to a group being systematically dehumanized (Pierce 1995). Changing this situation, Pierce believed, requires persuading the ordinary oppressor that relinquishing privilege is in their best interest.

Finally, by recognizing racism and sexism as public health challenges as Pierce (1995) insisted, a public health approach to understanding them requires asking the following: Who are the offenders and the offended? When does the offense occur? How does it occur? What are the appropriate responses? Answering these questions through Pierce's interest in the broader landscape of global health provides a rich opportunity for learning.

Global Psychiatry and the 2002 African Diaspora Meeting

Pierce's concluding thoughts in the Solomon Carter Fuller lecture included a call to serve the international community: "another opportunity to bring unity out of diversity would be for us to initiate more strong actions to bring our skill and education to other areas, even while we extend our resources to alleviate conditions in the U.S.A." (Pierce 1989, p. 310). By 1986, Pierce had long been a globally oriented scholar. Over the subsequent 15 years, as a professor in the Department of Psychiatry at Massachusetts General Hospital, he would operationalize his vision for global engagement of Black psychiatrists around shared population mental health concerns by convening The African Diaspora: Psychiatric Issues in 2002 (Organ 2002).

I (P.Y.C.) met Chester Pierce in Boston in 1999 while a fellow in the Department of Social Medicine at Harvard. My own career in what is now called *global mental health* had launched 5 years earlier. In 2002, Dr. Pierce invited me to serve as the U.S. delegate for the African Diaspora meeting, which he introduced as an event that would bring together representatives from 19 countries where Black people resided to discuss the commonalities and differences among the drivers of poor mental health.

I traveled to Boston in November 2002. After checking into my hotel, I held the elevator door for a man also staying in the hotel. He asked me what had brought me to Boston, and I explained that I was attending a meeting focused on mental health of the African Diaspora. He quickly told me that he was African, shook his head, and sighed, "My mother died of stress." He shared a snapshot of his early life and the heroic role his mother played in providing for him and the family. She was a woman merchant who traveled daily to market to sell vegetables and other goods on which the family subsisted. He witnessed his mother's exhaustion regularly, and he remembered his hunger and their frequent dependence on her siblings for food. The man's linking of his mother's mental health to her social circumstances and ultimately to her death foreshadowed themes that I and others would raise during the meeting.

Over the course of 5 days, 19 delegate psychiatrists from North, Central, and South America; the Caribbean; Africa; the South Pacific; and the United Kingdom presented richly detailed synopses of the leading challenges to mental health for Black communities in their countries in the company of dozens of additional participants from the community of Black psychiatry and social psychiatry in the United States. As noted in the proceedings (Organ 2002), two consistent topics arose across the presentations:

1. The need to diagnose and treat the insidious and destructive role that racism, through its local and global manifestations, continues to have on the mental health and well-being of people of African descent
2. The pervasive need for relevant and accurate evidence-based, empirical research and clinical intervention projects related to the mental health issues of people of African descent

Overarching Themes

COLONIALISM

The reflections of conference delegates on colonialism, racism, discrimination, and stigma in 2002 mirrored the impassioned discourse around similar themes in 2022. At the time of this writing in 2022, several factors had intensified discussions of racism in the United States and stimulated debate on decolonizing global health: the COVID-19 pandemic and its inequities in infections and deaths that disproportionately affected Black, Indigenous, and people of color; police violence against Black communities; and unequal access to vaccines that disadvantaged populations in Africa, Asia, and Latin America.

Conference delegates in 2002, however, provided firsthand accounts of the damaging effects of colonialism and its aftermath: unstable political systems that evolved from tensions between privileged groups under colonial rule and other groups seeking power (Organ 2002, p. 29), as well as destabilized cultural identities that colonialism effected (Organ 2002). In describing the religious heritage of Nigeria's people, Professor Oye Gureje noted that colonialism "left them in a psychological limbo:

unsure of where they are and uncomfortable with where they have come from" (Gureje et al. 2020, p. 29). Dr. Mohamed Zitouni described colonialism as the root of common mental health conditions in Morocco because it imposed a traumatizing "life between two worlds." He described the discordance of this life:

> The child, from the start, has the alternative of being born to fulfill his life, or to stray towards survival living a lesser life, in short, to accept himself as an inferior being, a lesser being, different from the masters, the colonizers. Such was the case of our coming into existence in North Africa.... [School] was a place of exile. Everything was different...I have used the words psychic trauma, exile and migration, because going to school threw us into a new, different, strange and threatening world, that was also compelling and even fascinating. And when one is fascinated one doesn't see anything for what it really is. (Zitouni 2002, pp. 71–72)

Professor Frederick Hickling's Jamaican psychohistoriography applied political and historical analysis of 500 years of European conquest and colonial rule. Using this method, he employed group psychodynamic principles to examine history in terms of events serving the interests of Black people and white people. Hickling concluded that racism was a persistent psychopathology observed among Europeans that drove the colonial project and the enslavement of Black people (Hickling 2019, 2002).

Black identities could also be protected and strengthened. Senegalese psychiatrist Omar Ndote viewed African cultural history as the dynamic and empowering antidote to the assaults of colonization and slavery. Africans had found strength through the ages in the "myths, gods, rhythms and values" of their cultural heritage whether on the continent or dispersed in diaspora (Organ 2002). Professor August Conceiçao's account of Brazilian communities in the northeastern city of Salvador, Bahia, expanded on the theme of community rejuvenation through reclaiming space for cultural heritage. Conceiçao reported on successful efforts in the preceding years to recover space for festivals, art, and other expressions of Black culture that provided sources of racial identity and economic activity.

RACISM, DISCRIMINATION, AND STIGMA

For Black Diaspora communities in the United Kingdom and the United States, racism and discrimination influenced life chances in most domains: infant mortality, education, economic stability, and criminal justice involvement (Hackett et al. 2020; Organ 2002; Williams et al. 2019).

As the U.S. delegate, I highlighted the implications for African Americans of membership in a stigmatized racial group, focusing on the concept of stigma. The process of stigma occurs when groups are labeled, stereotyped, separated, and demoted in status and when social forces are mobilized to create and maintain power over the identified group (Link and Phelan 2001). Broader in scope than racism alone, the concept of stigma captures multiple statuses or identities that a person can hold concurrently (Hatzenbuehler et al. 2013). A Black woman who is an undocumented immigrant likely experiences a distinct set of discriminatory behaviors that occur because of her race, sex, and legal status.

Black feminist theorists have explained how systems of oppression related to gender, class, race/ethnicity, and sexuality interact (Combahee River Collective 2002; Collins 2000; Lorde 1984), and Crenshaw's concept of intersectionality explains these complex systems of identities and oppressions (Collins et al. 2008b; Crenshaw 1991; Stewart and McDermott 2004). Intersectionality proposes that "people must be located in terms of social structures that capture the power relations implied by those structures" (Stewart and McDermott 2004, p. 532). The concept presumes that systems of power and oppression (which create differences along the axes of race, class, gender, and sexuality) are interlocking, and their effects can be explored only by taking all of these dimensions into account without prioritizing one form of oppression over another (Collins 1999).

These concepts have special relevance to health outcomes when mental illness is added to the systems of identity or oppression. Black people in the United States are more likely than white people to die in police encounters, and additional risks lie at the junction of mental illness, Black race, and law enforcement encounters (Jordan et al. 2021). Stigma processes and racism influence diagnostic accuracy for Black people and their subsequent trajectories of care. The criminalization of mental illness in communities already exposed to violence further traumatizes these communities, and the policing of these same communities more often ends in injury or death (Jordan et al. 2021). Male gender adds another dimension of risk of death. One cannot accurately assess the risk of dangerous outcomes without considering intersectionality.

Similarly, several delegates (United States, Uganda, Belize) at the conference raised the issue of the risk for HIV, which disproportionately affects Black populations globally. An intersectional approach to social stigma is useful for understanding this risk. For example, an unemployed Black woman with schizophrenia who immigrates to the United States from Cuba distinctly navigates the intersecting influences of poverty and the offenses of racism, sexism, and discrimination due to her diagnosis and symptoms of illness. Her employment, neighborhood, and housing options are shaped by these identities, as are her opportunities for relationships and her risk of exposure to HIV infection (Collins et al. 2008b). Furthermore, certain experiences of stigma related to mental illness and discrimination can be linked to HIV risk (Collins et al. 2008a). In a multiracial and multiethnic sample of women with mental illnesses, personal experiences of stigma attached to mental illness were associated with using substances before or during sex (Collins et al. 2008a). Experiences of discrimination associated with skin color, ethnicity, language, drug use, gender, sexual orientation, and other identities were linked to having a casual or exchange sex partner (Collins et al. 2008a).

Pierce noted that for victims of racism and sexism, as for people managing discrimination associated with having a severe mental illness, the relative lack of support defines the degree of stress they experience (Pierce 1995). Receiving needed support minimizes distress, and although maintaining access to adequate support and protection against racism and sexism requires persistent effort, it is essential (Pierce 1995). A robust social network is one feature associated with stigma resistance (i.e., the ability to counteract stigma) among people with schizophrenia (Sibitz et al. 2011).

What Is Global Mental Health?

Since the convening of psychiatrists of the African Diaspora 20 years ago, the field of global mental health has grown and evolved, redefining itself and raising the visibility of mental health as an integral part of global health. The shift had already begun by the time of the meeting. The 1990 Global Burden of Disease Study called attention to mental disorders as leading causes of disability around the world and more generally raised the issue of disability as the growing source of disease burden in future years (World Bank 1993). In 2001, the World Health Organization published the first World Health Report that focused on mental health (World Health Organization 2001). Its 10 recommendations included priorities that persist today, among them providing treatment in primary care; giving care in the community; involving communities, families, and consumers; linking with other sectors; and supporting more research (World Health Organization 2001). Six years later, the 2007 *Lancet* Series on Global Mental Health's galvanizing call to scale up mental health services globally (Chisholm et al. 2007), but especially in low- and middle-income countries, spurred a community of researchers, advocates, and funders to respond.

The *Lancet* series also echoed the second overarching theme of the 2002 Diaspora meeting: a call for more research and research investment. By 2009, the National Institute of Mental Health (NIMH) had committed to a larger role in global health and recruited new leadership to stimulate domestic and international research to reduce health inequities (Collins and Pringle 2016). I (P.Y.C.) joined NIMH to direct these efforts, and in 2010 we created the Office for Research on Disparities and Global Mental Health (ORDGMH), recognizing that globalization furthers new relationships and interconnectedness among people and nations (Pringle et al. 2019). The diversity of the United States is, in part, a reflection of global population shifts; consequently, any serious examination of mechanisms of and responses to mental health disparities cannot be limited to science within one country (Pringle et al. 2019). At the ORDGMH, we recognized that one route to mental health equity globally is through quality mental health research, and we developed initiatives that directly funded African investigators and institutions as well as researchers in Asia and Latin America and their regional collaborators. We created opportunities for building research capacity in settings previously underrepresented in National Institutes of Health research portfolios (Collins and Pringle 2016; da Silva et al. 2019; Pilowsky et al. 2016) and used these mechanisms to support mental health services research and implementation science (Rahman et al. 2020). The increased investment in mental health research in low- and middle-income countries from NIMH and other funders led to an expanded evidence base on effective interventions now being implemented in diverse sociocultural settings (Chibanda et al. 2016; Collins 2020).

Global diversity in mental health research is also needed for meaningful progress in the search for etiologies of mental illness. Recent African studies of the genetics of schizophrenia and bipolar disorders respond to the predominance of Northern European data in this area of research (Gulsuner et al. 2020; Martin et al. 2021). More is necessary: greater resources for research and capacity building provide opportunities for diverse ethnic and cultural populations to contribute to the evidence base and shape research questions and approaches, thereby increasing the likelihood that research outcomes will be of relevance to all of us (Collins 2020).

Although many efforts in global mental health have sought to address severe inequities by focusing on countries defined as low or middle income, global by definition includes the challenges faced by high-income countries as well (Collins et al. 2011). In fact, low-income and high-income settings exist within most countries. *Global* pertains to issues that affect multiple countries (e.g., shared determinants of health) and communicates the value of collaborative learning across countries and economies (Collins 2020). Such shared determinants of health include insufficient investment in mental health care, inadequate attention to prevention and treatment of mental disorders, and scarce human resources and, consequently, limited access and quality of care (Collins 2020). Equally important are upstream social determinants of mental health such as racism and other forms of discrimination, gender inequality, poverty, unplanned rapid urbanization, global economic downturns, forced migration, and complex humanitarian emergencies due to natural disasters and conflicts (Collins 2020). Neglect of quality education, investment in early child development, and safe and affordable housing is widespread around the world and ultimately affects mental health and well-being (Collins 2020). Said another way, "the global in global health refers to the scope of the problems, not their location" (Koplan et al. 2009, p. 1994).

To ensure that resources, leadership, and priorities match the needs of populations, the field of global health (and global mental health) continues to reckon with the power dynamics inherent in international relationships founded on colonial legacies and contemporary economic relationships (Collins 2020; Weine et al. 2020). Pierce recognized the danger of these power imbalances and complained that institutional racism and sexism lead to some fundamental problems: rarely is the viewpoint of the person with the stigmatized identity the focus of research; generally, the dominant group is the "gatekeeper and arbiter of what is published or taught, as well as when, where, and how it is published or taught" (Pierce 1995, p. 286). Addressing these persisting inequities must become more explicit.

Equity in mental health outcomes is more likely to occur with greater investments in the design and testing of interventions that tackle social problems (Burgess et al. 2020). Letting communities lead in identifying these priorities and integrating service users into the design of solutions could be features of these interventions (Burgess et al. 2020; Collins 2020).

Equity in the generation of global mental health evidence requires listening to, learning from, and responding to cultural perspectives in every setting (McKenzie 2019). Delegates from the African Diaspora meeting emphasized the need for a cultural psychiatry that values African cultural legacies. Although a growing body of new mental health services and epidemiological research examines healing and treatment approaches that integrate traditional African practices (Arias et al. 2016; Ayinde et al. 2021; Gureje et al. 2020; Nortje et al. 2016; Ojagbemi and Gureje 2020; van der Watt et al. 2017), a comprehensive treatment of African culture and mental health is needed. The Africa Global Mental Health Institute, the organization founded to fully realize Pierce's vision, could play a central role in further developing this body of knowledge.

Research examining cultural practices is not limited to religious or ritualistic practices, however. Even widely experienced movements in mental health service reform, such as deinstitutionalization, provide context-specific lessons about using political opportunities for advances in mental health (Collins 2020). Where deinstitutionalization has coincided with the end of military dictatorship or the start of democracy, each country has a unique story to tell. Jamaica used independence as the moment to expand culturally congruent mental health services (Hickling 2019). The Province of Rio Negro in Argentina used a similar political moment to legislate community mental health and close the psychiatric hospital (Collins 2008). These approaches to mental health care provide valuable lessons that are often not widely disseminated.

Call to Action

The reframing of the global mental health agenda presented by the *Lancet* Commission on Global Mental Health and Sustainable Development spotlights the centrality of people commonly neglected or tokenized in mental health research and service design: individuals with lived experience of mental health conditions (Patel et al. 2018). But specific calls for anticolonialism, antiracism, and mental health equity in global mental health must also be part of the reframed global mental health agenda (Hailemariam and Pathare 2020; Weine et al. 2020). We add these actions from the 2020 World Federation for Mental Health's Call to Action (Collins and Rao 2020):

1. Recognize and respond to racism in all its forms as a threat to health and well-being across the life span.
2. Stimulate and accelerate efforts to achieve sustainable development goal targets, which represent actions against social determinants of poor health.
3. Invest in social and behavioral interventions, including those that reduce stigma, bolster interpersonal relationships, and strengthen social supports and healthy social networks.
4. Ensure access to quality and affordable mental health care and primary care.
5. Reduce disparities in mental health care.

Global mental health recognizes a vastly intertwined world and values nurturing that interconnectedness for solving difficult problems through a diversity of perspectives. It is imperative that we use the resources and networks of the global mental health community to take these actions.

References

Alexander O: Okeechobee hurricane of 1928. Seattle, WA, BlackPast, 2021. Available at: www.blackpast.org/african-american-history/the-okeechobee-hurricane-of-1928. Accessed August 15, 2021.

Arias D, Taylor L, Ofori-Atta A, Bradley EH: Prayer camps and biomedical care in Ghana: is collaboration in mental health care possible? PLoS One 11(9):e0162305, 2016 27618551

Ayinde OO, Fadahunsi O, Kola L, et al: Explanatory models, illness, and treatment experiences of patients with psychosis using the services of traditional and faith healers in three African countries: similarities and discontinuities. Transcult Psychiatry Dec 16:13634615211064370, 2021 34913379

Bullard RD: Differential vulnerabilities: environmental inequality and government response to unnatural disasters. Soc Res (New York) 75:753–784, 2008

Burgess RA, Jain S, Petersen I, Lund C: Social interventions: a new era for global mental health? Lancet Psychiatry 7(2):118–119, 2020 31653556

Chibanda D, Weiss HA, Verhey R, et al: Effect of a primary care-based psychological intervention on symptoms of common mental disorders in Zimbabwe: a randomized clinical trial. JAMA 316(24):2618–2626, 2016 28027368

Chisholm D, Flisher AJ, Lund C, et al; Lancet Global Mental Health Group: Scale up services for mental disorders: a call for action. Lancet 370(9594):1241–1252, 2007 17804059

Collins PH: Learning from the outsider within: the sociological significance of Black feminist thought, in Feminist Approaches to Theory and Methodology: An Interdisciplinary Reader. Edited by Hesse-Biber S, Gilmartin C, Lydenberg R. New York Oxford University Press, 1999, pp 155–178

Collins PH: Black Feminist Thought: Knowledge, Consciousness, and the Politics of Empowerment, 2nd Edition. New York, Routledge, 2000

Collins PY: Waving the banner of the mental health revolution: psychiatric reform and community mental health in the Province of Rio Negro, Argentina, in Innovative Community Mental Health Services in Latin America and the Caribbean. Edited by Caldas de Almeida JM, Cohen A. Washington, DC, Pan American Health Organization, 2008, pp 1–32

Collins PY: What is global mental health? World Psychiatry 19(3):265–266, 2020 32931115

Collins PY, Pringle BA: Building a global mental health research workforce: perspectives from the National Institute of Mental Health. Acad Psychiatry 40(4):723–726, 2016 26586615

Collins PY, Rao D: World Mental Health Day 2020 call to action, in World Mental Health Day 2020: Mental Health for All: Greater Investment—Greater Access. World Federation for Mental Health, 2020, pp 151–156

Collins PY, Elkington KS, von Unger H, et al: Relationship of stigma and HIV risk behavior among women with mental illness. Am J Orthopsychiatry 78:498–506, 2008a 19123772

Collins PY, von Unger H, Armbrister A: Church ladies, good girls, and locas: stigma and the intersection of gender, ethnicity, mental illness, and sexuality in relation to HIV risk. Soc Sci Med 67(3):389–397, 2008b 18423828

Collins PY, Patel V, Joestl SS, et al; Scientific Advisory Board and the Executive Committee of the Grand Challenges on Global Mental Health: Grand challenges in global mental health. Nature 475(7354):27–30, 2011 21734685

Combahee River Collective: A Black feminist statement, in This Bridge Called My Back: Writings of Radical Women of Color. Edited by Moraga C, Anzaldúa G. Latham, NY, Kitchen Table, Women of Color Press, 2002, pp 234–244

Crenshaw KW: Mapping the margins: intersectionality, identity politics, and violence against women of color. Stanford Law Review 43(6): 1241–1299, 1991

da Silva ATC, Hanlon C, Susser E, et al: Enhancing mental health research capacity: emerging voices from the National Institute of Mental Health (NIMH) global hubs. Int J Ment Health Syst 13:21, 2019 30988696

Griffith EEH: Race and Excellence: My Dialogue With Chester Pierce. Washington, DC, American Psychiatric Association Publishing, 2023

Gulsuner S, Stein DJ, Susser ES, et al: Genetics of schizophrenia in the South African Xhosa. Science 367(6477):569–573, 2020 32001654

Gureje O, Appiah-Poku J, Bello T, et al: Effect of collaborative care between traditional and faith healers and primary health-care workers on psychosis outcomes in Nigeria and Ghana (COSIMPO): a cluster randomised controlled trial. Lancet 396(10251):612–622, 2020 32861306

Hackett RA, Ronaldson A, Bhui K, et al: Racial discrimination and health: a prospective study of ethnic minorities in the United Kingdom. BMC Public Health 20(1):1652, 2020 33203386

Hailemariam M, Pathare S: The missing global in global mental health. Lancet Psychiatry 7(12):1011–1012, 2020 33220190

Hatzenbuehler ML, Phelan JC, Link BG: Stigma as a fundamental cause of population health inequalities. Am J Public Health 103(5):813–821, 2013 23488505

Hickling FW: Owning our madness: contributions of Jamaican psychiatry to decolonizing global mental health. Transcult Psychiatry 57(1):19–31, 2019 31852387

Hickling FW: The African Renaissance and the struggle for mental health in the African Diaspora, in The African Diaspora: Psychiatric Issues—A Proceeding From the Meetings Held November 17–21, 2002. Edited by Organ PG. Boston, Department of Psychiatry, Massachusetts General Hospital, 2002, pp 123–134

Jordan A, Allsop AS, Collins PY: Decriminalising being Black with mental illness. Lancet Psychiatry 8(1):8–9, 2021 33341173

Koplan JP, Bond TC, Merson MH, et al; Consortium of Universities for Global Health Executive Board: Towards a common definition of global health. Lancet 373(9679):1993–1995 2009 19493564

Link BG, Phelan JC: Conceptualizing stigma. Annu Rev Sociol 27:363–385, 2001

Lorde A: Age, race, class, and sex: women redefining difference, in Sister Outsider. Freedom, CA, Crossing Press, 1984, pp 114–123

Mack W: The Chester, Pennsylvania race riot (1917). Seattle, WA, BlackPast, 2017. Available at: www.blackpast.org/african-american-history/1917-race-riot-chester-pennsylvania-1917. Accessed August 8, 2021.

Martin AR, Atkinson EG, Chapman SB, et al; NeuroGAP-Psychosis Study Team: Low-coverage sequencing cost-effectively detects known and novel variation in underrepresented populations. Am J Hum Genet 108(4):656–668, 2021 33770507

McKenzie K: Improving mental health services for immigrant, racialized, ethno-cultural and refugee groups. Healthc Pap 18(2):4–9, 2019 31596697

Momodu S: The Ocoee massacre (1920). Seattle, WA, BlackPast, 2020. Available at: www.blackpast.org/african-american-history/the-ocoee-massacre-1920. Accessed August 8, 2021.

Nortje G, Oladeji B, Gureje O, Seedat S: Effectiveness of traditional healers in treating mental disorders: a systematic review. Lancet Psychiatry 3(2):154–170, 2016 26851329

Ojagbemi A, Gureje O: The potential role of traditional medicine in the management of schizophrenia. Curr Psychiatry Rep 22(12):71, 2020 33089431

Organ PG (ed): The African Diaspora: Psychiatric Issues—A Proceeding From the Meetings Held November 17–21, 2002. Boston, Department of Psychiatry, Massachusetts General Hospital, 2002

Patel V, Saxena S, Lund C, et al: The Lancet Commission on Global Mental Health and Sustainable Development. Lancet 392(10157):1553–1598 2018 30314863

Pierce C: Offensive mechanisms, in The Black Seventies. Edited by Barbour FB. Boston, MA, Porter Sargent, 1970, pp 265–282

Pierce CM: Entitlement dysfunctions. Aust N Z J Psychiatry 12(4):215–219, 1978 283790

Pierce C: Unity in diversity: thirty-three years of stress, in Black Students: Psychosocial Issues and Academic Achievement. Edited by Berry GL, Asamen JK. Newbury Park, CA, Sage, 1989, pp 296–312

Pierce C: Stress analogs of racism and sexism: terrorism, torture, and disaster, in Mental Health, Racism, and Sexism. Edited by Willie CV, Rieker PP, Kramer BM, Brown BS. Pittsburgh, PA, University of Pittsburgh Press, 1995, pp 277–292

Pilowsky DJ, Rojas G, Price LN, et al: Building research capacity across and within low- and middle-income countries: the Collaborative Hubs for International Research on Mental Health. Acad Psychiatry 40(4):686–691, 2016 26895931

Pringle B, Williams M, Collins PY: Evidence for action: stimulating research to address the global mental health treatment gap, in Innovations in Global Mental Health. Edited by Okpaku SO. Cham, Switzerland, Springer, 2019, pp 63–88

Rahman A, Naslund JA, Betancourt TS, et al: The NIMH global mental health research community and COVID-19. Lancet Psychiatry 7(10):834–836, 2020 32846142

Sibitz I, Unger A, Woppmann A, et al: Stigma resistance in patients with schizophrenia. Schizophr Bull 37(2):316–323, 2011 19487336

Smith EL: The 1917 race riot in Chester, Pennsylvania. Pennsylvania History 75(2):171–196, 2008

Stewart AJ, McDermott C: Gender in psychology. Annu Rev Psychol 55:519–544, 2004 14744225

van der Watt ASJ, Nortje G, Kola L, et al: Collaboration between biomedical and complementary and alternative care providers: barriers and pathways. Qual Health Res 27(14):2177–2188, 2017 28901831

Weine S, Kohrt BA, Collins PY, et al: Justice for George Floyd and a reckoning for global mental health. Glob Ment Health (Camb) 7:e22, 2020 32963794

Williams DR, Lawrence JA, Davis BA: Racism and health: evidence and needed research. Annu Rev Public Health 40:105–125, 2019 30601726

Williams MT: Microaggressions: clarification, evidence, and impact. Perspect Psychol Sci 15(1):3–26, 2020 31418642

Williams MT, Skinta MD, Martin-Willett R: After Pierce and Sue: a revised racial microaggressions taxonomy. Perspect Psychol Sci 16(5):991–1007, 2021 34498518

World Bank: World development report 1993: investing in health. New York, World Bank, 1993. Available at: https://openknowledge.worldbank.org/handle/10986/5976. Accessed August 1, 2021.

World Health Organization: The World Health Report 2001: Mental Health: New understanding, new hope. Geneva, Switzerland, World Health Organization, 2001

Zitouni M: The psychopathology of acculturation, in The African Diaspora: Psychiatric Issues—A Proceeding From the Meetings Held November 17–21, 2002. Edited by Organ PG. Boston, Department of Psychiatry, Massachusetts General Hospital, 2002, pp 71–73

PART IV

Racism, Leadership, and Organized Psychiatry

Reflections on the Origin of the Black Psychiatrists of America

James P. Comer, M.D., M.P.H.

On May 20, 2019, I received a citation from the American Psychiatric Association (APA) in commemoration of the 50th anniversary of the date that a small delegation from the Black Caucus of the APA interrupted an annual meeting of the APA trustees to present a list of demands for change—in their focus, knowledge about, and need to address organizational and American racial policies and practices. I received a standing ovation on the occasion of the 50th anniversary, a climate and response far different from the angry, tense, anxious feelings and atmosphere at the time of the confrontation.

The last time, there were glares, avoidance, and a rare "I am with you." This time, there were congratulations all around at the meeting, in the hallways, and on the plane going home. But despite much change, there was evidence that although it is useful to acknowledge a flawed past and integrate it into our organizational and national histories and national life, it is still not easy.

The 50th commemoration was taking place as the first African American president of the APA, Dr. Altha Stewart, was finishing her term, a significant sign of progress. But continued discomfort was apparent in that she, not the organization, knew that I was a cofounder of the Black Psychiatrists of America (BPA) and the only one from the confrontation a half-century before who was present at this meeting (Comer 1973). Dr. Stewart remembered, and shortly before the meeting asked me to accept the citation for our Black Caucus group. This important benchmark moment was an almost forgotten organization event. In different ways and levels, such avoidance, denial, and reluctance have been the pattern of management of almost all things related to American racism as the nation struggles to absorb its history (Pierce 1970) and take corrective efforts.

The BPA-APA story is an important and informative slice of the American story. In this chapter, through my reflections on the origin of the BPA, I want to share my experiences: first, the impulses that led to its formation—when, why, and what we were trying to do—and then a discussion of what we learned and did. I describe how, in time and turn, these experiences affected my own career and life, and, finally, I discuss how I believe this work is a template for the kind of next-stage social structure change that must occur to address racism in America at its deepest level. It is this next level, structural change, that makes BPA and BPA-like work (supporting social justice) within the African American and progressive communities critically important and urgent. We suspected then and know now that truth, trust, fair play, and democracy are the only ways that racism can be paralyzed and that we can adequately promote good mental health.

Origin of the BPA

My message to the BPA in the organization's newsletter in the fall of 1973 after I had been elected the third president of the BPA is more helpful than my memory of 53 years ago. Thus, I quote and draw from it here.

The President's Message, Black Psychiatrists of America

After the historic 1963 March on Washington led by Dr. Martin Luther King, Jr., the minds of Black Americans were riveted on American racism, and the need to eliminate it, as they had never been before. In 1964, (the first year I attended the APA annual meeting) Black psychiatrists identified racism as a serious mental health problem and called for the mobilization of national resources to effect attitudinal change and significantly decrease prejudice. (Comer 1973, pp. 1, 5)

Dr. Chester Pierce, a Harvard-based senior psychiatrist and pioneer and my role model, was the major organizing force and leader of our group and became the first BPA president in 1968. Dr. Alfred Cannon was the second, and by 1973, I was a fifth-year Yale faculty member and became the third president. Dr. Pierce recommended this sequence of leadership to promote input and ownership by the younger psychiatrists for an effort that was going to require organizational growth and stability for a then yet to be determined program of action (Pierce 1959).

The self-proclaimed Black Caucus of the APA began an effort to educate Black and white professionals about the importance of responding to the problem of racism. As part of this effort, the federal government agencies concerned with and responsible for health, the Department of Health, Education, and Welfare and particularly the National Institute of Mental Health (NIMH), were identified and called on. The Falk Foundation supported some of this early work, and a pilot study grant was obtained from NIMH in 1968. Two national meetings of mostly senior Black psychiatrists were held in February and April 1968 in Kansas City and New York City, respectively.

By coincidence, the April 4, 1968, meeting was scheduled and held on the day of Dr. Martin Luther King Jr.'s assassination. His assassination was a huge and critical flex point in America. It was a horrific event for all Americans, a devastating setback for the principles of democracy, and a successful attack on African American and American progress, and it infused our April meeting room with an almost indescribable, surreal mixture of explosive outbursts of anger, rage, sadness, crying, and determination to keep going. The murder of Dr. King gave a much deeper appreciation not only of the reality and harm of racism but also of our discussion of the need for change through the formal organization of Black psychiatrists across the country.

A strategy of nonviolent protest had precipitated an unstoppable force for national change in which BPA became a small but important part. An executive committee was elected during our May 1968 BPA meeting. The committee, acting on behalf of its membership, called for an increase in the number of Blacks in responsible academic, clinical, and administrative positions within organized psychiatry and called for a decrease of racism in mental health programs and facilities across the country.

The first public action of our developing caucus of Black psychiatrists was the presentation of a panel at the May 1968 APA Annual Meeting in Boston, Massachusetts. During the 1969 APA Annual Meeting in Miami, our still self-proclaimed caucus group invaded and presented our demands for change at the APA Board of Trustees meeting. A number of activities were already under way, and more were initiated. The original BPA caucus became an ad hoc committee of the American Psychiatric Association and was eventually designated a caucus of the APA in 1977. As a part of our effort, Dr. Joseph Phillips was named head of an ad hoc committee of the BPA on Minority Group Affairs of NIMH. After delicate and difficult negotiations between Black psychiatrists (Alfred Cannon, Joe Phillips, and myself) and the leadership of NIMH, a Minority Group Center was established there in 1971. Dr. James Ralph, a Black psychiatrist, was named its first chief.

Although I was the youngest of the BPA cofounders in 1968, I may have been the only African American psychiatrist serving in any of the major mental health organizations and institutions at the time—the time of the long hot summers of 1967 and 1968, when angry protests and fires related to racial unrest erupted in more than 100 American cities (Gooden and Myers 2018; McLaughlin 2014). There were very few African Americans in academic psychiatry, in American psychiatry in general, or in mental health institutions, particularly at policy levels.

This might have been a contributing reason to the fact that a planned final year of my United States Public Health Service (USPHS)–sponsored training in child psychiatry at the Yale Child Study Center in 1967 was suddenly changed to the headquarters of NIMH in Washington, D.C. Nobody told me. I received orders. To my knowledge, I became the first African American officer so assigned. Interestingly, the only other African American mental health professional at the NIMH at the time was Frederick Douglass's grandson.

There was no racism-related research or intervention work plan or project for me at NIMH. In fact, I was still finishing my psychiatric residency. And the very expensive and vague intervention research project they were working to get off the ground, with no minority background input, as I arrived fell through when the six comparison group cities that had not had disturbances at the time soon had major racial disturbances. Grant applications to the institute from minority scholars were rare, and even more rarely successful, and were not being sought. In fact, there were few minority mental or public health scholars, and the pipeline for future scholars was all but empty. Although I was still an entry-level USPHS officer in 1967, I was able to roughly identify NIMH power programs, people, and the way the organization worked in order to support BPA's effort to promote inclusion and change.

The complex yet simple way in which such structural racism works was apparent in an early proposal to NIMH. A research group of the BPA, the Solomon Carter Fuller Institute, proposed a project that was to establish a fellowship to enable Black psychiatrists, in particular emerging trainees and scholars, to explore career possibilities with various established mental health organizations through residencies and projects. It was turned down. The reviewer comment was "That's old hat. We've done that." I pointed out that when "we" did it there were few to no African Americans anywhere in the pipeline.

The decision was reversed, and the program in time served as a major exposure and entryway to participation for Black psychiatrists. It was soon modified and expanded to include members from other mental health disciplines and all underrepresented minorities. That program contributed to the creation of the Division of Special Mental Health Programs. Dr. Jeanne Spurlock was appointed deputy director of the APA and provided an impressive 17 years of service, attending to minority and other interests from within the established structure of the APA, as the BPA caucus had supported and hoped.

This and other experiences deepened my awareness of structural racism and understanding of how it might be addressed. I still did not fully understand how the NIMH establishment did not know that there were no African Americans in positions of authority in that agency and why even learning about past conditions was not enough to motivate immediate corrective action at NIMH and in most of our mainstream institutions. The full reason, nationwide, turned out to be even more complex than I thought.

From the beginning, the budding BPA organization felt a need to support excellence in research and service. Out of this felt need, we created the Solomon Carter Fuller Institute, an effort led by Dr. Robert Sharpley. The institute honors the first Black psychiatrist in America, Solomon C. Fuller, who was from Liberia but spent his adult and professional life in the United States. His work was published in leading scientific and medical journals, and he was involved in dialogue with leading contemporaries of his day, such as Emil Kraepelin and Sigmund Freud.

A Solomon Carter Fuller Award for Distinguished Service was created by the BPA. Since 1975, the Solomon Carter Fuller Award and lecture has been presented by the APA to persons whose distinguished service has contributed positively to the mental health of Black Americans. Among the BPA and APA award recipients have been psychologist Dr. Kenneth Clark for his work cited in the U.S. Supreme Court school integration decision and psychiatrists Dr. Charles Prudhomme and Dr. Charles Wilkinson.

Black psychiatrists were active in support of Drs. Charles Prudhomme and Mildred Bateman in their elections to the position of vice president of the APA. And, as a result of BPA interest, Black psychiatrists have been named to the board of directors of foundations and editorial boards of professional and lay journals of significance. We have established contacts with Black psychiatrists in the Caribbean and Africa. We have identified the location and work of as many Black psychiatrists in America as possible.

The BPA developed a newsletter in order to maintain better communications among Black psychiatrists in America. This has led to a modern-day online communication network of Black psychiatrists who support each other and their interests and make their talents and services and what is known about psychiatry more available to the Black community and the nation.

As the BPA was being founded, many Black psychiatrists were making important contributions to African American mental health in the profession and the nation. In addition to the work of the individuals mentioned previously, this early work included Charles Pinderhughes, June Jackson Christmas, Hiawatha Harris, Alvin Poussaint, Billy Jones, Elizabeth Davis, Lloyd Elam, James Curtis, Hugh Butts, Mae McMullin, Annelle Primm, and Margaret Lawrence.

I felt we were off to a good start organizing and becoming more intentional and directional, and I was disappointed when Chester Pierce stepped back from his founder and leadership position after just one term. I felt a need for his experience and wise guidance. But he was positioning the BPA for the long haul, as he felt mandated to do. I had not fully anticipated a long haul. I had underestimated the deep structural nature, power, and pervasiveness of racism. I thought, maybe hoped, that it was a problem of ignorance and that it could be educated out of racists through schools and progressive economic and social policies and change.

Through my BPA work, particularly my term as president, I came to better understand the great magnitude and complexity of racism, individual and structural, and how difficult it is to change. Past and then present racism had wrestled change at a pace that was too slow to keep up with the requirements of a technology- and science-driven society. BPA activities and my intervention research in education work at the Yale Child Study Center grew out of efforts to quicken the pace.

In addition, by 1975 there was a new and intense pressure for greater representation of marginalized and underrepresented minority groups to participate as policy makers and mainstream civic leaders. Because of past neglect and exclusion, there were too few African Americans connected or known to mainstream policy and societal organizations. As a result of these situations, there was too much to be done and too few people in the mainstream pipelines to do the work.

I began to understand that these were cross-generational tasks of great magnitude and complexity, for which we would need to make continuous change, work where we were best suited and needed and could be most effective, and help prepare new people to carry on. I realized that my strength was in my intervention capacities and not organization leadership. I chose an opportunity to try to make deep structural change through my intervention work in public education rather than change through mental health organizational leadership. By 1975, while still connected to BPA and APA, I began to focus primarily on intervention through my public school–based university academic work. The Minority Center of NIMH, created through the advocacy of the BPA, eventually played a critical role in my academic intervention work, although I had no thought that it might.

The School Development Program (SDP) stuttered and almost stalled until we received a grant, Social Skills Curriculum for Inner-City Children (SSCICC), from the Minority Center that allowed schools to address structural shortcomings in education as well as meet the developmental needs of students, families, and school communities. This grant allowed our pioneering Whole Child development perspective, which included social and emotional learning and preparation for life, to survive and eventually flourish (Darling-Hammond et al. 2018). The BPA carried on the organization and advocacy work and remains a strong organizational force.

The SDP–BPA Connection

My academic research and intervention work began in 1968 when I joined the Yale Child Study Center faculty and founded the community-based SDP. My lifelong advocacy against racism found an institutional home when I first attended an APA Annual Meeting in 1964 and began to think more fully about how racism is the antithesis of good mental and public health. The concerns expressed by our group of Black psychiatrists and my work in public school education practices and policies that permitted and promoted racism were interconnected.

However, in the 1960s, most social and behavioral science research was focused on shortcomings and flaws in underachieving African American communities and culture—a deficit perspective. This perspective could not explain success among Blacks despite the magnitude of intentional exclusion and abuse throughout American history. In addition, little attention was given to understanding how flaws in our social structures and practices may have contributed to difficult academic and behavior problems or conditions for African Americans and all Americans. My BPA work on racial issues put the social structure flaws front and center, eventually providing a way for SDP to focus directly on deep-seated structural change and to contribute a model for paralyzing racism and promoting good education and mental health.

The focus on individual and group deficit in research is in line with our national narrative about what it takes to succeed: hard work and, in reference to success in school and education, good intelligence. My own life experience suggested that the narrative is simplistic and ignores well-documented biopsychosocial and public health research and knowledge. I consider this narrative, even now, to be a distraction and a part of a slave-based culture rationalization that is losing ground but still has strong ill effects in our culture of democracy. The Yale School Development Program was an effort to understand the complexity of school underachievement and remarkable resilience and success. My suspicion, supported by participation and observational evidence (Comer 1988), was that the students were able to succeed, and it was the societal social structures and systems that needed change.

Data of Another Kind

When I was being interviewed for the Yale School Development Program in 1967, I was asked what would make it possible for students who were underprepared for school to succeed in school. My reply: "a vital school community." I knew what I meant, but I did not know how to create it. The family I grew up in had created such a community, as did our church and other people and networks in which we felt belonging and/or entitlement (Comer 1988). I suspected that a well-functioning school could similarly create such a community, a school tied through networks back into families and on and out into other organizations and networks working to prepare students for school and life.

An experience I had in which families could not feel entitlement or belonging also helped me think about this need and challenge. While doing my required military service time for 2 years in the USPHS, I did volunteer work at Hospitality House in Washington, D.C., where I worked with mothers and children evicted from their housing project apartments for allegedly having a "man in the house." I directly observed and experienced the way they were demeaned, bullied, and abused. These were not promiscuous, bad, irresponsible, low-ability level, willfully underperforming young people who had not worked hard and had brought hardship on themselves and deserved it, as many argued. Congressman L. Mendel Rivers from South Carolina and his Deep South colleagues appeared to take delight in finding every platform they could to blame these women and children and make them feel bad for the "sins of their fathers." The women and their children were trapped by a complex American history and system that I would eventually come to understand as having been put and held in place by the force and power of racism. How might I work to give all families and young people the kind of opportunity networks and supports I had?

I gradually realized that my parents had made education and social life in a Black church–based primary culture our foundation and springboard for school readiness, functioning, and preparation for life. The social interactions, skills, and capacities my siblings and I gained at home prepared us for the expectations of school, and school was to further connect us to the mainstream culture and society and deepen, broaden, and enhance what we brought to it in order to continue to prepare us for life as family members, workers, and citizens of society.

All children need such preparatory experiences. This realization, which was based on powerful positive and negative experiences and modern biological, social, and behavioral research knowledge, led to our intervention research question: Could a program of in-school activities be created that would provide access to the capacities needed to be successful in school and life to students who are capable and to those who are not adequately developed? We were aware that nonreadiness and underdevelopment were traditionally considered to be faults or a lack of ability or, still worse, a sign of racial inferiority (Comer et al. 1987). The acute exacerbation of chronic racial turmoil after the assassination of the most iconic representation of antiracism, Martin Luther King Jr., made this more than an ordinary research question and called for an academic study approach that went beyond statistical studies.

SDP Intervention Research

Martin Luther King Jr. was assassinated in April 1968. When I arrived in New Haven in June 1968, the country was still reeling in the aftermath of the loss of an icon of hope for all Americans and for African Americans in particular. Our project schools, two largely African American elementary schools with difficult social conditions and the lowest academic achievements in the city, opened in September 1968. The almost palpable wish was that our work in schools could turn around the ill effects of great wrong in the nation and create opportunities for success. None of the organizations—university, foundation, school district, communities—involved had ever been in this situation before, and we were not ready. The start-up exploded, and within the first month we were almost shut down (Comer 1988, 1993). On the first day, the behavior of the students spiraled out of control. The well-meaning teachers, some still learning the latest new teaching method, did their best but were not prepared. Roles and responsibilities were unclear. The parents were furious and felt betrayed by the program sponsors—Yale, New Haven Schools, New Haven city. The local media made it prime time news (Comer 1980).

The scramble to survive was deeply difficult but led to a model for success of the project, greater opportunity for poor and marginalized families and children in other cities and potentially for society as a whole (Drake 1995). The first step was to engage the angry, disappointed-again parents with openness and truth and involve them in the change process as the situation allowed and required (Comer and Haynes 1991).

After many difficult and promising moments over the first 9 months, we had a summer reset and planning period. We were able to think holistically and interactively about what we all wanted for the students, parents, staff, the education enterprise, and the country; about the place and potential of education for making our dreams possible; and about a plan and process framework for making this happen. Most simply, we wanted the students to have a chance to be successful academically in school and in life as family members and citizens in a democratic society. Most adult participants (parents, teachers, custodians, administrators) agreed that they would need to work collaboratively to create the conditions in school to help make that possible (Comer 1986, 1987).

The SDP, which was embedded in the fabric of the two elementary schools in our pilot project, helped staff, parents, students, and the community create a nine-element school change process: three guidelines that influenced the behavior of all school participants, three teams that enabled all to contribute but not run over each other, and three operations that enabled the schools to carry out program, climate, and culture creation activities that motivated and supported teaching and learning in school and for life (Haynes and Comer 1996).

The three guidelines—consensus decision-making, no-fault problem-solving, and collaboration—served as behavior touchstones and generated a positive growth culture. The three teams—representatives of the key participant stakeholders, parents as a group, and support staff as a group—addressed management and made inclusion and a sense of ownership possible. The three operations—a comprehensive school plan (academic and social), staff development, and assessment and modification—directly promoted child development, behavior, and learning to create a school environment that was facilitative rather than disruptive and obstructive. These stakeholder principles, teams, and practices generated lever-like actions that turned human energy, sometimes free-floating and troublesome, into pleasure and achievement activities and outcomes (Ertz 2020).

Because all adult participants helped to design the process, they owned it. As they used their SDP process framework to address problems and create opportunities, they gradually created an in-school climate and culture similar to my own family and its primary social networks. But in the 5 years it took to create a school community of promise—a caring, motivated, vital, vibrant climate—test scores had gone up only slightly, and our generous foundation support ran out.

The turnaround in attitudes and behavior among all the participant groups was acknowledged and praised (Cauce et al. 1987), but the potential funders did not see the mental health or public health significance of what had happened until that point. The fact that the schools had moved from being greatly dysfunctional to functioning well was not thought of as a precursor to academic and personal development and preparation for life. Social, emotional, and developmental functions—the essence of our SDP work—were being ignored. Academic achievement as measured by test scores was thought of as an isolated cognitive ability function.

Because of the absence of significant test score gains, we received time to phase out the program but no continuation support. But we were not leaving. We pushed even more intentionally on social and emotional development and preparation for life by creating a project and proposal titled "Social Skills Curriculum for Inner-City Children" (SSCICC). This project was based on what parents told us they wanted for their children and the experiences and capacities our own lives and work suggested students would need to achieve them (Comer 1977).

One of the site visitors for our application from NIMH asked about the independent, intermediate, and dependent variables. One of the teachers on our school project team kept asking me, "What is he talking about?" and pointed out that you can see, feel, and touch the improvement to date. The site visitor needed measurable quantitative findings, and we were pointing to observable qualitative findings, which were precursors but were less measurable, and to some less scientific, indicators.

Nevertheless, one of the NIMH division chiefs thought our SDP demonstrated promise. Our previous proposal for a center that could have included our SSCICC project was favorably considered for support by all but one of the reviewers within the division he led. The objector, a psychiatrist who was the only African American on the review team, pointed out that there had been a directive to eliminate "demonstration" initiatives in order to support more biological research, which was believed to be more scientific and useful. Knowledge of this interest was fairly widespread and had been a part of my reason for leaving NIMH in the first place. I also knew of this interest in another way. The most vocal and influential advocate of a biological focus, who was one of my former supervisors and by then a colleague, had told me that he liked what SDP was doing, but too many demonstration projects were like patching potholes in the street. Once the other division reviewers were reminded of the directive, support for SSCICC was pulled away. We faced similar uncertainties and problems among other philanthropic and government funding sources.

Because of my part in advocating for the creation of the NIMH Minority Center as a BPA member, I had been reluctant to apply to the center. Dr. James Ralph, the Minority Center chief, heard about our proposal and encouraged me to apply. He felt that his diverse review committee could be objective and might be better equipped to understand the project's intent and possibilities. We applied and received a 3-year grant that eventually proved to be a critical proof point and an opportunity to open the door to a focus in education on social and emotional development, integrated with academics and preparation for life learning. The diverse review committee not only understood the research plan and method but offered their own life experiences in prediction of our success.

The SSCICC became a part of our SDP comprehensive school plan, one of the nine elements of the SDP process (Haynes et al. 1989). Four social skill project areas served to provide students with experiences and skills they would need to be successful in school and life: 1) business and economics, 2) politics and government, 3) health and nutrition, and 4) spiritual-leisure time and self-expression. Academic and social and emotional development opportunities were thoughtfully planned into each activity project unit by the educators and parents and the students themselves (Ramirez-Smith 1995).

The first project unit initiated, the politics and government unit, had a dramatic impact on the King School fourth graders, the entire school, and eventually the SDP. It was wrapped around and through a New Haven mayoral election. Using replicable methods, the unit took the students on discovery journeys into the city, brought city leadership (including the mayoral candidates) into the school, and engaged students in planning logistics and artistic performances and related academic activities (Darling-Hammond et al. 2018). The positive energy and excitement generated were vibrant and almost palpable.

In drama and music performances, school staff were surprised and delighted by the levels of ability and skill they saw in students who had not displayed them in the regular classroom. Students helped each other rather than ridiculing and abusing others. This strong school value was modeled in student and staff readiness to back up anyone who forgot their lines. Students', staff's, and parents' belief in themselves, each other, and their school grew. The spirit and momentum generated by the events did not go away but served to deepen the success culture of the school. Units in preparation for other life areas were all different but were also successful in helping students, staff, and parents achieve at a high level (Haynes et al. 1988).

At the end of the first SSCICC program year, annual test scores leaped dramatically after 7 months, and in 3 years both pilot schools were at and well over the national average in language arts and mathematics achievement. King School had no teacher turnover for 13 years, and even then it was for career advancement rather than because of discontent.

Implementation of the SSCICC within the SDP framework helped us understand how to generate the kind of vibrant culture that made a hoped-for level of development and learning possible where it had not been previously. After this success, our SDP pilot process was successfully field-tested in elementary, middle, and high schools. In the late 1980s the Rockefeller Foundation provided substantial funding for dissemination of the process. Implementation moved from 66 schools in three districts in 1988 to 80 districts and more than 650 schools by 1997 (Noblit et al. 2001). Rigorous evaluations have consistently shown impressive results when the SDP is faithfully implemented in schools and districts and is adequately understood and supported.

But for the BPA

The SDP outcomes have been widely reported and have helped to generate interest in the role of social and emotional learning or development in education. But what has not been given much attention is that but for the presence and action of the BPA in the 1960s, the SDP and other work that helped to change inaccurate and harmful understandings and behavior might well have died in project infancy. Such outcomes are costly and lead to nonalignment, patchwork success, bridges to nowhere, and a sense that problems that can be solved cannot be solved. Although there can be other reasons, racism embedded at the core of our social structures from the beginning of our nation creates conflict and tension that make change difficult even when both sides sense that change is needed.

I believe that our BPA-APA experience can be a model for bringing about the kind of next-stage social structure change that must occur in the United States. The social structure change process must intentionally focus on strengthening democracy while crippling generation-to-generation transmission of racism through universal human structures—families, school and/or education, political and economic policies and practices, and culture. Our SDP whole-child and whole-school development framework and our BPA-APA-NIMH ties worked in this way.

SDP was able to facilitate good family and school functioning through the use of integrated child development, education, and mental health principles and practices in schools. This reduced fear and anxiety, scapegoating, and other acting-out behaviors and conditions and constructively channeled aggression in ways that gave many students a greater chance for success in school and in life. These outcomes strengthened the potential of overcoming residual and latent aspects of our culture of slavery and tilled the soil of the culture of democracy by providing the kind of public school education that President John Adams and other Founding Fathers believed was necessary if the American experiment with democracy, "We the people" governance, was to succeed.

However, although this changed way of thinking and working was needed in the 1960s, it was late. Science- and technology-driven changes after World War II generated complex social and economic thinking, behavior, and conditions before many families and institutions across the spectrum of peoples could acquire capacities to manage them. African Americans had been targeted, abused, and denied the most. But this (our) group was slowly gaining the power and opportunity to resist effectively. As a result, during the 1960s, much of the nation's energy went into surfacing and addressing the ill effects of racism—particularly the denied opportunities and false narratives—rather than growing needed capacities to enable most people to survive and thrive. "These kids [Black kids] can't" was one of the most aggravating and limiting parts of the false narrative. Our SDP effort was part of the process needed to demonstrate that Black kids can succeed. And with an adequate sense of belonging and support for social, academic, and emotional development, many more kids did succeed. Two-thirds of the more than 600 schools that used SDP had outcomes from good to remarkable, sometimes with mostly white faculty and largely African American students.

As the SDP project was succeeding, the challenge became to help people select our development-centered education approach, or that of others, and make it widely and routinely possible, portable, and sustainable even with the natural conditions of human change and school staff turnover from illness, death, lack of preparation, economic issues, disagreements, or politics and the troublesome and powerful aspects of human nature that often played out through politics. We survived and thrived until the politics of the No Child Left Behind legislation in 2001 blocked our focus on child and adolescent development integrated into academic learning and preparation for life. This legislation took the education enterprise back to academic teaching in isolation, ignoring the science showing that academic learning and social and emotional development are inextricably linked and need to be addressed simultaneously and interactively.

But even before No Child Left Behind, education had moved too slowly to integrate whole-school and whole-child development and academic learning. Even when the model (SDP and others) provided the evidence of value and need, the country had not created an infrastructure of parents, educators, policy makers, practitioners, and the public that could adequately support the needs of the emerging and changing science- and technology-driven age. Racism played a powerful, almost invisible role in contributing to this situation.

For example, after one of the predominantly low-income African American schools used the SDP process and moved from last in the district to first in 3 years, the superintendent told the principal, "You know your kids can't do that well." By the time the students were retested and the state finally agreed there was no evidence of cheating, key people— disappointed, hopeless, and demoralized despite a Black community effort to blunt the trauma—had moved on to more supportive opportunities. The announcement of the retest results was minimized, whereas the initial question of possible cheating was a major focus of the news, contributing to the silence about, if not invisibility of, the success and the persistence of the false narrative (Glass 1996).

The students lost. The country lost. The people who struggled to do the right thing lost. And although this incident was more flagrant than others, it did not stand alone.

Nonetheless, as more students achieved well in places where many suspected it was not possible, public interest in and attention to support for child development in school increased. There is a growing level of understanding that students from all backgrounds can perform well under supportive conditions. Now there is a slowly emerging understanding that many determinants of academic learning are rooted in matters beyond each schoolhouse (e.g., educator and parent preparation, resources) and that moving toward an understanding that education policies and practice shortcomings in society contribute to underperformance of students and staff and need to be addressed. The COVID-19 pandemic has exposed long-standing racial and economic disparities dating back to the founding of the nation that contribute to the education difficulties of Black children and other children of color.

Intervention projects such as SDP and others are not enough. They show that positive and aspirational conditions can be generated for significant periods, even in communities experiencing difficult socioeconomic conditions, but aligning the cultural, political, and economic structures needed to sustain and grow these communities can be difficult to near impossible, even when the need is urgent. Such projects are vulnerable to the complex residual ill effects of our history and the culture of slavery. Again, but for the work of the BPA-APA-NIMH Minority Center in the 1960s, our in-school child development–focused education approach might not have survived to target and effectively demonstrate capacities and provide opportunities, especially for poor and marginalized communities. What we learned strongly suggests that an informed next-level structural change is needed, parts or all of which already exist but need to be thought about and tasked intentionally and differently.

Racism is a core problem, not a sole or silo problem. Aligning, connecting, and coordinating the sources of power and change in education and all our social structures are all needed. But doing so is difficult even at the small and single organization levels. And doing so is greatly difficult at the state and national levels because each of the 50 states usually operates much like a separate nation. Nonetheless, when faced with "must do" situations in the past, the federal government convened needed power sources, allocated money, and created megastructures and plans to overcome obstacles that threatened the country's present and future, resulting in the New Deal, the Tennessee Valley Authority, the Marshall Plan, the GI Bill, and the Apollo Program. And we did so with COVID-19, with Operation Warp Speed and other federal efforts to combat the virus.

These megastructures that enabled existing social structures that worked in silos to connect and work with common focus across boundaries to create mega plans and strategy were primarily economic-centered efforts. Today's urgent need is to make it possible for all people to achieve education or school success and mental health that prepare them to live in a democracy in a complex world. Therefore, today's mega plans must be designed to facilitate adequate family functioning, child and adolescent development, and preparation for youth to successfully participate in a democracy. This is different than in the past.

Through a federal government mega plan, the Tennessee Valley Authority changed a huge problematic area of the nation from poverty and social difficulty into an economic and social spark plug. But in all of its operations, the project was allowed to follow the rules of the Jim Crow South. Today's mega plan, with an economic core, must paralyze the expression of racism. That will require place-based models of how all five of our social systems—family, educational, economic, political, and cultural—can interact to support family and education experiences that can enable most people to succeed in school and in life and, in so doing, create and sustain a well-functioning democracy.

The pressure for change is a part of what the BPA-APA-NIMH Minority Center arrangement and work in the 1960s was about, but at the time it was an external element. The difference now is that the vision and pressure must be integral to planning. Such a mega plan can provide the needed magnitude of focus and power. Only the federal government can bring the public and private interests and the institutional and individual and group interests to the table with regard to problem management and problem-solving.

There is no easy recipe. A mega plan, much like the U.S. Constitution, is a living process, created as we live, learn, and participate in and make all our social systems work for all.

References

Cauce AM, Comer JP, Schwartz D: Long term effects of a systems-oriented school prevention program. Am J Orthopsychiatry 57(1):127–131, 1987 3826309

Comer JP: The president's message. Black Psychiatrists of America 2(2):1, 5, 1973

Comer JP: A social skills curriculum for inner city children: progress report, 1976–77. New Haven, CT, Yale University, 1977

Comer JP: Parent Participation in the Schools. Phi Delta Kappan 67(6):442–446, 1986

Comer JP: New Haven's school-community connection. Educ Leadersh 44(6):13–16, 1987

Comer JP: Maggie's American Dream: The Life and Times of a Black Family. Dutton Adult, 1988

Comer JP: School Power: Implications of an Intervention Project. New York, Free Press, 1993

Comer JP, Haynes NM: Parent involvement in schools: an ecological approach. Elem Sch J 91(3):271–277, 1991

Comer JP, Haynes NM, Hamilton-Lee M, et al: Dimensions of children's self-concept as predictors of social competence. J Soc Psychol 127(3):321–329, 1987

Darling-Hammond L, Cook-Harvey CM, Flook L, et al: With the whole child in mind: insights from the Comer School Development Program. Washington, DC, Association for Supervision and Curriculum Development, 2018

Drake DD: Student success and the family: using the Comer model for home-school connections. Clearing House 68(5):313–316, 1995

Ertz M: The Grawemeyer collection at the University of Louisville: descriptive statistics of the award's nominees and the collection's contents (1985–2020). Notes 77(1):33–55, 2020

Glass J: New testing validates high scores of 2 schools. Virginian-Pilot, August 5, 1996, p 1

Gooden ST, Myers SL: The Kerner commission report fifty years later: revisiting the American dream. RSF: The Russell Sage Foundation Journal of the Social Sciences 4(6):1–17, 2018

Haynes NM, Comer JP: Integrating schools, families, and communities through successful school reform: the school development program. School Psych Rev 25(4):501–506, 1996

Haynes NM, Comer JP, Hamilton-Lee M: The school development program: a model for school improvement. J Negro Educ 57(1):11–21, 1988

Haynes NM, Comer JP, Hamilton-Lee M: School climate enhancement through parental involvement. J Sch Psychol 27(1):87–90, 1989

McLaughlin M: The Long, Hot Summer of 1967: Urban Rebellion in America. New York, Springer, 2014

Noblit GW, Malloy WW, Malloy CE: The Kids Got Smarter: Case Studies of Successful Comer Schools: Understanding Education and Policy. Cresskill, NJ, Hampton Press, 2001

Pierce CM: A psychiatric approach to present day racial problems. J Natl Med Assoc 51(3):207–210, 1959 13655083

Pierce CM: Black psychiatry one year after Miami. J Natl Med Assoc 62(6):471–473, 1970 5493608

Ramirez-Smith C: Stopping the cycle of failure: the Comer Model. Educ Leadersh 52(5):14–19, 1995

The Urgency of Responsible Leadership in American Psychiatry

RACIAL BIAS AND THE BIOPSYCHOSOCIAL CRISES IMPACTING MENTAL HEALTH IN COMMUNITIES OF COLOR

Donna M. Norris, M.D.

The problem of the twentieth century is the problem of the color line.
W. E. B. Du Bois (1903)

In this chapter I highlight the roles of key Black psychiatrists and psychologists in America who sought to have positive influences on the mental health and well-being of African Americans and other marginalized communities through education and the expansion of the system of care offered by psychiatry. These reflections provide historical context and reveal firsthand experiences related to being a Black professional in this country. The struggle to rise above the limitations of racism and bias within the political structure of American psychiatry requires principled leadership under these constraints in order to make meaningful contributions to the field.

Kenneth B. Clark, Ph.D., the First Solomon Carter Fuller Awardee

In the early 1950s, a few Black psychiatrists began meeting among themselves at meetings of the National Medical Association (NMA) and the American Psychiatric Association (APA) and around the country seeking to address the inequities in the care offered to Blacks and other persons of color within psychiatric settings. In 1954, the Supreme Court's unanimous decision in *Brown v. Board of Education* opined that separate but equal was unconstitutional and violated the Equal Protection Clause of the 14th Amendment of the U.S. Constitution (*Brown v. Board of Education* 1954). The recipient of the first Solomon Carter Fuller Award was Kenneth B. Clark, Ph.D. The award was presented in 1970 by the Black Psychiatrists of America (BPA) for seminal research cited in this case. Although Clark was not able to be present for the meeting because of fragile health, he forwarded his written acceptance. Referencing the original brief argued by then attorney Thurgood Marshall signed by "thirty-two distinguished sociologists, psychologists, educators, and psychiatrists," Clark noted that "this brief could be used even today to answer many of our impatient young people who demand relevance. This was a most relevant document in the sense that it was concerned with issues of social justice, it was concerned with decency, humanity." Clark rejected the science of Daniel Patrick Moynihan, Christopher Jencks, and Arthur Jensen, who he noted "have become advocates of the continuation of segregated schools." He continued, stating that

> we, as concerned human beings, and as social scientists, psychologists, and psychiatrists, who happen to be black—we, together with our white colleagues who still maintain integrity and a primary loyalty to scientific objectivity and scientific concern with humans, cannot permit this new breed of social science reactionaries to prevail. We must continue to fight for justice and decency. We must continue to fight because we know and we believe that truth in science—truth—must always be on the side of morality. (Clark 1973, pp. 1–2)

Significantly, the records are less clear as to whether the American Psychological Association formally supported this legal argument before the Supreme Court for an end to segregation in schools (Benjamin et al. 2002). Charles Prudhomme, M.D., reported that he approached the American Psychological Association during this time and requested a brief amicus curiae in support of the *Brown v. Board of Education* matter. He was told by the association's leaders "to remain aloof from such a political issue," and his behavior was described as "acting out" (Prudhomme and Musto 1973). Nevertheless, the unanimity of this Supreme Court decision signaled the start of critical forces toward the establishment of equality in access to education for Black people and other marginalized groups. Most Black people benefited directly or indirectly from this greater access to education, including medical training.

Remembering Jeanne Spurlock, M.D. (1921–1999)

Jeanne Spurlock, M.D., was a child and adolescent psychiatrist; chief of the Child Psychiatry Unit, Michael Reese Hospital (1960–1968); chair of the Department of Psychiatry, Meharry Medical College (1968–1973); and deputy medical director of the APA until her retirement (1974–1991). Spurlock was a pioneering leader and mentor to hundreds of trainees in psychiatry and other mental health disciplines in the United States and internationally. She was also a mentor in my own career. The education and training of medical students and psychiatric residents were of primary importance to Dr. Spurlock and comprised the focus of her work throughout her entire professional life. Dr. Spurlock has four fellowships named in her honor: two fellowships for medical students offered by the American Academy of Child and Adolescent Psychiatry and two fellowships for psychiatric residents from the APA (the Jeanne Spurlock Congressional Fellowship and the Jeanne Spurlock, M.D. Minority Fellowship Achievement Award). Dr. Spurlock was the first Black American and first woman to receive the Edward A. Strecker, M.D. Award for excellence in psychiatry sponsored by the Pennsylvania Hospital, University of Pennsylvania Health Systems. She also received the Distinguished Service Award from the APA.

Less well known to some is the fact that Drs. Jeanne Spurlock and Elizabeth Davis Trussell, chairs at Meharry Medical College and Harlem Hospital, respectively, were among the women members of the Black Psychiatrists Think Tank during the 1960s (C. Pierce, personal communication, February 2010). They advocated for change within organized medicine and against discriminatory treatment of patients in major psychiatric institutions, including the National Institute of Mental Health (NIMH) and the APA. As a powerful critic of discrimination and stigma of all types—sexism, ageism, and racism—Spurlock encouraged her mentees to actively confront inequity wherever it emerged. Although colleagues considered her to be too blunt and straightforward in her strong advocacy for children and for women and others underrepresented in medicine, Spurlock was undeterred in her outspokenness against perceived injustice. At times, associates in professional meetings met Spurlock's comments with chilly receptions; nevertheless, she continued to be direct, challenging, and focused on the importance of addressing patients' mental health needs.

As a strong advocate for supporting the stability of Black families, Spurlock was particularly concerned about the impact on Black men and their families of the 1994 Crime Bill, which resulted in greater incarceration time and separation from their communities compared with that of white men with similar crimes (Spurlock 1994). Spurlock was also personally aware of the lasting impact of racism. In her 1988 Solomon Carter Fuller lecture, "Racism Revisited," she emphasized that race would remain of critical importance in this country going forward. Spurlock edited the book *Black Psychiatrists and American Psychiatry*, the first historical reference of the presence of Black psychiatrists and their work to make mental health services for Black Americans and other people of color more equitable (Spurlock 1999). For most African Americans, regardless of socioeconomic status, a measure of the combined factors of racism, unemployment/underemployment, and discrimination is always present and needs management throughout their life span (Spurlock and Norris 1991).

As a kindergartner, Spurlock recalled that color differences and racism presented obstacles to her friendships and play activities with classmates. White parents objected to her playing with their children on the basis of the color of her dark skin, which was an awakening to her. Spurlock recalled that her mother taught her and her siblings that there were no heights that they could not attain in this country "if you worked for it." It was only after the loss of Spurlock's brother to gun violence, in which the white murderer confessed to robbery and the shooting but did not face conviction, that her mother's viewpoint changed, and she recognized that racism was a systemic and pivotal factor in the murderer's release (Spurlock 1994). Today, use of firearms continues to have significant impacts on the lives of Black youth in America, with increased frequency when compared with the rates for white youths. Although poverty is one risk factor, being from a higher socioeconomic life circumstance does not necessarily offer any protective factor against injury and/or death by a firearm. Circumstances of geographic residence, mobility, and skin color within a racist society may augment this risk (Bell and Jenkins 1993; Caron 2021; Formica 2021; Watson-Coleman 2019).

Following medical school, Spurlock initially did not receive a psychiatric residency and training in psychoanalysis. For the latter, Spurlock received advice that it would not be useful training for her because "Blacks could not be analyzed." Spurlock understood that this was another discriminatory stereotype about Black people but persevered in her quest and moved forward to accomplish a distinguished career as a child psychiatrist and psychoanalyst. Although these were painful personal stories and never forgotten, Spurlock used these experiences as catalysts in her scholarship, in her encouragement of others, and in her lifelong advocacy for social and racial justice for families of color.

More than 50 years ago, Spurlock identified the array of root causes of turmoil that surrounded the lives of African American children and continue to be relevant today. These include racism and its devastating effects on self-esteem and the risks racism presents to the safety and future of young Black children living in violent and impoverished communities. The latter is a crucial factor, along with food and housing insecurity, that keeps disproportionate numbers of Black families in precarious financial states. Because of these conditions, many families are forced to continue to live in communities with almost daily exposures to gun violence, drugs, alcohol, and other substances as well as limited access to positive educational opportunities. Further, lack of adequate education jeopardizes the ability of these children to escape poverty and to move closer to a future of success. Under these circumstances, it may be easier for society to view these children as being a risk to others' safety and in need of court intervention rather than health and/or mental health services (Spurlock 1973, Spurlock 1994).

The COVID-19 pandemic has worsened the educational crisis for children of color because of the on-again/off-again pattern of frequent school closures related to the increasing virus prevalence. Even 2 years after the start of the pandemic, there were reports of children in communities of color who did not return to school and became part of the workforce to help provide support for their families (Fortin 2022). All of these factors remain significant challenges for future advocacy.

Family disruptions include the continuous migration patterns between the north and south as families seek gainful employment; family member loss due to the HIV/AIDS crisis, the opioid epidemic, and other substances of abuse; and more recently, the disproportionate effects of severe morbidities and increased excess deaths among Blacks and Hispanics due to the COVID-19 pandemic (Norris and Spurlock

1993; Span 2022; Treglia et al. 2021). Before the beginning of the COVID-19 pandemic, the poverty rate in the United States in 2019 was at its lowest since 1959 (10.5% for the United States, 18.8% for Black Americans, and 15.7% for Hispanic Americans), but with persistent inequities (Creamer 2020). During the pandemic, many groups, including Black Americans, lost even more ground, with 19.5% of Black people in the United States below the poverty line compared with 8.2% of white Americans (Center on Budget and Policy Priorities 2020).

Social Justice for Black Americans

Many of the Black psychiatrists of the 1950s and 1960s, including Spurlock, were political activists and worked side by side with the Freedom Riders in Tennessee, Mississippi, Alabama, and Georgia. Even before the 1963 March on Washington, they were in the forefront of the civil rights movement (C. Pierce, personal communication, February 2010). With this as background, Spurlock in her role as deputy medical director of the APA was familiar with questions regarding allegations of the abuse of human rights and psychiatry in mental health institutions.

In 1978 Spurlock accepted an invitation to join the APA's Committee to Visit South Africa with Alan Stone, M.D., chairperson; Charles Pinderhughes, M.D.; and Jack Weinstein, M.D. Their charge was to review allegations of abuse of Black people for political purposes and their placement in psychiatric facilities run by the Smith Mitchell organization (Stone et al. 1979). Key medical organizations, including the World Health Organization, the World Psychiatric Association, the APA, and the Committee of Black Psychiatrists, raised concerns in support of this investigation. The times were turbulent, and much of the world supported a boycott of South Africa because of apartheid. The use of boycotts had been a successful tactic during Martin Luther King Jr.'s work for equal rights throughout the southern states in the 1950s and 1960s. Among Black members of the APA and the BPA, there was significant support for the BPA to adhere to the boycott and not hold any international conferences in South Africa.

Charles Pinderhughes, M.D., elected as a member of the APA Board of Trustees in 1974, objected strongly to the Board of Trustees' reversal of its endorsement of the United Nations draft program Decade for Action to Combat Racism and Racial Discrimination (Spurlock 1999). During this time in the 1970s and 1980s, the boycott of South Africa was not a universally supported position in the United States, but there was regular discussion about it in psychiatric groups, especially following the APA's consultation. The report focused on Black people, but a concluding statement noted, "Apartheid, as we witnessed it in the Black townships, the squatter communities, and the homelands, as well as in the psychiatric facilities, has destructive implications for all the races of South Africa" (Stone et al. 1979, p. 1506).

While attending an APA meeting of mixed racial groups in the early 1980s, I indicated my support of the boycott, only to encounter a confrontation later in the hallway by a senior white APA leader who strongly objected to my position, angrily exclaiming, "You are wrong, you are wrong!" My thoughts now, as they were then, are that this was another example of a white man telling a Black person—and, in fact, an entire group of Black psychiatrists—that they were wrong in supporting these South African people and that he knew better than Black leadership in this country and in South Africa what was best for them. Significantly, it would be another 16 years after the APA consultation before Nelson Mandela would become the first democratically elected Black president of South Africa (1994–1999). Nevertheless, this was an important moment when leaders in psychiatry took a position to seek answers to whether there was an abuse of psychiatry against Black people.

Thirty years following the Stone group consultation and in preparation for my Solomon Carter Fuller lecture in 2012, I discussed with Dr. Stone the consultation group's findings and the sociopolitical atmosphere of the APA board of the 1970s. He recalled that he and like-minded colleagues on the board were social and political activists and "came (onto the board) with social issues on their agenda" (A. A. Stone, personal communication, October 2009). Dr. Stone described Dr. Jeanne Spurlock as a "big force in this" in her new role as deputy medical director. He knew that "she would speak her mind" and that for this consultation trip, she and Charles Pinderhughes, M.D., offered credibility for the delegation's work as they journeyed to South Africa to investigate the treatment of Black patients. During this same time in the United States, he noted, APA was more involved in addressing social concerns with legal cases dealing with segregation in psychiatric hospitals in the South and the inferior quality of mental health care for Black people. It was his view that social concerns have "taken a back seat to guild concerns," which he described as "more conservative."

In 2009, Stone described the current trends of the APA as a major change from the 1970s, when the Committee for Concerned Psychiatrists with leadership from Alfred Freedman, M.D.; John Spiegel, M.D.; and Lawrence Hartmann, M.D., focused on an agenda of social issues. Stone's professional scholarship addressed key advocacy concerns related to social justice and Black Americans. In 2019, in one of his last speaking occasions at an APA meeting, Stone presented a prelude to his lecture with a series of photographs of his memories of being on the 1947 Harvard football team, playing an integrated game at the University of Virginia with his teammates Chester Pierce, M.D., and Robert Kennedy. He recalled the role of social justice in this period of segregation in Southern areas of this country and the team's support of their sole Black teammate to defy these racial customs. Early personal friendships remained a vital component of his work toward equity, racial justice, and a consideration of values in appreciating others' experiences across the divide of race (A. Stone, personal communication, October 2009). During Stone's tenure on the APA board, homosexuality was eliminated as a mental disorder. In his presidential address, Stone attempted to demonstrate the complex relationship between psychiatry and morality as manifested in psychiatry's approach to racism, homosexuality, and female psychology (Stone 1980).

Racism and Apologies

In 2008, the American Medical Association (AMA) issued an apology statement to Black physicians "for more than a century of discriminatory policies that excluded Blacks from participating in a group long considered the voice of medicine" (American Medical Association 2008). More than a decade after the AMA's initial apology, a senior editor of their premier journal claimed that "no physician could be racist" and that "sociocultural factors, not structural racism, held back communities of color" (Mandavilli 2021). Another apology followed, and the AMA leadership proposed a 3-year plan to "dismantle structural racism" within the organization and within medicine. Notably, AMA members said that racism should be "taken out of the conversation" because its presence was offensive and was viewed as calling an individual "racist" (Mandavilli 2021).

In 2020, graphic media documentation showed full views of George Floyd's last moments of life, preceded and followed closely by the deaths of other young Black and brown people in this country. Medical organizations came out with antiracist messages and webinars as an urgent response to physician members and the public. In January 2021, the APA Board of Trustees issued a public apology in a press release "to its members, patients, their families, and the public for enabling discriminatory and prejudicial actions within the APA and racist practices within psychiatric treatment for Black, Indigenous, and People of Color (BIPOC)" (American Psychiatric Association 2021). Moreover, less than a year after the formal APA apology, the APA Board issued a statement to all members following a "derogatory" tweet by a former president of the association and chairperson of a department of psychiatry "reiterating its [APA's] position that racism and sexism harm the APA as an organization, the field of psychiatry, and the people and communities we serve" (Fadulu 2022).

These examples of racist utterances are negative stereotypes and are not minor events in the lives of Black Americans. They are examples of ingrained miseducation and misunderstanding about Black Americans. They tend to obscure the manner in which racism has become a part of everyday language, actions, and iterations, often without an individual's full awareness of the harm inflicted. *Microaggressions*, coined by Chester Pierce, are offensive mechanisms that appear as subtle insults directed at historically marginalized groups that communicate or engender hostility through actions that may be conscious or unconscious (Pierce 1970). Nevertheless, "micro" does not mean minor. In a racist society, these are repetitive mechanisms that cut deep and are often so disguised that the recipient is frequently confused about the real meaning of the verbal communications and actions received. Individuals of color experiencing microaggressions doubt their own sanity and ability to clearly understand these events, which may involve themselves or others.

Cognizance of the significance, depth, and complexities of racism is critical to the role and responsibilities of psychiatrists who provide mental health services to all people, regardless of color. For example, articles containing highly offensive racist and erroneous information are present throughout the scientific literature of the psychiatric profession. Is a blanket apology enough, or should these writings that were considered to be scholarly works be retracted specifically? Societal changes related to racism and discrimination are aspirational goals and are not likely to be quick accomplishments. Nevertheless, the overarching challenge is to attain equity and justice for all groups while demanding a commitment to a future of antiracist, thoughtful, and visionary leadership.

In 2001, *Mental Health: Culture, Race, and Ethnicity*, a supplement to the U.S. surgeon general's report, offered examples of such responsible leadership by addressing the impact of mental illnesses on Americans regardless of cultural and ethnic differences while recognizing the disparities in and barriers to mental health care that exist for diverse populations (Office of the Surgeon General 2001). Twenty years later, the APA began a series of webinars on racism and the role of organized psychiatry. The webinars provided information regarding this history, which may have been unknown by many in psychiatry. Historically, the misdiagnosis of Black Americans has a long history of voiced concerns by psychiatrists. In March 2022, the APA published a rigorous work, the *Diagnostic and Statistical Manual of Mental Disorders*, Fifth Edition, Text Revision, which presents an expanded and updated review of cultural formulations and appropriate language usage for diagnosis among diverse, ethnic, and cultural groups. It addresses the impact of culture, race, and racism on diagnosis and included expert reviewers in the field to better assist clinicians in improving accuracy and appropriate treatment planning (Moran 2022).

Diversity, Equity, and Inclusion

Leading psychiatric organizations in the United States and internationally are actively engaged in aligning relevant change in their structure and governance to promote diversity, equity, and inclusion efforts within their associations and in their missions (e.g., the American College of Psychiatrists, www.acpsych.org; the Association of American Medical Colleges, www.aamc.org/what-we-do/equity-diversity-inclusion). One of the most influential federal research agencies in the United States is NIMH. In the 1969 confrontational meeting of the BPA with the APA, "APA was encouraged to use its influence to help reduce the racism at the NIMH" (Pierce 1973, p. 538). Now more than 50 years have passed since that original Pierce report on NIMH, and there is significant policy planning in progress. Addressing the state of the agency, NIMH director Joshua Gordon, M.D., Ph.D., noted that "the death of George Floyd served as a wake-up call to me personally and to others in the NIMH community." Throughout the past year, the organization had been working to "identify and address the extent to which our policies, procedures, and culture serve to perpetuate the status quo and working to promote anti-racist ideas and actions" (Gordon 2022). Additionally, in an address to the scientific community at Harvard Medical School, Gordon reported on the NIMH Anti-Racism Task Force recommendations for culture change and new research planning on health disparities; improving the NIMH culture for equity, inclusion, and excellence; and changing policy, culture, and structure to promote workforce diversity (National Institute of Mental Health 2021). These policy changes offer new hope to younger people in the medicine workforce that they, too, can achieve career advancement in research, receive mentorship, and compete for and attain federal grant support at the NIMH as the organization notes future goals of becoming more inclusive and diverse in its workforce (Gordon 2022).

The Political Process and Psychiatry

In 2022, following thousands of media views of the violence perpetrated by law enforcement against people of color, the devastating differential effects of deaths and morbidity of the COVID-19 pandemic emerged. Although health care disparities have been present for generations, with lasting consequences on the health and welfare of Black people, a subset of people within parts of America and within psychiatry may be tired of discussing or working on issues of racism. These concerns may be overtly evident and displayed impatiently in public meetings. At other times, there may be neglect and silence in response to these matters despite their seriousness and lifelong impact on the lives of patients.

Over the years, Black leaders in American psychiatry sought elected positions within APA because they recognized that work regarding the mental health of Black and other marginalized groups was inadequate. The majority of these individuals were not successful in the APA political process but continued to provide exemplary commitment to the field and attained achievements in other mental health and/or professional medical organizations. Other leaders in American psychiatry also recognized that such inequities existed. Prior to my Solomon Carter Fuller lecture in 2010 titled "Racial Politics in American Psychiatry," I conducted interviews of a select group of Black and white psychiatrists who had sought and/or held elected office in the APA. These psychiatrists included Drs. Chester Pierce, George Mallory, Hugh Butts, June Jackson Christmas, Phyllis Harrison-Ross, Hiawatha Harris, James Comer, Alfred Freedman, Alan Stone, Felton Earls, Michelle Clark, and Mildred Mitchell-Bateman. Questions focused on their insights regarding the influence of American psychiatry, including the APA, on social concerns regarding race and disparities in mental health care for patients of color. In the following sections I present highlights from interviews with Mildred Mitchell-Bateman, M.D., who was the first woman and first Black psychiatrist elected vice president of the APA in 1973 and who later ran for APA president, and Michelle Clark, M.D., a distinguished Black psychiatrist leader.

Mildred Mitchell-Bateman, M.D. (1922–2012)

In my discussions with Dr. Mitchell-Bateman, she recalled that Black psychiatrists were active on social concerns long before the group had any involvement with the APA. They worked tirelessly on civil rights and projects for improvement of the mental health of Black Americans; however, they were not actively engaged in the political process within the APA. Initially, these Black psychiatrists met separately at the time of either NMA or APA meetings. However, as their numbers increased, they formed their own organization (BPA) and met alone. She stated that this was a similar path to that followed by women psychiatrists, who established a separate organization, the Association of Women Psychiatrists, independent of the APA. Although most Black women aligned with the Caucus of Black Psychiatrists, Mitchell-Bateman found that Black women had to choose an affinity group within the APA, that is, a designation as Black or as a woman. She chose to divide her time between the two groups.

Mitchell-Bateman's psychiatric career included serving as the commissioner of mental health for the state of West Virginia for 15 years and as chair of psychiatry at Marshall University (Mitchell-Bateman 1999). Her view was that the office of vice president was considered to be a "Black seat" and "tokenism," with its effectiveness dependent on who sat there. She and others recalled that the "old boy's network" was a factor in the political process to "break up succession" and "to open up the APA to broader representation in all levels" (A. Freedman, personal communication, May 2010; M. Mitchell-Bateman, personal communication, February 2010). When Mitchell-Bateman expressed an interest in and ran for APA president in 1976, she did not expect universal support in the political process. Women allies among the group of white psychiatrists supported her, but others stated that it was not timely for her to run because the APA had already had three women presidents, and with her soft voice, she was not "a forceful enough person" to speak up for women. Of note is the problem that often accompanies women who strive for leadership: Sex-based discriminatory stereotypes often surface to limit their progress. As an example, one may hear, "You don't look like a president or a chief executive officer." The opposition for Mitchell-Bateman came from other quarters as well. A Black psychiatrist advised her to drop out of the race because she could not win against a white man.

Mitchell-Bateman reported that it was later determined that a white man was to be the opponent, and he was a strong advocate against efforts to develop a national health plan. As commissioner of mental health for the state of West Virginia, Mitchell-Bateman supported a public health plan option. Looking back on history, this was ahead of the times for the majority of physicians in medicine; the AMA had not been fully supportive of Medicare legislation in the 1960s (Cohen 1985). Although both white men and women supported Mitchell-Bateman's run for office, she recalled that many spoke against it, noting that in her position on the public option, she could not fully represent the APA, which at that time was against a national health insurance plan. Mitchell-Bateman addressed her greatest concern that her candidacy would split the cohesion among the women's group.

When the APA held its 1981 annual meeting in Louisiana, a state that did not ratify the Equal Rights Amendment, some women psychiatrists refused to attend. Others suggested to Mitchell-Bateman that they had made an error in judgment in not supporting her earlier campaign and that she should consider another run for office. However, by this time, Mitchell-Bateman noted that her workload was too busy for her to campaign again (Mitchell-Bateman, personal communication, February 2010). In 2016, almost 50 years after Black psychiatrists confronted the APA Board of Trustees with concerns about unmet mental health needs of Black patients, the membership elected Dr. Altha Stewart, the first Black president of the APA.

Black Psychiatrists and Organized Psychiatry: Michelle O. Clark, M.D.

In this time of great need a/nd with a crisis in mental health service delivery systems across the country, young, gifted Black psychiatrists are choosing to disengage from the APA, the largest major association for psychiatrists. This exodus is not a recent phenomenon; however, it is more visible because these young psychiatrists have held high-profile positions within the organization. My Solomon Carter Fuller presentation included a brief career snapshot of one of these leaders, Michelle O. Clark, M.D.

Clark is a former chair of the APA Committee of Black Psychiatrists, a former APA/NIMH fellowship awardee for 3 years, and a psychiatry section chair of the NMA. A graduate of Columbia University Medical School, she advanced to distinguished fellow within the APA prior to her resignation. As chair of the Committee of Black Psychiatrists, she sat on the Board of Trustees in a nonvoting seat and felt it important to be there and be ever vigilant to address concerns of disparities and other mental health challenges that have impacts on older adults, children, and minority groups (M. Clark, personal communication, January 2010, April 2022). She guided the committee work to coauthor an APA curriculum text for the treatment of Black patients. When asked why, after 27 years, she left the APA, Clark responded that the organization was "not relevant to minority concerns, not for patients, and not for communities of color." Initially, Clark recalled her enthusiasm in joining the APA, which she thought would provide opportunities to gain knowledge and hear different points of view about mental health care. However, there was a "political side," which she thought was more representative of "payback" for friends of those in leadership who seemed more interested in positions of influence on committees rather than rewarding competence or merit (M. Clark, personal communication, January 2010, April 2022). Since that time, other young Black psychiatrists have become disillusioned with the rate of progress in diversity and equity within the organization. There will never be enough Black psychiatrists to provide optimal care for the entire Black and brown communities in this country. Therefore, it is imperative that we mentor and support young Black psychiatrists to stay in the forefront of organized psychiatry and help them to prepare for leadership and scholarship in the field. The departures of young Black psychiatrists from the organization represent a warning sign of the developing crisis that the field faces to maintain readiness to address the inequities of service delivery needs and to meet the career aspirations and goals of our young professional colleagues.

Reflections of an Elected Black APA Officer: Donna M. Norris, M.D.

Starting my tenure in the APA Assembly, I was a representative for Black psychiatrists, for the Massachusetts District Branch, then as a leader for Area 1 (New England states of Maine, New Hampshire, Massachusetts, Vermont, and Rhode Island and eastern Canada). Later, I became the first African American and first woman speaker of the APA Assembly and achieved election as APA secretary-treasurer. I received three presidential citations from APA presidents, and I was fortunate to collaborate with psychiatrist colleagues from a variety of races, cultures, and subspecialties. We were allies and were united in our joint work and mission to serve our patients and offered professional and personal supports to each other. Whether we agreed or not, there was a respectful discussion of concerns.

In my speech to the APA Assembly more than 20 years ago, I discussed the challenges for the future of psychiatry. We knew then that violence was at crisis proportions and likely to escalate. "Violence and the upsurge in racist theories and practices are social issues that are destructive to the spirit of all individuals and negatively affect mental health and well-being" (Norris 1999, p. 1479). Projected increases in numbers of minority populations in this country and racial discriminatory practices in medicine and their impact on medical care were among the examples of additional future challenges. It became clear to me that members among the APA leadership group did not want the APA to continue its commitment to articulating advocacy for underserved and underrepresented groups. There were challenges regarding the continued support of underrepresented groups as being too expensive and having little documented evidence of results. Eventually, minority and underrepresented committees that had met twice a year at the September Component Meetings and at the APA Annual Meeting were discontinued and replaced by APA caucus groups that met only once yearly with uneven administrative support.

The political atmosphere of retrenchment from the past was returning to the forefront. When I arrived in Boston in the 1970s as a resident, a group of senior Black psychiatrists was already engaged in offering bimonthly group mentorship to young Black trainees in the area. The majority of my fellow resident colleagues were the only persons of color in their respective programs, and for most, this was their only opportunity to discuss psychiatry with senior and/or junior Black professionals. Leaders such as Drs. Charles Pinderhughes, Chester Pierce, Frances Bonner, Alvin Poussaint, Orlando Lightfoot, Anne Bell, and Dorothea Simmons offered their expertise and advice about how to successfully navigate training in these majority white academic centers. The group was representative of academic, research, and clinical expertise, was known nationally and internationally, and was active at all levels of leadership. These psychiatrists had played important roles in protests for social justice and civil rights activities of the 1950s and 1960s.

With this as a backdrop, few African Americans in this area or across the nation held leadership roles in American psychiatric organizations, particularly within the APA, a group I had only recently joined with encouragement from my department chief. During the APA Annual Meetings, Black psychiatrists spoke eloquently in presentations on scientific programs. I began to notice that few in this group ever attained elective office. Almost 40 years later, I returned to this question and interviewed African American and white psychiatrists in preparation for my Solomon Carter Fuller lecture. One of the psychiatrists I interviewed was Chester Pierce, M.D. (C. Pierce, personal communication, February 2010). He recalled that even before Selma and Dr. King's marches in Alabama, Black physicians in Oklahoma were leading sit-ins and protests for equal rights. Further, he recalled his work as an Assembly representative to the APA from Oklahoma. Pierce noted that the state then was a "vibrant place" and "ahead of the times." As an example, Pierce recalled that Dr. Wolf, the chief of medicine at the Oklahoma Veterans Administration Hospital, observed Black patients lying in the hallways when there were empty beds in rooms with white patients. He moved the Black patients into the empty beds in rooms with white patents until their discharge, after which all hospital wards were integrated a decade before the Civil Rights Act of 1964, which outlawed segregation in public facilities. Significantly, Pierce noted that the civil rights movement had a group of white friends, even though they were "poles apart politically." He identified Charlton Heston, president of the Screen Actors Guild, and actor Paul Newman as friends of the movement whose presence and voice made a difference.

More than 50 years have now passed since a small group of Black psychiatrist leaders confronted the APA Board regarding the pernicious impact of the racist practices perpetrated against Black Americans by ignoring social issues, such as poverty, segregated mental health hospitals, and poor diagnostic rigor regarding mental health needs of Black patients. The 1970 Waggoner presidential address, "Cultural Dissonance and Psychiatry," gingerly considered that psychiatry should more fully address social concerns: "overcrowding in our cities [which] can be a partial explanation for the increase in social aggression and crime" and the "problem of racism" (Waggoner 1970, p. 45). Since then, others have acknowledged that the entire psychiatric system of care has been affected by racist practices and, at times, has resulted in limited access for Black Americans, children and adults, to needed care from a specialty already in short supply in this country (Romano 1990; Sabshin et al. 1970). These reported system failures have forced people into the legal system, leaving them with minimal or no mental health services. Today, greater numbers of persons experiencing acute and chronic mental illnesses are dependent on limited community supports. This places people at risk of becoming homeless and becoming victims on America's streets.

Racial Politics

Racial politics refers to a process by which one group exploits or impedes the progress of another group on the basis of race—consciously or unconsciously—with a personal or organizational agenda. Issues related to the dimensions of racism, interracial practice patterns, the complexities of social change, and the power dynamics between diverse groups often masked in a racist society remain unresolved and have a profound influence on care for the patients we serve (Bernard 1972; Harrison and Butts 1970). With the country's changing demographics, Black people and other people of color are moving toward a majority status. This anticipated change is a potential opportunity for new leadership to enhance the strength of organized psychiatry. Chester Pierce, M.D., signed his communications with "Yours in the struggle." This is a critical message to all Black and white psychiatrists who are committed to the mission of equity in mental health care for patients and for the profession. This is not an easy straight path toward change. There are starts and stops along the way that require patience. The ultimate goal is the attainment of a profession sustained by equity, diversity, and quality service for all that embodies the Hippocratic oath of physicians.

Summary

In this chapter I have reviewed select professionals in mental health and their career experiences in organized medicine as they sought to provide equitable mental health care for Black patients and other patients of color. Although there were challenges associated with their positions of leadership within psychiatry, their personal abilities to identify allies in the field with whom they worked collaboratively enhanced their effectiveness in improving mental health services. As exemplified by Kenneth Clark, the fight for justice may seem long, disjointed, and without a clear upward trajectory at times. His leadership in education, with limited professional organizational supports, provided so many Black people and other groups of color in this country the impetus to change the courts and attain a legal right to equal education.

The slow pace of change is disheartening for young people as well as older generations. Nevertheless, withdrawing from this struggle and refusing to engage in this fight for system change would portend a bleak future for the profession. It is important for concerned psychiatric professionals to have an active presence in organized medicine focused on striving for objectivity, social justice, and integrity while addressing scientific concerns. In 2022, there is a fierce competition among departments of psychiatry throughout the country for underrepresented groups in medicine to join their residency training programs. These young physicians know they want psychiatric training that values diversity and provides culturally sensitive supervision for their work with patients. They demand a nonracist environment of support and mentorship to build on achieving their career goals. These future psychiatrists deserve an educational and professional environment that is inclusive and relevant to best serving their patients and allows them to flourish in their own personal development and leadership trajectory.

To our young colleagues: Focus your efforts on developing an expertise and consider what contributions you will make to augment the future of the profession and care for the patients who need mental health services. Retain your humility in service to your patients and remain true to your values. Despite the efforts of others who may not fully appreciate these efforts, find ways to continue to be engaged in the decision-making processes, at the system level, about the mental health care of Black patients and other patients under your care. Build connections with other professional networks and professional organizations. Always seek to challenge the status quo, especially when it does not address the needs of patients. Work to improve the systems and science of the field. Do not permit the biased opinions or actions of others to distract you from your professionalism or compromise your values. Continue to work hard and persevere even in the midst of institutional racism.

References

American Medical Association: AMA apologizes to black doctors for racism. NBC News, July 10, 2008. Available at: www.nbcnews.com/health/health-news/ama-apologizes-black-doctors-racism-flna1C9461472. Accessed April 20, 2022.

American Psychiatric Association: APA apologizes for its support of racism in psychiatry. Washington, DC, American Psychiatric Association, January 18, 2021. Available at: www.psychiatry.org/newsroom/apa-apology-for-its-support-of-structural-racism-in-psychiatry. Accessed April 20, 2022.

Bell CC, Jenkins EJ: Community violence and children on Chicago's southside. Psychiatry 56(1):46–54, 1993 8488212

Benjamin LT Jr, Crouse EM; American Psychological Association: The American Psychological Association's response to Brown v. Board of Education: the case of Kenneth B. Clark. Am Psychol 57(1):38–50, 2002 11885301

Bernard VW: Interracial practice in the midst of change. Am J Psychiatry 128(8):978–984, 1972 5058118

Brown v Board of Education of Topeka: Opinion, May 17, 1954. Records of the Supreme Court of the United States Record Group 267. Washington, DC, National Archives, 1954. Available at: www.archives.gov/milestone-documents/brown-v-board-of-education. Accessed April 22, 2022.

Caron C: Why are more Black kids suicidal? A search for answers. New York Times, November 18, 2021. Available at: www.nytimes.com/2021/11/18/well/mind/suicide-black-kids.html. Accessed April 6, 2022.

Center on Budget and Policy Priorities: Tracking the COVID-19 economy's effects on food, housing, and employment hardships. Washington, DC, Center on Budget and Policy Priorities, August 13, 2020. Available at: www.cbpp.org/research/poverty-and-inequality/tracking-the-covid-19-economys-effects-on-food-housing-and. Accessed March 22, 2022.

Clark KB: Clark acceptance speech for the Solomon Carter Fuller Award. Black Psychiatrists of America Newsletter Fall 2(2):1–2, 1973

Cohen WJ: Reflections on the enactment of Medicare and Medicaid. Health Care Financ Rev suppl(suppl): 3–11, 1985 10311372

Creamer J: Inequity persists despite decline in poverty for all major race and Hispanic origin groups. Suitland, MD, U.S. Census Bureau, September 15, 2020

Du Bois WEB: The Souls of Black Folk. Chicago, IL, A.C. McClurg, 1903

Fadulu L: Columbia psychiatry chair suspended after tweet about dark-skinned model. New York Times, February 23, 2022. Available at: www.nytimes.com/2022/02/23/nyregion/columbia-jeffrey-lieberman.html. Accessed February 23, 2022.

Formica MK: An eye on disparities, health equity, and racism—the case of firearm injuries in urban youth in the United States and globally. Pediatr Clin North Am 68(2):389–399, 2021 33678293

Fortin J: More pandemic fallout: the chronically absent student. New York Times, April 20, 2022. Available at: www.nytimes.com/2022/04/20/us/school-absence-attendance-rate-covid.html. Accessed April 22, 2022.

Gordon J: Steps toward equity at NIMH: an update. Bethesda, MD, National Institute of Mental Health, April 20, 2022. Available at: www.nimh.nih.gov/about/director/messages/2022/steps-toward-equity-at-nimh-an-update. Accessed April 22, 2022.

Harrison PA, Butts HF: White psychiatrist's racism in referral practices to Black psychiatrists. J Natl Med Assoc 62(4):278–282, 1970 5423387

Mandavilli A: Editor of JAMA leaves after outcry over colleague's remarks on racism. New York Times, June 1, 2021. Available at: www.nytimes.com/2021/06/01/health/jama-bauchner-racism.html. Accessed November 4, 2021.

Mitchell-Bateman M: Reflections of a commissioner of mental health and a head of a department of psychiatry, in Black Psychiatrists and American Psychiatry. Edited by Jeanne Spurlock. Washington, DC, American Psychiatric Publishing, 1999, pp 179–186

Moran M: Impact of culture, race, social determinants reflected throughout new DSM-5-TR. Psychiatr News, February 24, 2022. Available at: https://psychnews.psychiatryonline.org/doi/10.1176/appi.pn.2022.03.3.20. Accessed May 5, 2022.

National Institute of Mental Health: NIMH director's statement: our commitment to ending structural racism in biomedical research. Bethesda, MD, National Institute of Mental Health, March 1, 2021. Available at: www.nimh.nih.gov/news/science-news/2021/nimh-directors-statement-our-commitment-to-ending-structural-racism-in-biomedical-research. Accessed April 21, 2022.

Norris DM: Report of the speaker: APA official actions. Am J Psychiatry 156(9):1478–1479, 1999

Norris DM, Spurlock J: Separation and loss in African American children: clinical perspectives, in Culture, Ethnicity, and Mental Illness. Edited by Gaw AC. Washington, DC, American Psychiatric Press, 1993, pp 175–188

Office of the Surgeon General: Culture, Race, and Ethnicity: A Supplement to Mental Health: A Report of the Surgeon General. Rockville, MD, Substance Abuse and Mental Health Services Administration, 2001

Pierce C: Offensive mechanisms, in The Black Seventies. Edited by Barbour FB. Boston, MA, Porter Sargent, 1970, pp 265–282

Pierce C: The formation of the Black Psychiatrists of America, in Racism and Mental Health. Edited by Willie CV, Kramer BM, Brown BS. Pittsburgh, PA, University of Pittsburgh Press, 1973, pp 525–554

Prudhomme C, Musto DF: Historical perspectives on mental health and racism, in Racism and Mental Health. Edited by Willie CV, Kramer BM, Brown BS. Pittsburgh, PA, University of Pittsburgh Press, 1973, pp 47

Romano J: Reminiscences: 1938 and since. Am J Psychiatry 147(6):785–792, 1990 2188515

Sabshin M, Diesenhaus H, Wilkerson R: Dimensions of institutional racism in psychiatry. Am J Psychiatry 127(6):787–793, 1970 5482872

Span P: As families grieve, grandparents step up. New York Times, April 12, 2022. Available at: www.nytimes.com/interactive/2022/04/12/well/family/covid-deaths-parents-grandparents.html. Accessed April 13, 2022.

Spurlock J: Some consequences of racism for mental health of children, in Racism and Mental Health. Edited by Willie CV, Kramer BM, Brown BS. Pittsburgh, PA, University of Pittsburgh Press, 1973, pp 147–163

Spurlock J: The Andrea Delgado, M.D. Transcultural Conference Lecture: African American Children in Turmoil, unpublished manuscript, 1994

Spurlock J: Videotape interview. Washington, DC, Academy of Child and Adolescent Psychiatry, October 28, 1994. Accessed July 2021.

Spurlock J (ed): Black Psychiatrists and American Psychiatry. Washington DC, American Psychiatric Press, 1999

Spurlock J, Norris DM: The impact of culture and race on the development of African Americans, in American Psychiatric Press Review of Psychiatry. Edited by Tasman A, Goldfinger SM. Washington, DC, American Psychiatric Press, 1991, pp 594–607

Stone AA: Presidential address: conceptual ambiguity and morality in modern psychiatry. Am J Psychiatry 137(8):887–891, 1980 7416289

Stone AA, Pinderhughes C, Spurlock J, et al; American Psychiatric Association Committee to Visit South Africa: Report of the Committee to Visit South Africa. Am J Psychiatry 136:(11):1498–1506, 1979 11643507

Treglia D, Cutuli JJ, Aratesh KJ, et al: Hidden pain: children who lost a parent or caregiver to COVID-19 and what the nation can do to help them. COVID Collaborative, December 2021. Available at: www.covidcollaborative.us/assets/uploads/img/HIDDEN-PAIN-FINAL.pdf. Accessed April 13, 2022.

Waggoner RW Sr: The presidential address: cultural dissonance and psychiatry. Am J Psychiatry 127(1):1–8, 1970 5426242

Watson-Coleman B: Ring the alarm: the crisis of Black youth suicide in America: a report to Congress from the Congressional Black Caucus. Washington, DC, Congressional Black Caucus, December 20, 2019. Available at: https://watsoncoleman.house.gov/suicidetaskforce. Accessed March 7, 2023.

The Caravan Moves On

FROM SOLOMON CARTER FULLER TO PSYCHIATRY IN THE TWENTY-FIRST CENTURY

Altha J. Stewart, M.D.

The life of Solomon Carter Fuller is, according to biographer Mary Kaplan, "the story of an African American who would not permit the racism of the early twentieth century to quench his resolve and commitment to a productive life in medicine and scientific research" (Kaplan 2005, p. ix). And for me, a student of the history of psychiatry, that is more than enough reason to want to know more about the man who, despite the obstacles of a racist society, pursued his dreams and made significant contributions to science in the fields of neurology, medicine, and psychiatry. In looking at his life, I am reminded of a quote by Ralph Ellison from his 1964 book *Shadow and Act*: "Can a people…live and develop over three hundred years simply by reacting? Are American Negroes simply the creation of white men, or have they at least helped to create themselves out of what they found around them?" (Ellison 1964, p. 315).

Fuller was certainly not simply reacting to things around him as he created a life's work of accomplishments that made him a role model for psychiatrists today. Unfortunately, many psychiatrists today do not fully understand the significance of his contributions to neuroscience and psychiatric disorders, which helped move the field from the pseudoscience of Drs. Samuel Cartwright (1851) and Benjamin Rush (1799) to what we now understand to be the foundational work of neuroscience in our understanding of the brain and what we know to be the neurological basis of psychiatric disorders.

Dr. Fuller began his life in Africa, went to college and received his early medical and postgraduate training in the United States, received early career training and worked in Germany in the laboratory of Alois Alzheimer, and then returned to the United States, where he ended his career in the Boston area. His work aligns in many ways with that of later clinicians, scholars, and researchers who shared his passion as a teacher, clinician, and researcher. His life and achievements can be discussed in the context of conversations on structural racism in psychiatry, acknowledging a new appreciation for his contributions to medicine, pathology, neurology, and psychiatry.

Solomon Carter Fuller's life does not fit the stereotype often assumed to be the life story of some Blacks in medicine; he did not start life as poor or "disadvantaged." When Fuller was born in 1872, America was recovering from the Civil War, which had ended a mere half decade earlier, and was entering a period of racial oppression that extended enslavement of Blacks without the continued legal practice of chattel slavery. This period, euphemistically called "Reconstruction," proved to have long-term negative consequences for generations of African Americans, including the creation of many of the social, economic, and health disparities we see today. Dr. Fuller's grandfather, John Lewis Fuller, had been enslaved in Virginia, and after buying his freedom, he emigrated with his wife to Liberia. It has been reported that the Fuller family may be in possession of documents suggesting that there may be a connection between Benjamin Rush and Solomon Carter Fuller (Willie et al. 1973). In "Benjamin Rush and the Negro," author Betty Plummer (1970) suggested that the slave Rush described in his abolitionist papers may have been an ancestor of Fuller's, based on the area in Virginia where Fuller's family was enslaved.

Fuller's grandfather built a tobacco and brickmaking business and worked his way to prosperity. His son, the first Solomon Fuller, became a landowner and government official in Liberia, and Dr. Solomon Carter Fuller grew up under privileged circumstances. His entry into medicine and then psychiatry 3 years later is a story of a man who achieved in the face of the adversity of the late 1800s and early 1900s, when rights gained by Blacks during Reconstruction were stripped away.

After graduating Livingstone College in 1893, Fuller entered Long Island College Hospital Medical School for a short time before transferring to Boston University School of Medicine, where he earned his medical degree. After a 2-year internship, Fuller joined the staff at Westborough State Hospital and subsequently developed an interest in the mental and neurological conditions of psychiatric patients. To gain fuller knowledge about the underlying nature of diseases he observed clinically, Fuller performed autopsies to collect and analyze tissue sections from deceased mental patients. He was appointed pathologist to the hospital and became an instructor of pathology at Boston University, gaining notoriety as an esteemed practicing neuropsychiatrist and teacher in the Boston area (Kaplan and Henderson 2000).

Dr. Fuller's academic research career is well documented in Kaplan's biography (Kaplan 2005), but medical research was viewed as a luxury at the time, and opportunities for advanced research in the neurological aspects of senile dementia were minimal at the turn of the century. However, Dr. Fuller wanted to advance his technical skills in the origin, nature, and course of brain diseases, so he turned to Edward K. Dunham at Bellevue Hospital Medical Center in New York City to gain further training in bacteriology and autopsy. Encouraged by Dr. Dunham, Fuller soon saw the advantages of study abroad and joined the more than 15,000 Americans who journeyed to Germany and Austria for progressive medical education and training between 1870 and 1914 (Kaplan and Henderson 2000).

In 1904, Fuller traveled abroad to study at the University of Munich with Professors Emil Kraepelin and Alois Alzheimer, as well as at the Pathological Institute of the University of Munich with Professors Otto Bollinger and Hans Schmaus. Little documentation of his experiences in Germany is available because assistants spent their time immersed in work in hospitals and laboratories conducting research, receiving no credit for their work. Fuller took every advantage to learn and described Alzheimer as "a delightful unassuming person who was a poor lecturer, but when you spend time with him in the lab and on the wards, you learned the stuff" (Kaplan and Henderson 2000, p. 254). Fuller led the science, neuroscience, and neuropathology research in senile dementia (Alzheimer's disease), and it was his work that led to the discovery of neurofibrillary tendrils and amyloid plaques. The biographer Kaplan's father observed that but for the fact that Fuller was Black, the disease might have been named Alzheimer-Fuller Syndrome (Kaplan 2005, p. x).

Returning to the United States and the Boston University School of Medicine, Fuller rose from instructor in 1909 to emeritus professor of neurology by 1933. He was a member of the American Medical Association, the Massachusetts Medical Society, the New England Medical Society, the American Psychiatric Association (APA), the New England Psychiatric Association, and the Boston Society of Psychiatry and Neurology. In fact, APA archival records indicate that he was a dues paying member in the early 1900s.

Fuller appeared on the cover of the *Journal of the National Medical Association* in 1954, and the volume included an article with a brief personal and professional biography and a discussion of his landmark work in Alzheimer's disease and other areas of neurological and psychiatric research. The article noted that Fuller was one of the first Negro physicians to serve on the faculty of an American medical school other than Howard or Meharry and included a recounting of his work during World War I as a member of Advisory Medical Board No. 17. It described how in 1943 he returned to his alma mater, Livingstone College, to receive the honorary degree of doctor of science. While there, he was interviewed in a radio broadcast on the impact of World War II on the mental and nervous energies of combatants and civilians. He believed that adequate precautions were taken to ensure that men experiencing nervous or mental disease did not reach combat service and were discharged from the Armed Forces when their condition was ascertained by authorities. He expressed the opinion that the government's program was adequate to weed out such cases, and that, moreover, advanced developments in the field of psychiatry could be expected to rehabilitate a much greater percentage of mentally diseased combatants in this war than had been possible in other times of combat stress (Kaplan and Henderson 2000).

On November 30, 1953, a memorial resolution honoring Dr. Solomon Carter Fuller was read by Dr. James B. Ayer and entered into the official record of the Boston Society of Psychiatry and Neurology, and it was published in the *New England Journal of Medicine* on January 21, 1954 (Ayer 1954). The resolution began "Dr. Fuller's life story is well worth summarizing, for it represents the progressive rise of a man, handicapped by alien birth, by poverty and absence of friends, to a position of trust and competence:—a story which we like to believe can only happen in America" (Ayer 1954, p. 127). The resolution chronicled Dr. Fuller's personal and professional experiences over the 82 years of his life. Highlights included excerpts of his early life in Liberia, where his grandfather migrated after buying his freedom, his return to the United States to study at Livingstone College and later Boston University School of Medicine, and his work with Alzheimer and Kraepelin during his time in Europe in the early twentieth century. The presentation also listed the numerous honors and memberships in the prestigious medical societies of his day. Dr. Ayer's presentation ended with, "I saw and talked with him: though blind, his memory was excellent, his speech flawless, his interests alive. He knew he had not long to live, but accepted the fact in his usual philosophical manner, like the perfect gentleman he was" (Cobb 1954, p. 127).

Yet most psychiatrists know little of Fuller's true contributions to the field of psychiatry and the role his work played in laying the foundation for our understanding of psychiatric illnesses as brain disorders. His work was in an area that we take for granted today, and it began with the work of a Black man who made connections between the changes in the brain at the neuroanatomical level that led to an understanding of diseases we recognize and treat today. Compare his scientific research with Alzheimer to the pseudoscience-based diagnoses of drapetomania by Cartwright (1851), Rush's theories of leprosy as the basis for Black skin color (Rush 1799), and the work of those who misused data in their interpretation of the 1840 census that allegedly "proved" that enslavement was a protective factor for mental health in Blacks because freedom and movement north were clear "evidence" for continuing the institution of slavery (Jarvis 1844; Litwack 1958). Although we know little of the breadth of Dr. Fuller's work life in his early years, we do know that he conducted some of the seminal work that went on to make one of the men he worked with a household name.

In addition to senile dementia and degenerative brain disorders, Fuller also studied pernicious anemia in people with mental illness and the effects of chronic alcoholism on the brain and conducted early research on bipolar disorder. One must wonder if researchers had followed up on his work in pernicious anemia, would we still have a 25-year difference in life span for individuals with mental illness? On the basis of his work in this area, might we have created the precursor to what has now become the integrated care model? Would we still be dealing with the pattern of mental health disparity that exists today? If his work on the effects of alcohol on the brain had been followed up sooner, would there have been such a gap in time between his research and Dr. Carl Bell's work in fetal alcohol spectrum disorder?

Over the course of Dr. Fuller's career, his role in what might be described as advocacy was underrecognized and undervalued. He was often the first and only Black psychiatrist in many professional settings and recognized that there might be limitations to what he could expect to accomplish. He was the only Black in the group at the historic Clark University Psychology, Pedagogy and School Hygiene Conference, arranged in honor of Sigmund Freud's only visit to the United States in

1909. The conference participants included a "who's who" of pioneers in psychiatry and psychology, including Freud, Jung, and, of course, Solomon Carter Fuller, who lectured on "Cerebral Histology With Special Reference to Histopathology of the Psychosis." His laboratory at Westborough State Hospital was described by a successor as "the best place in the country to study the histopathology of the cerebral cortex and the latest pathological findings in severe mental illness" (S. Benjamin, personal communication, February 2021).

An article in the *Washington Post* noted that it was Fuller's work in the early stages of Alzheimer's research that arguably did the most to reveal the true nature of the disease. Fuller reported on the significance of neurofibrillary tangles 5 months before Alzheimer did, and his discovery identified a physically observable basis for this affliction, which so decimates the memories of its victims. Ultimately, the results of Fuller's research helped to confirm that the condition known as Alzheimer's disease was the result not of insanity but rather a physical disease of the brain. He also went on to publish the first comprehensive review of this disease. In 1905, when Fuller returned to Westborough State Hospital, where he resumed his duties as a pathologist with a special focus on Alzheimer's disease, he used his proficiency in German to produce the first English-language translations of much of Alzheimer's work (Cavanaugh 2021).

I believe there is an arc that extends from Dr. Fuller's life and career in the early days of the twentieth century to today's twenty-first-century Black psychiatrists that is particularly relevant. This is most apparent in today's Black psychiatrists, whether they work in academic medicine and research or clinical practice. As Black physicians work to address the challenges of health disparities, health inequity, social injustice, social determinants of mental health, and poor access to and quality of care, many of them have experiences like those of Dr. Fuller as they navigate in a system that is no longer governed by legal discrimination but that is certainly based on a foundation of systemic racism, which creates an environment not unlike the one Fuller experienced. These contemporary challenges create environments much like the unwelcoming ones that Fuller was exposed to in his career. For some physicians, their responses to these challenges manifest as the courage and commitment to call out the structural racism in the profession, often at great risk to their own career success. For others, the often hostile culture in which they work proves to be too toxic and unhealthy for them to succeed and thrive, causing them to depart to pursue other opportunities outside the academic experiences that include clinical care, education, or research in psychiatry. In some cases, however, the overwhelming trauma and exhaustion of trying to work in some of the challenging settings creates intolerable toxic conditions, and we are seeing many leave the profession altogether.

Today, many early and mid-career Black psychiatrists have directed their energy and efforts outside the systems chosen by Fuller to work on issues confronting Blacks in psychiatry. Several are well known from their lectures and publications on topics relevant to the dismantling of structural racism in psychiatry, improving clinical treatment and intervention services to address the specific needs of Black people (including those related to the impact of racism, racial trauma, and associated social determinants), and research that is more inclusive and responsive to the needs of Black people. Similar to Fuller's arrival at the dawn of the twentieth century, in the early days of the twenty-first century we now hear the names Ruth Shim, Sarah Vinson, Jessica Isom, Danielle Hairston, Ayana Jordan, Kevin Simon, Kali Cyrus, Morgan Medlock, and others as they tackle some of the challenging issues of structural racism in psychiatry. Many of them are finding ways to go on to have successful academic careers built on professional excellence, personal confidence, and courage, just as Fuller did.

Fuller had to deal with what we now call *structural racism* in academic medicine, and he once decided to resign a position rather than work under a younger and less experienced white colleague at a stage in his career when he would have been promoted to the job if he were white. And although Fuller sometimes had to remain silent in the face of obvious racist acts, in his work and actions he continued to be present, representing a type of protest against the social mores of the day through his expressions of quiet but undeniable professional excellence. Other twentieth-century Black psychiatrists who demonstrated a similar, if less quiet, protest behavior professionally include Drs. Alvin Poussaint, James Comer, William Grier, Charles Prudhomme, George Mallory, Jeanne Spurlock, Alyce Gullattee, Chester Pierce, Frances Cress Welsing, Carl Bell, and Patricia Newton, to name a few. The list also includes a group of rising stars in the profession, some of whose names were mentioned earlier and who will, I believe, serve as bold navigators to a more just and equitable psychiatry over the next century.

Fuller's legacy of work connects him to many contemporary psychiatrists of African descent when his life is viewed through the lens of science, training, education, research, and advocacy. His accomplishments, passion for the work, and humility about not having to receive credit are reminiscent of some of the physicians who followed him in doing work to "improve the quality of life for Black people in America" (Cavanaugh 2021). Fuller displayed a great deal of grace and professionalism throughout his career in the face of racism and other adversity. I consider him to be a role model and predecessor for psychiatrist-researchers such as Carl Bell, whose research on fetal alcohol syndrome disorder, perhaps an extension of Fuller's own work in this area, provided an understanding of how alcohol consumption by young mothers early in pregnancy created some of the health and mental health issues that led to so many Black children being directed into special education and justice systems instead of appropriate prevention and treatment interventions. And Fuller's commitment to the study of the neurology of the brain and its relationship to psychiatric disorders seems consistent with the career pursuits of other well-known Black psychiatrists, including the following:

- Dr. Frances Cress Welsing and her work on the impact of white supremacy and the culture of racism on the psychological health of Black people laid the groundwork for much of the work to eliminate structural racism and antiracist psychiatry that is under way today. She also is a major source of support and understanding for many Black mental health professionals in their work with Black patients. And although we do not think of Dr. Cress Welsing as a researcher in the same way we do Fuller, her work to observe practices and behaviors in whites and to describe the psychological impact and outcome of racism on Blacks has proven to be critical to understanding the importance of a cultural framework for addressing the true mental health needs of the Black community.
- Dr. Jeanne Spurlock worked to ensure that children; racial, ethnic, and sexual minorities; and other disenfranchised populations have equitable access to available mental health resources by developing training programs and other opportunities to promote culturally competent care. Dr. Spurlock's pioneering initiatives advocating for better clinical treatment and her strong advocacy for marginalized people and communities laid a tremendous foundation for work that continues today in the areas of addressing social determinants of mental health, dismantling structural racism in psychiatry, and creating antiracist psychiatric practices.
- Dr. Chester Pierce and his work on racism and mental health and the impact of racism in media images on the psychological health of Blacks, along with his efforts to increase the understanding by mainstream psychiatry of the importance of these issues, are notable in truly addressing racism in society and psychiatry. His introduction of the term *microaggressions* into the country's lexicon has provided a language and framework for some of the discussions we are hav-

ing now regarding structural racism in psychiatric training and clinical treatment.

- Dr. Alvin Poussaint stands out for his work to combat racism in psychiatry, to change how the media portray Blacks, and to promote the importance of psychiatry and psychiatric treatment in the Black community at a time when most whites in leadership positions in psychiatry were unwilling to address significant issues affecting the mental health and well-being of Black Americans. By calling out racism in psychiatry in the 1970s and 1980s as an issue that the field must address, he stood at the forefront in the early discussions on this issue. And although he was dismissed by white psychiatrists who also sought to discredit him at the time, Dr. Poussaint has continued to make the case that racism must be addressed in order to have an environment in this country that supports psychological wellness in Black people. A new generation of Black psychiatrists is working in this area today.

Black psychiatrists such as Frantz Fanon from Martinique and Fred Hickling from Jamaica who were not born in the United States clearly understood the importance of identifying issues directly related to the colonial-based racial structure that create psychological distress in their home countries. Such issues are part of the creation of the racist foundation of this nation as well. Fanon and Hickling both wrote about these phenomena from their own cultural perspectives and in psychological terms that are relevant to the work of Fuller as well as the other notable psychiatrists included here.

In retrospect, my APA presidential term in 2018 can be viewed in a similar way. The election of a Black person as president after so many medical societies (both large and small) had long ago achieved that goal was highly celebrated by many who had waited so long for that day. And there were certainly many reasons to celebrate this milestone in the APA organization. I remember with fondness the receptions organized by the Caucus of Black Psychiatrists and the Black Psychiatrists of Greater New York. Both gave me a chance to socialize with friends old and new and thank the coalitions of supporters who made my election possible. The opening session in May 2018 gave me an opportunity to share my goals for the year, including working to address diversity, equity, and inclusion in the organization and tie them to the APA strategic plan and 1970 blueprint for action created by former APA medical director Melvin Sabshin (Sabshin et al. 1970). I was energized by the young psychiatrists I had met during the campaign who pointed to these and other social justice issues as being important to them, and I hosted what I considered to be a successful presidential retreat on the topics of diversity, equity, and inclusion in psychiatry.

I was proud to be part of editing two books during this period, *Black Mental Health: Patients, Providers, and Systems* (which included a chapter on my journey to becoming the first Black president of APA) and the special volume of *Psychiatric Clinics of North America* on *Achieving Mental Health Equity*, both of which included a mix of more senior Black psychiatrist contributors and some members of that new vanguard of young and exceptionally talented Black psychiatrists mentioned earlier (Griffith et al. 2018; Stewart and Shim 2020). And as most who know me understand, I have what my dear friend Allie Symonds called "an expansive personality," so although I did not see a need to make the issue of mental health equity a sole focus at the start of my term, it was clearly part of many president's columns, was mentioned at most official APA events, and was the theme for both educational conferences during my presidential year.

I suppose it was naive to assume that because I was comfortable with the topics of race and culture in psychiatry, others would become comfortable having these difficult conversations as well. My involvement in APA over the years had included many such conversations at the intersections of race and gender, which meant that I had credibility on my side personally and a long-standing commitment to the organization professionally. Certainly, my passion and willingness to lead in this area would be enough to make things happen. Unfortunately, shortly after I took office, it became clear to me that the symbolism reflected in the election of a Black president was just that for some people in APA leadership. It became clear that my hope that APA would take seriously the work we needed to do on the issues first raised by Black psychiatrists in 1969 would not be realized.

I wonder if we might have been better prepared for the series of events that transpired in 2020 had we followed up on the demands of the Black psychiatrists who challenged the APA Board of Trustees in 1969, Dr. Sabshin's blueprint in the *American Journal of Psychiatry* in 1970, and the incomplete work on the APA's 2015 strategic plan on institutional racism. Would the APA's position on and plan for addressing this issue have been clearer to members leading into the start of the syndemic of COVID-19, racial killings, and calls to eliminate structural racism that came crashing down nationally and on the APA? The growing unrest, especially among our early and mid-career Black psychiatrists, was similar to the unrest that led to the 1969 disruption of that Board of Trustees meeting. Unlike in 1969, however, today's psychiatrists have access to a range of digital and social platforms to mobilize quickly to express publicly their dissatisfaction with leadership.

By virtue of my role as a senior Black psychiatrist and past APA president, it seemed that the growing dissension and dissatisfaction among a segment of the membership was an ideal way for me to contribute. After all, past presidents are often recalled to service when they have a valuable skill or style that is needed at a point in time by the organization. However, I did not fully appreciate at the time the challenge I represented for APA's leadership regarding how they would deal with these challenges and the challengers. Over the remainder of 2020, I was accused of encouraging members to express their dissatisfaction, anger, and frustration over the APA's responses to a variety of issues important to them, in ways that were considered disrespectful and even threatening to members of the leadership team. In the aftermath of the public resignation of one of our most respected psychiatrist colleagues, I was questioned by the president about my role in her decision. There seemed to be a kind of "magical thinking" that I had influenced young Black psychiatrists to leave the organization they described as no longer serving their needs and requiring too high a minority tax to remain. That the question and other allegations were even posed made 2020 the year I will remember for the huge minority tax I paid for being the first Black president of APA.

Although Fuller might often have had to remain silent, his biography includes examples of his efforts to mitigate racial disparities in mental health care by training young Black psychiatrists to treat Black veterans of World War I. But he could not overcome the medical profession's racial workforce inequities and discriminatory culture and practices. For example, as a professor at Boston University, he was paid less than his white colleagues, and despite carrying out the duties of the head of the neurology department, he never received the title of chair or even a full professorship. He once remarked, "With the sort of work that I have done, I might have gone farther and reached a higher plane had it not been for the color of my skin" (Kaplan 2005, p. 68). I believe he saw his work as needing to be "present" on occasions when his presence was a reminder that Black professionals of excellence were a part of the evolving field of psychiatry, neurology, and pathology. This legacy continues through the American Psychiatric Association's named award created in his honor in 1969, which coincides with the date of the meeting where Black psychiatrists presented demands for change to the APA Board of Trustees. Recipients of the APA's Solomon Carter Fuller award are selected to honor work that "has significantly improved the quality of life for Black people" (American Psychiatric Association 2022).

I will remember Fuller as the man who stood beside me during the year of my historic APA presidency. The portrait of the first Black psychiatrist hung above the desk in the office assigned to APA presidents in the Washington, D.C., headquarters during that year. I have not been to the offices since early 2020, several months after my immediate past-president term ended, so I cannot say if the portrait is still hanging there. However, the constant presence of his portrait during my presidency gave me the opportunity to reflect on my own place in the history of the field of psychiatry.

It was around that time that I began to see myself as someone who shares many of the characteristics and experiences I saw in Fuller. The historic nature of my role as the first Black president of the world's largest psychiatric organization and this nation's oldest medical society meant that, like Fuller, I could be "present" in places where my presence might create the framework for having much needed conversations, no matter how personally painful they might be. And being present in those moments was reminiscent of how Fuller might have felt so often in his life, although I can only imagine what being the "only one" must have felt like for him. We know little of the time he spent lecturing at Harvard Medical School, where he was remembered by medical student Karl Menninger as his teacher, or what happened after he was rejected by Johns Hopkins for a position because he was a "colored man," although he was recommended by Adolf Meyer and then APA president Karl Bowman. This is an experience that we see repeated today for many aspiring Black academicians who are not silent on the need for system change to diversify the workforce, eliminate disparities, and create more equity in health care. Similarly, most people today know very little about some of the interactions I experienced or witnessed during and after my tenure as president of the APA, some of which are much too painful to recount in full at this time.

Finally, one of the reasons I will always view Fuller as an early protest psychiatrist is his work to recruit more Black people into the mental health profession at a time when this was not popular. It was also evident in his work to change the system that deemed Black veterans to be ineligible for veterans benefits because of diagnoses of "behavior disorders" or "bad conduct cases" by the Veterans Health Administration (allegedly arising as sequelae from CNS syphilis). Dr. Fuller used his clinical and laboratory work to challenge that system so that mentally ill Black veterans could receive their rightful benefits, another classic example of how he protested to overcome some of the racist practices of his day. And certainly, I consider the number and type of racially motivated incidents involving Black psychiatrists (including those I experienced) over the past five decades to be minor compared with those he endured, but each one leaves its own indelible mark on the community of Black psychiatrists and is a painful reminder of how much work there still is to be done.

My goal in presenting the 2021 Solomon Carter Fuller lecture was to articulate how Fuller's work ethic and process of engaging those around him were based on not simply reacting to what was going on around him but creating from what was around him. He appears to have been comfortable with what some would call a "different-ness"—personally, as an African-born American who lived, studied, and worked in multiple locations, and professionally, as a scientist who excelled in multiple disciplines. He had an inner confidence that, despite the realities of when he lived, allowed him to remain centered and focused and to have hope and envision a future that included Black doctors, better care for Black people, and a more just and equitable life for Black people.

And I can now see parallels in my own life and career accomplishments where I also did not simply react to what was going on around me but tried to create something that I hope will be part of a better future for Black people. The most recent examples include recruiting and encouraging young psychiatrists to work in the field as leaders, advocates, and innovators to create the profession we need for the future. Another is the creation of the Center for Health in Justice Involved Youth (now the Center for Youth Advocacy and Well-Being) at the University of Tennessee Health Science Center, where we work with one of the most stigmatized groups in our society—young (10–19 years old), mostly Black males directed into the cradle-to-prison pipeline at birth because of poverty, poor educational opportunities, multigenerational trauma, and a host of other social challenges—youth who are not just "bad kids." Assuring that they have access to trauma-informed health and behavioral health treatment instead of out-of-home placement or detention is an example of creating and not just reacting to what is going on around us.

Other examples are evident in how many of today's Black psychiatrists approach their work to achieve a more equitable mental health system by working against a health care system that supports "weaponizing" racist tactics against Black professionals and other professionals of color, often using overt racially discriminatory actions to deny them professional opportunities. The work of Black psychiatrists in pursuit of creating innovative and effective approaches to providing culturally appropriate care, improving education and training methods, and working to eliminate structurally racist systems of care are reminiscent of Fuller's passion as he studied senile dementia and degenerative brain disorders, pernicious anemia in people with mental illness, the effects of chronic alcoholism on the brain, and bipolar disorder. And much like

Fuller and his input on the impact of war on the military and civilians during WWII, many of today's Black psychiatrists are quite vocal on one of the most challenging issues of our time, the impact of structural racism on all aspects of Black life.

I want to thank the members of the American Psychiatric Association's Caucus of Black Psychiatrists, who selected me as the 2021 Solomon Carter Fuller awardee. Finally, I offer my sincere gratitude to Dr. Solomon Carter Fuller for being a tremendous role model. In reviewing his life story, I am reminded of the analogy of the house in need of repairs used by Isabel Wilkerson at the start of her book *Caste: The Origins of Our Discontents* (Wilkerson 2020). She described how although the house's current residents may not have caused the problems in the structure, they are responsible for addressing the problems now. In that vein, I believe we are responsible for carrying on the work that Dr. Fuller began with his noble efforts to ensure that Black psychiatrists can thrive and are involved in the great work in which psychiatry is engaged in the twenty-first century. And although his legacy may not be truly understood by all, his contributions to move psychiatry from the medical specialty we knew in the late nineteenth and early twentieth centuries will be forever remembered as an important part of the foundation of the field of psychiatry.

References

American Psychiatric Association: Solomon Carter Fuller award. Washington, DC, American Psychiatric Association, 2022. Available at: www.psychiatry.org/psychiatrists/awards-leadership-opportunities/awards/fuller-award. Accessed November 21, 2022.

Ayer JB: Solomon Carter Fuller—1872–1953. N Engl J Med 250(3):127, 1954

Cartwright SA: Report on the diseases and physical peculiarities of the Negro race. New Orleans Med Surg J 11:691–715, 1851

Cavanaugh R: On World Alzheimer's Day, the Black doctor who helped decode the disease. Washington Post, September 21, 2021. Available at: www.washingtonpost.com/history/2021/09/21/world-alzheimers-day-solomon-carter-fuller. Accessed March 9, 2023.

Cobb WM: Solomon Carter Fuller, 1872–1953. J Natl Med Assoc 46(5):370–372, 1954 20893712

Ellison R: Shadow and Act. New York, Random House, 1964

Griffith EH, Jones BE, Stewart AJ (eds): Black Mental Health: Patients, Providers, and Systems. Washington, DC, American Psychiatric Association Publishing, 2018

Jarvis E: Insanity among the coloured population of the free states. Philadelphia, PA, T.K. and P.G. Collins, 1844. Available at: https://collections.nlm.nih.gov/ext/mhl/101475758/PDF/101475758.pdf. Accessed November 21, 2021.

Kaplan M: Solomon Carter Fuller: Where My Caravan Has Rested. Lanham, MD, University Press of America, January 1, 2005

Kaplan M, Henderson AR: Solomon Carter Fuller, M.D. (1872–1953): American pioneer in Alzheimer's disease research. J Hist Neurosci 9(3):250–261, 2000 11232367

Litwack LF: The federal government and the free Negro, 1790–1860. J Negro Hist 43(4):261–278, 1958

Plummer BL: Benjamin Rush and the Negro. Am J Psychiatry 127(6):793–798, 1970 4921620

Rush B: Observations intended to favour a supposition that the black color (as it is called) of the Negroes is derived from the leprosy. Am Philos Soc Trans 4:289–297, 1799

Sabshin M, Diesenhaus H, Wilkerson R: Dimensions of institutional racism in psychiatry. Am J Psychiatry 127(6):787–793, 1970 5482872

Stewart AJ, Shim RS: Achieving mental health equity. Psychiatr Clin N Am 43(3):xiii–xiv, 2020 32773083

Wilkerson I: Caste: The Origins of Our Discontents. New York, Random House, 2020

Willie CV, Kramer BM, Brown BS (eds): Racism and Mental Health. Pittsburgh, PA, University of Pittsburgh Press, 1973

15

Nigrescence and the Future of American Psychiatry

Stephen A. McLeod-Bryant, M.D.

Ruth Shim reminds us that the leadership of the American Psychiatric Association (APA) once exhorted psychiatry, and specifically white psychiatrists, to dismantle racism within psychiatry (Shim 2021). As Sabshin noted,

> We are asking white psychiatrists to become increasingly aware of how their everyday practices continue to perpetuate institutional white racism in psychiatry and to support the search for realistic solutions to providing psychiatric services to black people. We ask white psychiatrists to provide strong sanction and support to these efforts. This means making available the necessary resources of money, manpower, and authority— and not just in the current token amounts. It means not defending the vested white interests in old institutional forms of professionalism when new strategies and roles are suggested; it means a significant reduction in economic barriers to psychiatric care; it means relinquishing negative stereotypes of the black patient; it means truly sharing administrative decision making with black colleagues and black communities. (Sabshin et al. 1970, p. 792)

Yet, more than 50 years later, organized psychiatry has been called to task because of continuing vestiges of structural racism. Sabshin et al.'s exhortation may have fallen short because, in part, more attention was paid to what white psychiatrists must give up, as opposed to how to share "administrative decision making with black colleagues and black communities" (Sabshin et al. 1970, p. 792). By the same token, some Black psychiatrists may have read Sabshin's statement and waited for established psychiatry to begin providing resources, granting authority, and sharing decision-making in new ways. What appears underappreciated is how Black psychiatrists, or Black people more generally, reach the point of demanding a seat at the decision-making table where meaningful change can be produced when they have been excluded for so long.

When I was awarded the APA's Solomon Carter Fuller Award in 2020 and was asked to provide its accompanying lecture, it was initially difficult for me to grasp how I embodied the award, which "honors a black citizen who has pioneered in an area that has significantly improved the quality of life for black people" (APA, www.psychiatry.org/membership/awards-leadership-opportunities/awards/fuller-award). This was made more difficult when comparing myself with the great Black psychiatrists who had been honored with the award in the past: Drs. Chester Pierce, Nancy Boyd-Franklin, James Comer, Alvin Poussaint, Phyllis Harrison-Ross, Carl Bell, and Patricia Newton, to name a few. But, on reflection, I realized I shared a common pathway with my ancestors and contemporaries in discovering how I could improve the practice of psychiatry for Black psychiatrists and the care of Black people with mental illness. In this chapter I will review the pathway of nigrescence as exemplified in my work over 13 years as a representative of the Caucus of Black Psychiatrists to the APA Assembly. It is nigrescence, a personal evolution of Blackness, that informs the efforts of all Black psychiatrists in achieving social justice and striving for an antiracist world.

Theory of Nigrescence

There is…no way of correcting perfectly the lens through which an individual autobiographer sees the world or the hearing aid through which the storyteller first hears the facts from his subject.
Ezra E.H. Griffith (2023, pp. xiv–xv)

William Cross (1994) began characterizing normative Black American self-identity development beginning in the late 1960s in Chicago and continued his observations at Cornell University. He noted W.E.B. Du

Bois's autobiographical affirmation of becoming a Negro while a student at Fisk University, a historically Black college, in the late nineteenth century as being one of the earliest recorded descriptions of this development. Dr. Cross observed five stages along the pathway of Black identity formation in the United States, which he labeled as *pre-change, encounter, transition, internalization,* and *rapprochement.* Although Cross first proposed the stages as a linear process for forming the Black American identity, he later refined his theory, noting that ongoing encounters may lead to regression along the path and reformulation of previously achieved stages. He also noted that Black identity formation could be somewhat independent of the socially assigned race (i.e., the apparent race based on stereotypical external cues [Jones et al. 2008]), with "Blackness" not being the primary cultural identity of a person despite appearances otherwise.

The pathway of my Black identity is illustrative of Cross's five stages.

PRE-CHANGE

Pre-change is a period when race has little constructive relevance to the individual. Cross suggested that with respect to being Black, the individual might experience self-hatred or denial of their Blackness or might feel that other determinants of their cultural identity, such as gender or sexual orientation, are more important.

Growing up in rural upstate New York in the 1960s, I found myself living in a neighborhood where my brother and I were the only Black children. As a toddler, preschooler, then kindergartner, I do not recall having any conflicts due to my race being different from all of my white counterparts. I played in the homes and yards of my friends and they came over to my house. I was not conscious of being Black.

ENCOUNTER

The encounter is an event during which a person who appears to have power will make an individual's Blackness consciously relevant. This is typically through an act of prejudice, discrimination, or overt racism directed toward the Black individual.

My encounter occurred in the small rural elementary school where my brother and I were the only Black students. The encounter occurred while I was in the second grade. "Phil" became enraged at me after we accidentally bumped into each other in the boys' restroom of the school. He yelled the N-word at me, his fists balled in rage.

To the best of my knowledge, this was the first time I recalled hearing the N-word directed at me. Although I did not know what it meant,

I had the awareness it was not meant as a term of endearment. Later that day, after escaping from Phil and finishing my school day, I spoke with my mother. As was her habit, she asked me how my day had gone at school. When I told her of my encounter with Phil, she drew a heavy sigh, as if, against all hope, she had resigned herself to the inevitability of this day. She then began to pointedly instruct me, using the news media and publications of the day, on the differences in how Blacks and whites were being treated in America. She tried to make clear that I was Black and would be treated differently by others because I was Black. That was my first encounter.

TRANSITION

My first encounter did not turn me into a Black person. I struggled with the notion that I was different because of the color of my skin, something over which I had no control. Initially, I thought my parents were mistaken. After all, this was then the Age of Aquarius. Many songs were being sung and many words were being spoken about how we were all brothers and sisters. However, many more encounters of exclusion, derision, and marginalization followed my first encounter in elementary school into my middle school and high school years. (I was one of but 6 Black students in a high school of 1,800 students.) I became convinced I could not, would not be accepted in the dominant racial group, and therefore, if I was to survive with a sense of self, I would need to immerse myself and gain strength from my Blackness.

Cross noted the experience of many Black Americans, particularly in college, where they immerse themselves in Blackness and avoid activities that proclaim whiteness. At the University of Rochester, where I was 1 of 150 Black students among an undergraduate population of 4,000, I sat at the "Black" table during meals, became a member of the Black Student Union, and went to predominantly Black parties for social release. I became more familiar with soul and funk music and the writings of Dr. Martin Luther King Jr., Malcolm X, and Akbar. At the same time, I questioned my learned precepts regarding patriotism, democracy, capitalism, and Christianity.

INTERNALIZATION

Over the 8 years of my time at the University of Rochester, my comfort with and acceptance of being Black in America grew and matured with the help of a community that embraced and supported me despite the efforts of the dominant culture to marginalize us. Cross describes this stage as a period of building a coherent sense of oneself as a Black person able to withstand racist assaults. It is what kept me going despite being the only Black student in my medical school class or the only student who was interested in going into psychiatry, despite Rochester's rich history in providing leaders in psychiatry.

RAPPROCHEMENT

Cross observed in many of the individuals who spent time in the stage of internalization that there was a maturation in thought regarding Black-white issues and a softening of the sharp demarcation between Black being good and white being evil. Cross labeled this stage *rapprochement*, noting that people in this stage tend to be committed to actions that today would be considered antiracist (Kendi 2019) rather than be wholly pro-Black or anti-white. My continuing experiences in medical school and then residency led me to explore my rapprochement as a member-in-training in the APA.

Historical Context and the Legacy of Notable Black American Psychiatrists

Having described the stages of nigrescence in autobiographical fashion, and before describing my expression of rapprochement in the APA, it is important to understand the context I stepped into that was created by Black psychiatrists before me in the APA. Solomon Carter Fuller was the first African to become a psychiatrist in America (Spurlock 1999). His grandfather, John Lewis Fuller, bought his freedom from slavery in Virginia and moved his family to Liberia, where Solomon was raised. He came to the United States at age 17 to attend Livingstone College in North Carolina. He may have had his first encounter in Black identity formation during his efforts to enter college in the United States. There is scant written evidence of the maturation of his racial identity, but given the climate of American race relations in the late nineteenth century, it is easy to imagine his internalization occurring during his years in the United States. Despite the racism existing in America, he received his medical degree from Boston University in 1897 and began his training as a pathologist and psychiatrist at Westborough State Hospital. He applied for postdoctoral training in the United States but was accepted only at the University of Munich under the tutelage of Dr. Alois Alzheimer at Emil Kraepelin's clinic.

Dr. Fuller researched the organic causes of Alzheimer's disease, bipolar disorder, and schizophrenia. He was an avid student of brain pathology, neuropathology, and aging. It is noteworthy that he lectured in 1909 at a conference held at Clark University when Sigmund Freud made his only visit to America to attend this same conference. In a paper written in 1912, Dr. Fuller set the course for current research in Alzheimer's disease when he wondered about the significance of plaques and neurofibrillary changes seen on histological slides of brains afflicted with Alzheimer's disease. His pathway laid the groundwork for many Black psychiatrists in the United States as he became the first black APA member, fellow, and author to publish in the *American Journal of Psychiatry*.

Another trailblazer in Black psychiatry who gave context to my participation in the APA was Dr. Chester Pierce (Griffith 2023). Dr. Pierce grew up as a "minority" in Glen Cove, New York, where there were 800 Black residents among 8,000 inhabitants. Although it is not clearly documented what his first encounter was in Glen Cove, it is clear that he had many encounters in which he was marginalized as a Black person. As he grew through his stages of transition, internalization, and rapprochement, he became the founding president of the Black Psychiatrists of America and led a group of Black members of the APA to demand that the APA confront the racism preventing Black psychiatrists and Black patients from having their needs addressed. He later coined the term that helped Black people articulate one of the subtler forms of racism: *microaggressions*, the experience of someone from the dominant group slighting, insulting, or otherwise marginalizing Black people (Pierce 1970).

Under Dr. Pierce's leadership, Black psychiatrists pushed the APA at its 1969 Annual Meeting in Miami to confront and resolve its racism. The Caucus of Black Psychiatrists was formed as a component to officially keep Black issues in the forefront of the APA's consciousness. In addition, APA's leadership accepted the demand of having a nonvoting Black observer at the Board of Trustees' meetings. This observer had the dual role of serving as a "conscience" to APA's leadership and serving as a source of information to educate Black psychiatrists who had been marginalized from the inner workings of APA's leadership.

Dr. Pierce's efforts also led to the hiring of a director of minority group programs, which was the forerunner of the medical director for minority/national affairs, which then became the deputy medical director for the Office of Minority/National Affairs and later evolved into the director of Diversity and Health Equity. This position was intended to keep an active Black presence within the administrative bureaucracy of the APA, where the needs of Black psychiatrists and Black patients would also be kept at the forefront.

In addition, Dr. Pierce encouraged Black psychiatrists to engage in scholarship and publish their thoughts and findings regarding improving the lives of Black people. He was one of the first psychiatrists to recognize the importance of bringing together psychiatrists of African descent from around the world to better understand the mental health needs of Black people from a global perspective. He was also an expert on the effects of extreme environments (e.g., Antarctica, outer space) on mental and physical health and wrote extensively in this area. His interest and encouragement led to a number of Black psychiatrists engaging in research and publishing (see, e.g., Adebimpe 1981; Hickling 1975; Jones et al. 1981; Lawson et al. 1984; Pinderhughes 1971).

My Pathway and the APA

My involvement in the APA began as an APA/National Institute of Mental Health minority fellow, meeting and learning from the greats in Black psychiatry who participated in the work of the APA and discussing with my peers what it meant to be a Black psychiatrist in America. Naive with respect to my identity as a Black psychiatrist, I was stimulated to return to the stages of transition, internalization, and rapprochement. This evolution in my cultural identity was also informed by my growing exposure to administrative psychiatry and the question as to how bureaucracies could be reshaped to effect positive change.

In 1999, I was selected to join the Committee of Black Psychiatrists and then, in 2003, under the mentorship and encouragement of Dr. John Gaston, also a Solomon Carter Fuller Award winner, accepted the role of representative to the APA Assembly on behalf of the Caucus of Black Psychiatrists. The Assembly is the representative body of the APA tasked with advising the Board of Trustees in the positions and policies the organization should take regarding the various challenges facing the organization.

I became the chief advocate on the floor of the Assembly regarding a position statement drafted by the Committee of Black Psychiatrists, "Position Statement on Resolution Against Racism and Racial Discrimination and Their Adverse Impacts on Mental Health" (American Psychiatric Association Council on Minority Mental Health and Health Disparities 2018). Members of the committee who drafted this resolution were Drs. Sandra Walker, Lisa Green-Paden, Napoleon Higgins, James Lee, Saundra Maass-Robinson, Sherri Simpson, Kalaya Okereke, O.C. White, Marketa Wills, Rahn Bailey, Carl Bell, and William Lawson, the majority of whom are still quite active in established psychiatry today. As an advocate for this resolution before my colleagues within the Assembly, I encountered resistance to accepting this resolution when told that the APA was a "scientific" and "clinical" body that had little or no business wading into social or political conflicts. However, support was found within my caucus and with allied white psychiatrists to see the effort through, and we succeeded in having the position statement passed (it was more recently revised in 2019). The immersion within my caucus was critical. Late night conversations strategizing with Drs. Carl Bell, John Gaston, Altha Stewart, Annelle Primm, Donna Norris, and Ledro Justice were seminal in challenging and informing my attempts to effect change.

A subsequent encounter I experienced as representative to the Assembly occurred in 2009 when the APA had a fiscal crisis in which decisions were made to drastically reduce administrative expenditures. One of the decisions made by leadership was to dissolve the minority/underrepresented committees. Most significantly, this meant that the Committee of Black Psychiatrists, APA's concrete expenditure of funds and staffing to support psychiatrists meeting to address Black issues within the organization, was being eliminated. Although the medical director of the Office of Minority/National Affairs was Black at the time, her role was to address interests of psychiatrists and patients of color, and she could not focus just on the concerns of Black psychiatrists and patients.

This left the Caucus of Black Psychiatrists as the lone body within the APA to specifically address the concerns and issues of Black people within the organization. The caucus, being a volunteer organization with limited APA staff support and no funding from the general organization to conduct its business, was hard-pressed to address issues of structural racism within the APA. A position statement was drafted on behalf of the caucus requesting financial and staff support to conduct its business meetings twice per year, once at the May Annual Meeting and once at the Institute for Psychiatric Services meeting in October. In addition, it was requested that at least one Black psychiatrist be an administrative department director within the central office of APA to provide input to leadership and resources for membership. At that time, Dr. Annelle Primm served in that role as medical director of the Office of Minority/National Affairs. This experience of rapprochement led to support for Caucus of Black Psychiatrist meetings twice a year and for Dr. Primm maintaining her presence within the central office.

Observations in Continued Engagement With the APA

There was another encounter a few years later when the office of medical director for the APA became open when Dr. James Scully retired. Dr.

Primm was a finalist for this position, but she was not selected. Despite her decade of efforts within the APA as medical director for the Office of Minority/National Affairs and her concrete activities building APA resources for the mental health and treatment of people of color, she was not chosen. Moreover, the process that led to her not being chosen reminded many Black psychiatrists of the microaggressions we felt within the organization, including the defeats experienced by Dr. Donna Norris as she attempted to become the first Black president of the organization. Dr. Primm's rejection was also in the context of the lack of Black representation throughout the leadership of the governance structure of the APA. Personally, it was another encounter, a reminder of my marginalization as a psychiatrist because of my Blackness.

Because of our concerns in the Caucus of Black Psychiatrists, I approached APA leadership as Assembly representative of the caucus and arranged a meeting during the 2013 APA Annual Meeting in San Francisco with then president Dr. Dilip Jeste, incoming president Dr. Jeffrey Lieberman, and president-elect Dr. Paul Summergrad to discuss with Caucus of Black Psychiatrists representatives, as well as with other leaders of APA minority/underrepresented caucuses, our experiences of structural racism within the APA. At that time, I felt the support of Black psychiatric leaders Drs. William Lawson, Carl Bell, Ezra Griffith, Rahn Bailey, and Altha Stewart, among others. This attempt at rapprochement embodied Cross's definition of reaching out to Black and white leaders to seek justice. This discussion led Dr. Lieberman to appoint Dr. Maria Oquendo to lead a Board of Trustees–Assembly Ad Hoc Workgroup on Minority/Underrepresented Psychiatry. She was tasked with engaging all minority/underrepresented caucuses in frank discussions about how to better represent their concerns within the APA. After extensive discussions and deliberation, the Ad Hoc Workgroup proposed that the APA ensure the election of a Black or Native American/American Indian president by nominating candidates only of those races. This eventually led to the election of Dr. Altha Stewart as the first Black president of the APA.

However, despite this and other changes implemented on recommendation of the work group, as my engagement with the APA continued, so did my encounters with racism. Police violence visited on Black men became thrust on the national consciousness after several horrifying examples were filmed, broadcast, and circulated on social and televised media. In 2015, with the help of members within the Caucus of Black Psychiatrists, I proposed an action paper, "Improving APA Support of the Mental Health of African-American Males," to the Assembly, seeking approval for a number of actions the APA could take to support the mental health of African American males at that time. However, only one of the proposed actions was approved by the Assembly: The Council on Medical Education and Lifelong Learning was instructed to "investigate how to provide training opportunities for psychiatrists and collaboration experts to provide community-based, culturally competent therapeutic interventions for traumatized African American communities." Of note was the criticism of the proposal provided by the Council on Research: "The primary problem I have with the draft is the assumption [police violence] is related to race without supporting research…. The title of the action paper [also] shows a bias."

My Nigrescence's Denouement With the APA

Soon after this last encounter, I decided that I had had enough. After 13 years of effort, my energy and resolve were flagging, and my peers within the Caucus of Black Psychiatrists were generating new ideas and energy that could make a greater impact in future encounters with the structural racism within the APA. COVID-19, the murder of George Floyd and continuing violence of police and other armed Americans against Black citizens, and climate change and natural disasters, all of which affect Black communities disproportionately, have highlighted the APA's limited responsiveness to crises within the Black community. A new generation of leaders, each having traveled their own pathways to rapprochement in nigrescence, are ready to carry the torch in bringing about change in the APA and throughout the world of health care and social justice. It is incumbent on the APA to embrace all of its members and what their unique experiences and intellects have to offer to solve these crucial problems. The ideas and recommendations of Black psychiatrists such as Drs. Frank Clark, Ericka Goodwin, Kimberly Gordon, Danielle Hairston, Dionne Hart, Napoleon Higgins, Jessica Isom, Ayana Jordan, Morgan Medlock, Dionne Powell, Steven Starks, Sarah Vinson, Cheryl Wills, and others must be heard and incorporated into the evolving direction of the APA if there is to be effective change for all psychiatrists and their patients.

It is the process of nigrescence, the forming of Black identity in a sometimes hostile social environment, that shaped me and my Black colleagues into being who we are. It is this process that leads us to push back against the structural racism we see around us and demand and fight for change. This process has been indirectly affecting the APA since the 1960s and continues to shape and reshape the APA today. The recent Task Force on Racism in the APA chaired by Cheryl Wills and recent Assembly actions to concretely address white privilege within the organization are the results of this continuing evolution of Black psychiatrists realizing their rapprochement.

"…[T]ruly sharing administrative decision making with black colleagues and black communities," which Sabshin et al. (1970, p. 792) asked of their white colleagues, is easier said than done. The pathways that bring whites and Blacks together to try to share in decision-making are strewn with the pain and misunderstandings from past encounters. The very act of sitting down together may trigger flashbacks of past trauma. But the future success of the APA will depend on its ability to constructively engage and support this evolving nigrescence in its Black members. The future success of the APA will depend on the rapprochement of its Black members in constructively engaging with (and sometimes demanding of) its white membership.

Finally, hearkening back to the statement by Dr. Griffith regarding the lens of the autobiographer and the hearing aid of the storyteller, my reflections on my personal pathway in discovering my Blackness and how that affected my work within the APA illustrate my imperfections in recalling the past without bias. This places me in the same boat as critics and allies alike, imperfect humans struggling to do what is right. In the case of race relations and the struggle to end racism, it is better to reflect back on our path to cultural identity, despite our imperfections, than never to look back and be unaware of our contributions to the problem or the solution.

References

Adebimpe VR: Overview: white norms and psychiatric diagnosis of black patients. Am J Psychiatry 138(3):279–285, 1981 7008631

American Psychiatric Association Council on Minority Mental Health and Health Disparities: Position statement on resolution against racism and racial discrimination and their adverse impacts on mental health. Washington, DC, American Psychiatric Association, 2018. Available at: www.psychiatry.org/File%20Library/About-APA/Organization-Documents-Policies/Policies/Position-2018-Resolution-Against-Racism-and-Racial-Discrimination.pdf. Accessed December 1, 2021.

Cross WE Jr: Nigrescence theory: historical and explanatory notes. J Vocat Behav 44:119123, 1994

Griffith EEH: Race and Excellence: My Dialogue With Chester Pierce. Washington, DC, American Psychiatric Association Publishing, 2023

Hickling FW: Social class and mental illness in a general hospital psychiatric unit in Jamaica. West Indian Med J 24(2):76–83, 1975 1189411

Jones BE, Gray BA, Parson EB: Manic-depressive illness among poor urban Blacks. Am J Psychiatry 138(5):654–657, 1981 7235063

Jones CP, Truman BI, Elam-Evans LD, et al: Using "socially assigned race" to probe white advantages in health status. Ethn Dis 18(4):496–504, 2008 19157256

Kendi IX: How to Be an Antiracist. New York, Random House, 2019

Lawson WB, Yesavage JA, Werner PD: Race, violence, and psychopathology. J Clin Psychiatry 45(7):294–297, 1984 6735988

Pierce C: Offensive mechanisms, in The Black Seventies. Edited by Barbour FB. Boston, MA, Porter Sargent, 1970, pp 265–282

Pinderhughes CA: Psychological and physiological origins of racism and other social discrimination. J Natl Med Assoc 63(1):25–29, 1971 5165382

Sabshin M, Diesenhaus H, Wilkerson R: Dimensions of institutional racism in psychiatry. Am J Psychiatry 127(6):787–793, 1970 5482872

Shim RS: Dismantling structural racism in psychiatry: a path to mental health equity. Am J Psychiatry 178(7):592–598, 2021 34270343

Spurlock J: Black Psychiatrists and American Psychiatry. Washington, DC, American Psychiatric Press, 1999

Appendix

Solomon Carter Fuller Award Lecturers

The Solomon Carter Fuller Award and Lecture was established by the Black Psychiatrists of America in 1969 to honor a Black citizen who has pioneered in an area that has significantly benefited the quality of life for Black people. Starting in 1975, the award lecturers were selected either by the American Psychiatric Association (APA) Committee of Black Psychiatrists or the APA Caucus of Black Psychiatrists.

Table A–1.   Solomon Carter Fuller Award Lecturers, 1973–2021

Year	Lecture Title	Lecturer/Recipient
1973	Acceptance Speech for Solomon Fuller Award	Kenneth B. Clark, Ph.D.[a]
1974	No lecture given	
1975	Government and the Black Family	The Hon. Mervyn M. Dymally
1976	Toward a Second American Revolution	John Hope Franklin, Ph.D.
1977	Handling Aggression by Blacks and Other Subordinated Groups	Allison Davis, Ph.D.
1978	Epidemiological Aspects of Mental Illness Among Older Black Women and Men	Jacquelyne J. Jackson, Ph.D.
1979	Affirmative Action	Eleanor Holmes Norton L.L.B.
1980	The Rights of Prisoners and Patients	The Hon. Constance Baker Motley
1981	Tomorrow's Psychiatrists: A Black Leader's Perspective	Ambassador Andrew Young
1982	Torn Between Two Systems	Charles A. Pinderhughes, M.D.
1983	Minority Access to Medicine Revisited	George I. Lythcott, M.D.
1984	Education for Psychiatry	Luther D. Robinson, M.D.
1985	Opening our Hearts and Our Hearths	Rev. George H. Clements
1986	Unity in Diversity: 33 Years of Stress	Chester M. Pierce, M.D.
1987	The Challenge of Blackness	Lerone Bennett Jr.
1988	Racism Revisited	Jeanne Spurlock, M.D.
1989	A Plan for the 90s	Tony Brown
1990	Education and the American Future	James P. Comer, M.D.
1991	Our Children: Miles to Go, Promises	Evelyn K. Moore, M.A.
1992	Black Monday's Children: A Multi-Cultural Agenda for the 21st Century	Gloria Johnson Powell, M.D.

Table A–1. Solomon Carter Fuller Award Lecturers, 1973–2021 *(continued)*

Year	Lecture Title	Lecturer/Recipient
1993	No lecture given	Marian Wright Edelman
1994	Our Heritage, Our Future: Comments on Medical and Psychiatric Education	Dewitt C. Alfred Jr., M.D.
1995	Can Psychiatry Serve Tomorrow's Black Families: Challenges for a Profession in Transition	June Jackson Christmas, M.D.
1996	Blacks, the Media and Mental Health	Alvin F. Poussaint, M.D.
1997	Future Challenges and Opportunities in Public Health	David Satcher M.D., Ph.D.
1998	Violence Prevention: A Public Health Mandate to Save Our Children	Deborah B. Prothrow Stith, M.D.
1999	Substance Abuse Treatment in Multi-Cultural Communities: A National Perspective	H. Westley Clark, M.D., M.B.A., J.D.
2000	Authentic Representation, Belonging, and the Narrative of Self-Identification	Ezra E.H. Griffith, M.D.
2003	Culture/Racism and Ethnic Diversity With Past Corrective Actions Successes, and Failures	James H. Carter, M.D.
2004	I Am a Fact, Not a Fiction	Phyllis Harrison-Ross, M.D.
2005	The Treatment of African American Clients and Families	Nancy Boyd-Franklin, Ph.D.
2006	History of and Corrective Proposals for Disparities in Mental Health Care	Milton C. Hollar, M.D.
2007	From Psychopharmacology to Ethnopsychopharmacology	David C. Henderson, M.D.
2008	Mental Health Services: Still a Challenge	Mildred Mitchell-Bateman, M.D.
2009	Pills to Treat Alcoholism	Bankole A. Johnson, M.D.

Table A-1.   Solomon Carter Fuller Award Lecturers, 1973–2021 (continued)

Year	Lecture Title	Lecturer/Recipient
2010	Solomon Carter Fuller: What Would He Say About Racial Politics in American Psychiatry Today	Donna M. Norris, M.D.
2011	Public Health Efforts: Successful and Failed	Carl Bell, M.D.
2012	Racial and Ethnic Influences on Mental Health: The Evolving Evidence	James S. Jackson, M.D.
2013	Policy to Practice: Challenges for Effective Mental Health Care	John O. Gaston, M.D.
2014	MAD vs. BAD: Linking Mental Health Disparities and Public Health Consequences	William B. Lawson, M.D., Ph.D.
2015	Transforming Race in Medicine: Body and Mind, Heart and Soul	Dorothy E. Roberts, J.D.
2016	The Sweet Enchantment of "Post-Racial" Racism in America	Eduardo Bonilla-Silva, Ph.D.
2017	No lecture given	Damon S. Tweedy, M.D.
2018	Mental Health Challenges Facing Patients and Providers of African Descent	Patricia A. Newton, M.D., M.P.H., M.A.
2019	"What Were You Thinking?" A Keystone Question for Emotional Fitness	Loma Kaye Flowers, M.D.
2020	Nigrescence and the Future of American Psychiatry	Stephen McLeod-Bryant, M.D.
2021	The Caravan Moves On: From Solomon Carter Fuller to Psychiatry in the 21st Century	Altha Stewart, M.D.

[a]Award issued by Black Psychiatrists of America.

INDEX

Page numbers printed in **boldface** *type refer to figures and tables.*